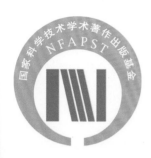

国家科学技术学术著作出版基金资助出版

Supported by the National Fund for Academic
Publication in Science and Technology

颅内动脉粥样硬化性狭窄血管内介入治疗

Endovascular Therapy for Intracranial Atherosclerotic Stenosis

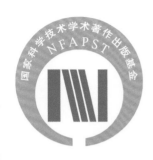

Supported by the National Fund for Academic
Publication in Science and Technology

颅内动脉粥样硬化性狭窄
血管内介入治疗

Endovascular Therapy for Intracranial
Atherosclerotic Stenosis

主　编　马　宁
主　审　缪中荣　王拥军

LUNEI DONGMAI ZHOUYANG YINGHUAXING XIAZHAI XUEGUANNEI JIERU ZHILIAO

图书在版编目（CIP）数据

颅内动脉粥样硬化性狭窄血管内介入治疗 / 马宁主编 . —北京：
北京大学医学出版社，2023.7
ISBN 978-7-5659-2696-9

Ⅰ. ①颅… Ⅱ. ①马… Ⅲ. ①脑动脉硬化－动脉粥样
硬化－介入性治疗 Ⅳ. ① R743.1

中国版本图书馆 CIP 数据核字（2022）第 136033 号

颅内动脉粥样硬化性狭窄血管内介入治疗

主　　编：马　宁
出版发行：北京大学医学出版社
地　　址：（100191）北京市海淀区学院路 38 号　北京大学医学部院内
电　　话：发行部 010-82802230；图书邮购 010-82802495
网　　址：http://www.pumpress.com.cn
E - m a i l：booksale@bjmu.edu.cn
印　　刷：北京金康利印刷有限公司
经　　销：新华书店
责任编辑：畅晓燕　　责任校对：靳新强　　责任印制：李　啸
开　　本：889 mm×1194 mm　1/16　印张：26.75　字数：820 千字
版　　次：2023 年 7 月第 1 版　2023 年 7 月第 1 次印刷
书　　号：ISBN 978-7-5659-2696-9
定　　价：238.00 元
版权所有，违者必究
（凡属质量问题请与本社发行部联系退换）

编者名单

主编　马　宁
主审　缪中荣　王拥军

编者及译者（按姓名汉语拼音排序）

陈涵丰　浙江大学医学院附属第一医院
陈林考　台州市中心医院（台州学院附属医院）
陈　旺　临沂市人民医院
陈　湘　北京航天总医院
成　涛　山西省心血管病医院
崔　凯　内蒙古林业总医院
崔荣荣　北京市大兴区人民医院
邓一鸣　首都医科大学附属北京天坛医院
董欢欢　湖北省中医院（湖北中医药大学附属医院）
Ferdinard K. Hui　The Queen's Medical Center, Honolulu, Hawaii
付伟伦　首都医科大学附属北京天坛医院
顾燕忠　杭州市余杭区第二人民医院
韩　明　衡水市第四人民医院
何　勇　山西省心血管病医院
何子骏　首都医科大学附属北京天坛医院
贺红卫　首都医科大学附属北京天坛医院
洪全龙　福建省泉州市第一医院
侯志凯　首都医科大学附属北京天坛医院
胡　琼　山西省心血管病医院
胡彦君　香港大学深圳医院
黄　睿　台州市中心医院（台州学院附属医院）
霍晓川　首都医科大学附属北京天坛医院
计仁杰　浙江大学医学院附属第一医院
贾白雪　首都医科大学附属北京天坛医院
姜铃先　首都医科大学附属北京天坛医院
姜　鹏　首都医科大学附属北京天坛医院
江裕华　首都医科大学附属北京天坛医院
康开江　首都医科大学附属北京天坛医院
蒯　东　山西省心血管病医院

Lei Feng　Kaiser Permanente Los Angeles Medical Center
李红闪　保定市第一中心医院
李康悦　首都医科大学附属北京天坛医院
李　强　衡水市第四人民医院
李晓青　首都医科大学附属北京天坛医院
李　鑫　三河燕郊福合第一医院
李新明　南昌市第一医院
李郁芳　北京航天总医院
连　瑜　内蒙古科技大学包头医学院第一附属医院
刘深龙　沧州市人民医院
刘亚辉　三河燕郊福合第一医院
刘一凡　山西白求恩医院（山西医学科学院）
刘泽辰　Harvard T.H. Chan School of Public Health
雒东江　北京航天总医院
马　宁　首都医科大学附属北京天坛医院
毛更生　中国人民解放军总医院第三医学中心
苗春芝　唐山市工人医院
缪中荣　首都医科大学附属北京天坛医院
聂庆彬　中国人民解放军总医院第三医学中心
秦桂萍　北京市房山区良乡医院（首都医科大学良乡教学医院）
秦舒森　首都医科大学附属北京天坛医院
水新俊　山西省心血管病医院
宋　佳　河北省沧州中西医结合医院
宋立刚　首都医科大学附属北京天坛医院
孙洪扬　临沂市人民医院
孙立倩　首都医科大学附属北京天坛医院
孙　瑄　首都医科大学附属北京天坛医院

孙　勇　三河燕郊福合第一医院

王　坤　首都医科大学附属北京天坛医院

王　嵘　首都医科大学附属北京天坛医院

王天保　广西中医药大学第一附属医院

王贤军　临沂市人民医院

王现旺　邯郸市第一医院

王拥军　首都医科大学附属北京天坛医院

王玉峰　山西省心血管病医院

吴岩峰　南京医科大学第二附属医院

徐子奇　浙江大学医学院附属第一医院

阎　龙　首都医科大学附属北京天坛医院

杨　波　北京市健宫医院

杨冬旭　济宁医学院附属医院

杨海华　北京市大兴区人民医院

杨家宝　首都医科大学附属北京天坛医院

杨　炯　巴彦淖尔市医院

杨连琦　承德市中心医院

杨　明　首都医科大学附属北京天坛医院

杨新健　首都医科大学附属北京天坛医院

杨　樟　贵州医科大学附属医院

姚丽娜　保定市第二中心医院

姚　亮　辽宁中医药大学附属第二医院

尤吉栋　银川市第一人民医院

于江华　河北医科大学第二医院

俞妮妮　三门县人民医院

余　莹　首都医科大学附属北京天坛医院

袁景林　北京市大兴区人民医院

张义森　首都医科大学附属北京天坛医院

张增权　三河燕郊福合第一医院

朱其义　临沂市人民医院

左凤同　沧州市中心医院

序言一

颅内动脉粥样硬化性狭窄（intracranial athero-sclerotic stenosis，ICAS）是中国人群卒中发病的重要原因之一，与40%～60%的颅内大血管闭塞有关，因此有关ICAS的治疗具有非常重要的意义。虽然强化药物治疗能够降低一部分伴有ICAS患者的卒中复发率，但是对于侧支循环较差的患者，强化药物治疗效果欠佳，因此需要血运重建手术来改善狭窄程度，预防卒中复发。

血管内介入治疗是目前血运重建手术的重要手段，在临床上已经被广泛应用，但是由于地区性或个人的技术差异，对于ICAS的介入治疗还存在诸多问题。马宁教授在ICAS的介入治疗方面已经深耕十多年，积累了丰富的经验，他的每一个病例都经过认真的评估和挑选，大部分病例都是自己亲自上阵，保证了手术的质量，取得了显著疗效。本书积累了他和同道们多年来手术的典型病例，在术前评估、手术技术、材料选择等方面都进行了详细的解读，供初学者或业内同行们参考。

在这里我衷心祝愿马宁教授团队在今后的ICAS治疗方面再创佳绩！

缪中荣

Foreword I

Intracranial atherosclerotic stenosis (ICAS) is a leading cause of ischemic stroke in China, accounting for approximately 40%–60% of intracranial large vessel occlusions. Therefore, the treatment approach for ICAS is of great significance. Aggressive medical treatment, including dual-antiplatelet regimens and intensive atherosclerosis risk factor control, can reduce stroke recurrence in certain patients with ICAS. However, the stroke recurrence rate remains high, particularly in patients with inadequate collateral circulation. Endovascular revascularization can increase the diameter of stenosed vessels and improve brain perfusion, ultimately resulting in reduced stroke recurrence.

Endovascular treatment is an essential approach to revascularization that has been widely adopted in clinical practice. However, there are still challenges in the endovascular treatment of ICAS due to regional disparities and individual technical differences. Professor Ma Ning has devoted more than a decade to the endovascular treatment of ICAS, amassing a wealth of experience. Each case has been meticulously selected and evaluated, with most procedures performed by Professor Ma himself, ensuring the quality of operations and achieving outstanding therapeutic effects. This book outlines the expertise of Professor Ma and his colleagues in preoperative assessment, endovascular treatment techniques, and device selection, and highlights their achievements in managing typical cases of ICAS.

I sincerely hope that Professor Ma Ning and his team will continue to make remarkable achievements in the treatment of ICAS in the future.

Zhongrong Miao

序言二

颅内动脉粥样硬化性狭窄（ICAS）一致被认为是东亚人群缺血性脑血管病的主要病因，流行病学发现接近一半的中国缺血性脑血管病患者合并中度及以上的颅内动脉狭窄。因此理论上讲，对于颅内动脉狭窄患者应该采取积极的治疗措施，给予更大程度的关注。

然而，大型临床试验并不支持对于症状性和非症状性颅内动脉狭窄进行血管内介入治疗，介入治疗存在很多争议。究其原因，既有已发表研究的种族代表性、研究设计和研究质量的问题，也有参与研究者的手术技巧造成的研究结果偏差。从临床角度而言，患者的选择和手术技巧是非常重要的临床问题，有时比研究设计和质量更为重要。为此，马宁教授组织编写了这本《颅内动脉粥样硬化性狭窄血管内介入治疗》一书。

本书采用病例报告的形式，系统描述了不同狭窄部位、不同临床情况下，介入治疗的技巧和成功经验，也包括手术并发症的处理。全部病例来自临床一线，对于临床指导非常难得，我相信临床一线的介入治疗医师一定会从中获取丰富的营养。

非常高兴把此书推荐给大家。

王拥军

Foreword II

Intracranial atherosclerotic stenosis (ICAS) is widely regarded as the major cause of ischemic stroke in East Asian populations. Epidemiological studies have found that nearly half of Chinese patients with ischemic stroke also have moderate to severe intracranial arterial stenosis. In theory, more aggressive treatment measures and increased attention should be given to intracranial arterial stenosis.

However, large-scale clinical trials do not support endovascular treatment for symptomatic and asymptomatic ICAS, and the endovascular treatment itself remains controversial. The reasons for this controversy include issues of racial representation, study design, and study quality, as well as biases in research results caused by the endovascular treatment skills of study participants. From a clinical perspective, patient selection and endovascular treatment techniques are very important clinical issues, sometimes more important than study design and quality. To address these concerns, Professor Ning Ma organized and edited the book *"Endovascular Therapy for Intracranial Atherosclerotic Stenosis"*.

This book employs a case report format to systematically describe the techniques and experiences of endovascular treatment for different stenosis locations and various clinical situations, as well as the management of peri-procedural complications. All cases are from the frontline of clinical practice, which is very valuable for clinical guidance. I believe that neuro-interventionists at the frontline of clinical practice will benefit greatly from this resource.

I am delighted to recommend this book to you.

Yongjun Wang

前　言

颅内动脉粥样硬化性狭窄（ICAS）是导致缺血性卒中的主要原因之一。不同种族之间 ICAS 患病率有明显差异，亚裔缺血性卒中患者占 30%～50%，而北美人群仅占 5%～10%。中国颅内动脉粥样硬化（Chinese Intracranial Atherosclerosis，CICAS）研究结果表明急性缺血性卒中和（或）短暂性脑缺血发作（TIA）患者合并 ICAS 的比例高达 46.6%，且伴有 ICAS 的患者卒中复发率更高。因此，探讨"如何降低 ICAS 所致缺血性卒中的致残率、致死率和复发率，提高患病人群的生活质量和延长寿命"，已成为我国重大慢性疾病防治的优先战略。

作为内科药物干预无效的症状性 ICAS 患者的重要治疗手段，近十余年迅猛发展的血管内治疗技术因能有效血运重建和预防卒中复发而备受瞩目，但由于在介入治疗适应证、介入器械选择、围术期并发症、支架内再狭窄等方面存在诸多临床问题而限制了其推广应用。

本书总结了 ICAS 的研究进展，展示了各位编者在临床工作中有关 ICAS 血管内治疗的精选病例，包括患者围术期药物准备、治疗技术、器械选择策略以及远期疗效，旨在加深读者对 ICAS 的理解，并加强高流量卒中介入中心临床操作经验的推广。

本书采用中英文双语对照形式，不仅有利于国内读者提高专业英文水平，也有助于与国际同行交流国内 ICAS 治疗现状及经验。

本书能获国家科学技术学术著作出版基金的资助，感谢刘玉清院士、邱贵兴院士、乔杰院士的推荐。本书能顺利成稿，感谢所有患者的信任！感谢从业路上我的指导老师的帮助！感谢所有编者及译者的付出！感谢妻子、女儿和父母的支持！

最后衷心希望读者能从阅读本书获益！中英文内容难以避免存在错误，也请广大读者批评指正！

马　宁

Preface

Intracranial atherosclerotic stenosis (ICAS) is one of the major causes of ischemic stroke. There is a marked racial disparity in the prevalence of ICAS, which is 30%–50% among the Asian patients with ischemic stroke but only 5%–10% among North American patients. The Chinese Intracranial Atherosclerosis (CICAS) study showed that the prevalence of ICAS in individuals with acute ischemic stroke and/or transient ischemic attacks (TIA) was 46.6%. Furthermore, patients with ICAS had a higher risk of stroke recurrence compared with those without intracranial arterial stenosis. Consequently, the issue of "how to reduce the morbidity, mortality, and recurrence of symptomatic ICAS, as well as improve patients' living quality and life expectancy" has been considered as a primary strategy for preventing major chronic diseases in China.

Endovascular treatment for ICAS, an effective approach to blood flow reconstruction and stroke recurrence prevention, has emerged as a promising approach for treating symptomatic ICAS patients who are refractory to medical treatment. However, it remains uncertain in some clinical issues such as endovascular treatment indications, interventional device selection, periprocedural complications, and long-term in-stent restenosis. These uncertainties have impeded its clinical application.

In this book, we summarize the recent advances in ICAS and demonstrate the selected cases of endovascular treatment for ICAS. These cases are presented through detailed displays of periprocedural medical management, endovascular treatment strategies, interventional device selection, and long-term prognosis. It aims to get a better understanding of ICAS and facilitate introduction of the clinical experiences in high-volume stroke intervention centers to more neuro-interventionalist.

This book is presented in a bilingual format in Chinese and English. This not only helps domestic readers improve their professional English level but also facilitates communication with international counterparts regarding endovascular treatment for ICAS.

This book has been supported by the National Fund for Academic Publication in Science and Technology. I am grateful for the endorsement of distinguished Academician Yuqing Liu, Academician Guixing Qiu, and Academician Jie Qiao. I owe a debt of gratitude to all the patients who trusted us, to the guidance of my mentors on my professional journey, and to all the authors and translators who have contributed to this book. I would also like to express my appreciation for the support of my wife, daughter, and parents.

Lastly, we sincerely hope that readers can benefit from reading this book. We recognize that errors may exist in both the Chinese and English versions, and we welcome criticisms or corrections from our readers.

Ning Ma

缩略语

AA	花生四烯酸	arachidonic acid
ADP	腺苷二磷酸	adenosine diphosphate
AICA	小脑前下动脉	anterior inferior cerebellar artery
ASL	动脉自旋标记	arterial spin labeling
BA	基底动脉	basilar artery
cAMP	环磷酸腺苷	cyclic adenosine monophosphate
CBF	脑血流量	cerebral blood flow
CBV	脑血容量	cerebral blood volume
cGMP	环磷酸鸟苷	cyclic guanosine monophosphate
COX-1	环氧合酶 -1	cyclooxygenase-1
CT	计算机断层成像	computed tomography
CTA	CT 血管成像	CT angiography
CTP	CT 灌注成像	CT perfusion
CVR	脑血管反应性	cerebrovascular reactivity
DSA	数字减影血管造影	digital subtraction angiography
ESR	红细胞沉降率	erythrocyte sedimentation rate
HRMRI	高分辨率磁共振成像	high-resolution MRI
ICAS	颅内动脉粥样硬化性狭窄	intracranial atherosclerotic stenosis
INR	国际标准化比值	international normalized ratio
LDL-C	低密度脂蛋白胆固醇	low-density lipoprotein cholesterol
MCA	大脑中动脉	middle cerebral artery
MRA	磁共振血管成像	magnetic resonance angiography
MRI	磁共振成像	magnetic resonance imaging
mRS	改良 Rankin 量表	modified Rankin scale
mTICI	改良脑梗死溶栓分级	modified thrombolysis in cerebral infarction
MTT	平均通过时间	mean transit time
NIHSS	美国国立卫生研究院卒中量表	National Institutes of Health Stroke Scale
OEF	氧摄取分数	oxygen extraction fraction
PDE	磷酸二酯酶	phosphodiesterase
PDWI	质子密度加权成像	proton density-weighted imaging
PET	正电子发射断层显像	positron emission tomography
PICA	小脑后下动脉	posterior inferior cerebellar artery

STA	颞浅动脉	superficial temporal artery
SWI	磁敏感加权成像	susceptibility-weighted imaging
TCD	经颅多普勒（超声）	transcranial Doppler
TG	甘油三酯	triglyceride
TIA	短暂性脑缺血发作	transient ischemic attack
TTP	达峰时间	time to peak
TXA$_2$	血栓素 A$_2$	thromboxane A$_2$

目　录

CONTENTS

第一部分

颅内动脉粥样硬化

动脉粥样硬化是一种全身性疾病，颅内动脉是动脉粥样硬化的好发部位之一。在所有缺血性卒中患者中，8% ~ 10%是由于颅内动脉粥样硬化性狭窄（intracranial atherosclerotic stenosis，ICAS）所致[1]。研究显示在我国缺血性脑血管病中颅内动脉狭窄的检出率高达39.3%[2]。由于颅内动脉自身解剖结构的特点与外周动脉不同，其动脉粥样硬化的发生、发展与外周动脉的区别目前仍存在争论。随着研究的不断深入，对颅内动脉粥样硬化的认识也不断加深。为此，我们在总结临床经验、荟萃文献的基础上，依次对颅内动脉粥样硬化的流行病学、病理生理以及治疗进展进行探讨。

Part I

Intracranial Atherosclerosis

As a systemic disease, atherosclerosis often involves the intracranial arteries. Of all patients with ischemic stroke, 8%–10% are due to intracranial atherosclerotic stenosis (ICAS).[1] Studies have shown that the detection rate of intracranial arterial stenosis in ischemic cerebrovascular disease is as high as 39.3% in China.[2] Because the anatomical characteristics of intracranial arteries are different from those of peripheral arteries, the differences of the occurrence and development of atherosclerosis between intracranial and peripheral arteries are still under debate. With continuous deepening of the relevant research, the understanding of intracranial atherosclerosis is also deepening. For this reason, by summarizing the clinical experience and meta-analysis, we will discuss the epidemiology, pathophysiology, and treatment progress of intracranial atherosclerosis.

第一章

流行病学

在过去40年间中国作为中低收入国家，卒中发病率增加100%，颅内动脉粥样硬化是卒中高发病率的重要原因[3]。

早在1962年，Bauer等[4]就发现动脉粥样硬化的分布可能存在人种差异，随后的研究发现白种人颅外血管病变的发病率较高，而亚洲人群颅内血管狭窄的发病率较高[5]。

1974年Brust等[6]对侨居在夏威夷的不同人种卒中患者的动脉粥样硬化分布进行研究时，首次提及中国人群颅内外动脉粥样硬化的分布情况。

黄一宁等[7]发起了中国最早的一项有关健康人群颅内动脉粥样硬化的调查，他们应用无创的经颅多普勒超声（transcranial Doppler，TCD）对北京市1574例40岁以上人群进行筛查，发现其中2.9%有颅内动脉狭窄或闭塞。

高山等[8]报道了北京协和医院96例短暂性脑缺血发作（transient ischemic attack，TIA）患者的TCD、颈动脉彩色超声和数字减影血管造影（digital subtraction angiography，DSA），结果发现51%的患者有颅内血管狭窄或闭塞，19%有颅外血管病变，颅内血管病变中以大脑中动脉（middle cerebral artery，MCA）受累最为多见，高达66%。

2000年Wong等[9]对连续的705例因急性卒中住院的中国患者进行TCD检查，发现48.9%的患者有大动脉狭窄或闭塞性病变，其中36.6%为单纯颅内血管病变，2.3%仅为颅外血管病变，10.1%同时存在颅内和颅外血管病变。颅内血管狭窄的好发部位分布依次为：MCA（73.3%）、椎基底动脉（40.3%）和大脑前动脉（35.9%）。

王桂红等[10]对171例伴发卒中或TIA的脑血管狭窄患者的DSA进行解读，结果显示颅内动脉狭窄性病变的发病率为80.7%，明显高于颅外动脉的56.1%[11]。

李尧等[12]在2005年利用TCD对北京东城区40岁以上的居民进行调查研究发现，在1782例受调查者中颅内动脉狭窄发病率为6.6%，颅外动脉狭窄发病率为2.0%，颅内外动脉均狭窄的发病率为1.6%。

由此可见，颅内动脉粥样硬化在中国人群中的发生率明显高于欧美人群，且颅内动脉狭窄的发生率高于颅外动脉。

（杨波）

Chapter 1

Epidemiology

The incidence of stroke has increased by 100% in China during the past 40 years, and intracranial atherosclerosis is an important cause of the high incidence of stroke.[3]

As early as 1962, Bauer et al[4] found possible racial differences in the distribution of atherosclerosis, and subsequent studies found a higher incidence of extracranial vascular lesions in whites, while the incidence of intracranial vascular stenosis was higher in Asian populations.[5]

In 1974, Brust et al[6] first mentioned the distribution of intracranial and extracranial atherosclerosis in the Chinese population when they studied the distribution of atherosclerosis in stroke patients of different races living in Hawaii.

Huang Yining et al[7] initiated the earliest survey of intracranial atherosclerosis in healthy people in China. They screened 1574 people over 40 years old in Beijing by transcranial Doppler (TCD) and found that 2.9% of people had intracranial artery stenosis or occlusion.

Gao Shan et al[8] reported the results of TCD, carotid artery color ultrasound and digital subtraction angiography (DSA) in 96 patients with transient ischemic attack (TIA) in Peking Union Medical College Hospital and found that 51% of patients had intracranial vascular stenosis or occlusion, and 19% of patients had extracranial vascular disease. The middle cerebral artery (MCA) is most frequently involved in intracranial vascular disease, which is up to 66%.

In 2000, Wong et al[9] performed TCD in 705 consecutive Chinese patients admitted to the hospital with acute stroke and found that 48.9% of patients had large artery steno-occlusive disease, of which 36.6% had simple intracranial vascular disease, 2.3% had extracranial vascular disease, and 10.1% had both intracranial and extracranial vascular disease. Common affected locations of intracranial stenosis were MCA (73.3%), vertebro-basilar artery (40.3%) and anterior cerebral artery (ACA) (35.9%).

Wang Guihong et al[10] interpreted the DSA in 171 patients with cerebrovascular stenosis associated with stroke or TIA, and the results showed that the incidence of intracranial arterial stenotic lesions was 80.7%, which was significantly higher than 56.1% of extracranial artery.[11]

In 2005, Li Yao et al[12] investigated residents over 40 years old who had completed TCD examination in Dongcheng District of Beijing and found that the incidence of intracranial artery stenosis was 6.6%, the incidence of extracranial artery stenosis was 2.0%, and the incidence of both intracranial and extracranial artery stenosis was 1.6%, among 1782 respondents.

Thus, the incidence of intracranial atherosclerosis in the Chinese population is more significant than that in the European and American populations, and the incidence of intracranial arterial stenosis is higher than that in the extracranial artery.

(Translated by Bo Yang)

第二章

病理生理学

动脉粥样硬化是一种全身性疾病，主要累及大、中动脉，包括冠状动脉、脑动脉和外周动脉。研究已经证实氧化型低密度脂蛋白在动脉粥样硬化过程中发挥关键作用[13]。动脉粥样硬化使得血管内膜增厚或斑块形成，致使血管管腔逐渐狭窄乃至闭塞。

最近的研究表明，解剖学位置是影响动脉粥样硬化斑块形成的重要因素，前循环动脉粥样硬化与后循环动脉粥样硬化在危险因素、患病率以及卒中机制等方面存在差异。颈内动脉的解剖研究发现，外弹力膜存在于颈内动脉岩段近端，至海绵窦段后逐步消失。海绵窦段是颈内动脉最狭窄的部位，外弹力膜消失，血管壁弹性改变，可能是诱发动脉粥样硬化的易感因素[14]。相比之下，基底动脉（basilar artery，BA）片段状的外弹力膜对其抵御动脉粥样硬化，起到了一定的作用[15]（图2.1）。

动脉粥样硬化好发于40岁以后，随着年龄的增长，其发病率以及严重程度逐渐增加[16]。修订的美国心脏协会标准[17]将动脉粥样硬化分为三个

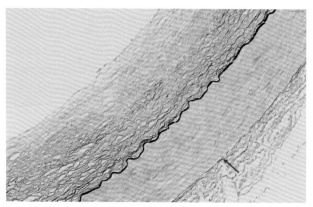

图 2.1　基底动脉外弹力膜（箭头）

阶段：①非动脉粥样硬化性内膜病变，无内膜增厚；②早期斑块，平滑肌细胞聚集（内膜增厚），泡沫细胞沉积（内膜黄色瘤）（图2.2 A），平滑肌细胞和细胞外脂质沉积于富含蛋白多糖的基质中（病理性内膜增厚）（图2.2 B）；③晚期斑块，坏死核心形成，上覆纤维帽（纤维帽粥瘤）（图2.3），随着病变的发展，纤维帽变薄，其内可见巨噬细胞和淋巴细胞浸润（薄纤维帽粥瘤），斑块进一步纤维化、

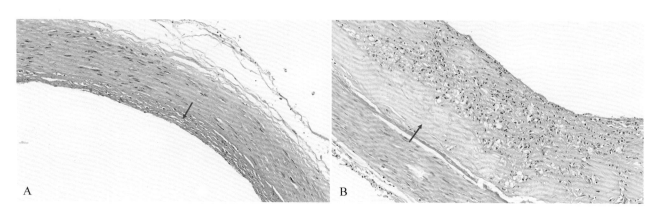

图 2.2　早期斑块内可见平滑肌细胞、泡沫细胞（**A**，箭头），以及富含蛋白多糖的基质（**B**，箭头）

Chapter 2

Pathophysiology

Atherosclerosis is a systemic disease that primarily affects large and medium arteries, including the coronary, cerebral, and peripheral arteries. Studies have confirmed the key role of oxidized low-density lipoprotein in the process of atherosclerosis,[13] which causes vascular intimal thickening or plaque formation, resulting in gradual lumen stenosis to occlusion.

Recent studies have shown that anatomical location is an important factor in plaque formation of atherosclerosis, and anterior circulation atherosclerosis differs from posterior circulation atherosclerosis in risk factors, prevalence, and stroke mechanisms. An anatomical study of the internal carotid artery revealed that the external elastic membrane existed in the petrous segment of the internal carotid artery and gradually disappeared after the cavernous segment. Arterial wall elasticity change is considered to be a factor predisposing to atherosclerosis.[14] In contrast, the segmental external elastic membrane of the basilar artery (BA) plays a certain role in resisting atherosclerosis (Fig. 2.1).[15]

Since the age of 40 years, the incidence and severity of cerebral atherosclerosis have increased gradually with the age.[16] According to the revised American Heart Association criteria,[17] the atherosclerosis lesions were classified into three stages: (1) nonatherosclerotic intimal lesions, without intimal

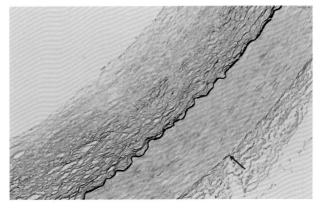

Fig. 2.1 External elastic membrane in the basilar artery (arrow)

thickening; (2) early plaques, accumulation of smooth muscle cells (intimal thickening), foam cells (intimal xanthoma) (Fig. 2.2 A), and proteoglycan-rich matrix (pathological intimal thickening) (Fig. 2.2 B); (3) advanced plaques, well-formed necrotic core with an overlying fibrous cap (fibrous cap atheroma) (Fig. 2.3), with the development of the lesion, the fibrous cap becomes thinner, and infiltrated by macrophages and lymphocytes (thin fibrous cap atheroma), plaque is fibrotic and calcified further (fibrocalcific plaque); (4) complicated advanced plaques, erosion, plaque rupture, luminal thrombus and intraplaque hemorrhage. The

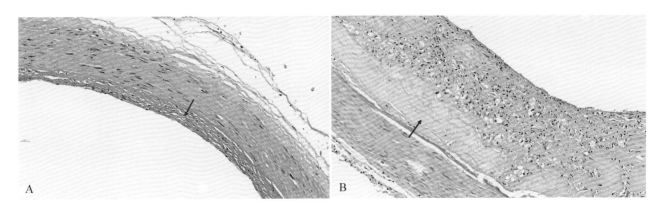

Fig. 2.2 Smooth muscle cells, foam cells (**A**, arrow), and proteoglycan-rich matrix (**B**, arrow) were accumulated in early plaques

钙化（纤维钙化斑块）；④复杂的晚期斑块，糜烂，斑块破裂，管腔血栓和斑块内出血。斑块病理形态学分型在前循环动脉和后循环动脉间没有显著差异，斑块成分类似，均很少检出复杂的晚期斑块，也很少观察到斑块溃疡和斑块内出血[16]。但目前的研究表明，前循环和后循环动脉粥样硬化斑块对血管壁的影响有明显差异，前循环管腔狭窄明显，且多为偏心性斑块；而后循环管腔狭窄较轻，但容易形成血栓[18]。

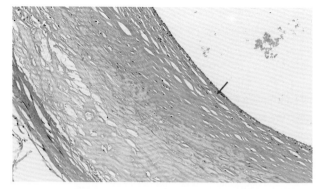

图 2.3　晚期斑块可见坏死核心形成，上覆纤维帽（箭头）

（秦桂萍）

plaque phenotype does not display significant difference between anterior and posterior circulation arteries, and the components of plaques were detected similarly between anterior and posterior circulation. Complicated advanced plaques were infrequently detected, and the plaque ulceration and intraplaque hemorrhage were observed seldomly in the anterior and posterior circulation arteries.[16] However, the current study showed that there are significant differences in the influence of atherosclerotic plaques on the vascular wall between anterior and posterior circulation. The plaques are mostly eccentric and often lead to obvious lumen stenosis in the anterior circulation, while in the posterior circulation, the stenosis is milder but prone to thrombosis.[18]

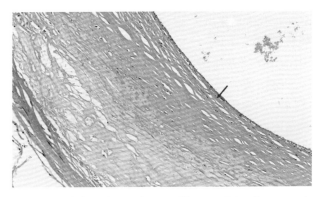

Fig. 2.3 Well-formed necrotic core with an overlying fibrous cap in advanced plaques (arrow)

(Translated by Guiping Qin)

第三章

干预治疗

颅内动脉粥样硬化是中国缺血性卒中的重要病因。来自中国国家卒中登记（China National Stroke Registry，CNSR）的数据显示，颅内大动脉粥样硬化性卒中约占所有缺血性卒中的 45%[19]。目前关于症状性颅内动脉粥样硬化的治疗尚存在一些争议。大量国内外高质量的临床研究陆续发表，为症状性颅内动脉粥样硬化的治疗提供了指导。颅内动脉粥样硬化的治疗手段主要包括内科治疗、外科治疗和血管内介入治疗。

第一节　内科治疗

症状性颅内动脉粥样硬化的药物治疗是一项综合的管理措施，包括抗血小板药物的选择、他汀类药物治疗以及危险因素的控制等，现分述如下。

一、抗血小板药物

（一）抗血小板药物的作用机制

1. 阿司匹林

阿司匹林通过乙酰化丝氨酸 -530，不可逆地抑制位于血小板和内皮细胞上的环氧合酶 -1（cyclooxygenase-1，COX-1），防止花生四烯酸转换为血栓素 A_2（thromboxane A_2，TXA_2）。阿司匹林通过阻止 TXA_2 的产生，抑制血小板聚集。

2. 噻吩吡啶类药物

$P2Y_{12}$ 受体是血小板上的一种腺苷二磷酸（adenosine diphosphate，ADP）受体，与血小板聚集和分泌的放大有关[20-21]。噻吩吡啶类药物（如氯吡格雷和普拉格雷）不可逆地阻断 $P2Y_{12}$ 受体，抑制 ADP 介导的血小板活化。替格瑞洛是一种新型噻吩吡啶类药物，可逆地抑制 ADP 介导的血小板活化。

3. 磷酸二酯酶抑制剂

磷酸二酯酶（phosphodiesterase，PDE）是前列环素和一氧化氮受体激动剂系统中调节糖蛋白 IIb-IIIa 激活的关键酶。双嘧达莫通过抑制磷酸二酯酶，增加环磷酸鸟苷（cyclic guanosine monophosphate，cGMP）浓度，抑制腺苷的细胞摄取和代谢，间接升高环磷酸腺苷（cyclic adenosine monophosphate，cAMP）水平，从而抑制血小板功能。西洛他唑通过抑制磷酸二酯酶，增加环磷酸腺苷浓度，抑制血小板功能。

4. 糖蛋白 IIb-IIIa 受体拮抗剂

糖蛋白 IIb-IIIa 受体是与血小板聚集过程有关的主要血小板表面受体，糖蛋白 IIb-IIIa 受体拮抗剂通过与血小板表面 IIb-IIIa 受体可逆性结合，达到快速抑制血小板聚集的作用。糖蛋白 IIb-IIIa 受体拮抗剂包括阿昔单抗、替罗非班、依替巴肽。

（二）抗血小板的单药治疗

1. 阿司匹林

根据 20 世纪 70 年代和 80 年代进行的临床试验，研究人员在 1988 年得出结论认为阿司匹林在血管性疾病的二级预防中是有效的[22-23]。但阿司匹林单药的疗效有限。在服用常规剂量阿司匹林的患者中，有相当一部分人的血小板活化没有受到足够的抑制，这样会降低阿司匹林预防卒中的疗效[24-25]。

Chapter 3

Therapeutic Approaches

Intracranial atherosclerosis is an important cause of ischemic stroke in China. Data from China National Stroke Registry (CNSR) showed that intracranial large artery atherosclerotic strokes account for approximately 45% of all ischemic strokes.[19] At present, there are still some controversies about the treatment of symptomatic intracranial atherosclerosis. Plenty of high-quality clinical studies have been published successively to provide guidance for the treatment of symptomatic intracranial atherosclerosis. The treatment of intracranial atherosclerosis mainly includes medical therapy, surgical therapy, and endovascular therapy.

Section 1   Medical Therapy

Medical therapy of symptomatic intracranial athero-sclerosis is a comprehensive management measure, including the choice of antiplatelet drugs, statin therapy, and the control of risk factors. It is described as follows.

1. Antiplatelet agents

1.1 Action mechanism of antiplatelet agents

1.1.1 Aspirin

Aspirin irreversibly inhibits cyclooxygenase-1 located on platelets and endothelial cells by acetylation of serine-530, preventing the conversion of arachidonic acid to thromboxane A_2 (TXA_2) and prostacyclin. Aspirin inhibits platelet aggregation by preventing TXA_2 production.

1.1.2 $P2Y_{12}$

$P2Y_{12}$ receptor is an adenosine diphosphate (ADP) receptor on platelets, which is related to the amplification of platelet aggregation and secretion,[20, 21] and thienopyridines (such as clopidogrel and prasugrel) irreversibly block $P2Y_{12}$ receptor and inhibit ADP-mediated platelet activation. Ticagrelor is a novel thienopyridine that reversibly inhibits ADP-mediated platelet activation.

1.1.3 Phosphodiesterase inhibitor

Phosphodiesterase (PDE) is a key enzyme in the prostacyclin and nitric oxide receptor agonist systems that regulates the activation of glycoprotein Ⅱb-Ⅲa. Dipyridamole inhibits platelet function by inhibiting phosphodiesterase, increasing the concentration of cyclic guanosine monophosphate, inhibiting the cellular uptake and metabolism of adenosine, and indirectly increasing the level of cyclic adenosine monophosphate. Cilostazol inhibits platelet function by inhibiting phosphodiesterase and increasing cyclic adenosine monophosphate concentration.

1.1.4 Glycoprotein Ⅱb-Ⅲa receptor antagonists

Glycoprotein Ⅱb-Ⅲa receptor is the main platelet surface receptor related to the process of platelet aggregation. Glycoprotein Ⅱb-Ⅲa receptor antagonists achieve rapid inhibition of platelet aggregation by reversibly binding to Ⅱb-Ⅲa receptor on the platelet surface. Glycoprotein Ⅱb-Ⅲa receptor antagonists include abciximab, tirofiban, and eptifibatide.

1.2 Single antiplatelet therapy

1.2.1 Aspirin

According to clinical trials conducted in the 1970s and 1980s, the investigators concluded that aspirin was effective in the secondary prevention of vascular diseases in 1988.[22, 23] However, the efficacy of aspirin was limited. A significant proportion of patients taking conventional doses of aspirin did not have sufficient inhibition of platelet activation, which reduced the efficacy of aspirin in preventing stroke.[24, 25]

"华法林-阿司匹林治疗症状性颅内动脉疾病（WASID）"研究[26]表明对于症状性颅内动脉狭窄>70%的患者，使用阿司匹林与使用华法林的临床疗效类似，但阿司匹林更安全，从而确立了阿司匹林在颅内动脉狭窄治疗中的临床地位。然而，尽管使用阿司匹林抗血小板治疗，第1年的卒中复发风险仍高达18%。一项针对稳定性心血管疾病患者的前瞻性研究发现阿司匹林降低死亡、心肌梗死或卒中风险达3倍以上[27]。目前研究发现低剂量阿司匹林（75～150 mg/d）是一种有效的适合长期使用的抗血小板疗法，然而，为增加预防效果盲目增加阿司匹林剂量可使患者的净获益被增加的出血风险抵消[28]。

2. 氯吡格雷和替格瑞洛

"氯吡格雷与阿司匹林在缺血事件风险患者中的比较（CAPRIE）"研究[29]发现，氯吡格雷组每年发生脑血管意外、心肌梗死或血管性死亡的风险略低于阿司匹林组（5.32% *vs.* 5.83%）。由于氯吡格雷治疗的患者很少出现严重不良反应，其已成为一种广泛应用于预防心脑血管事件的抗血小板药物。氯吡格雷是一种前体药物，通过被肝细胞色素P450-3A4（CYP3A4）激活而发挥作用，因CYP3A4活性不同，氯吡格雷抑制血小板的程度存在明显个体差异[30]。CYP2C19功能缺失等位基因［*2和（或）*3］携带者是氯吡格雷无效的强预测因子，因遗传变异导致氯吡格雷抵抗的症状性颅内动脉粥样硬化患者可能有更高的卒中复发风险。在亚洲人群中，CYP2C19功能缺失等位基因的携带者所占比例高达58.8%[31]，因此需要寻找替代治疗方案。

替格瑞洛不经肝CYP2C19代谢，故不受CYP2C19基因多态性的影响，有望成为氯吡格雷抵抗患者的有效替代药物。目前，由于新型抗血小板药物（包括普拉格雷和替格瑞洛）增加出血风险，并没有广泛应用于缺血性卒中的治疗，原因可能是出血事件抵消了其所带来的临床获益。因此，需要更多的临床研究探索新型抗血小板药物的有效性和安全性。

（三）双联抗血小板治疗

抗血小板治疗过程中替代通路的激活是导致抗血小板药物不敏感或抵抗的重要原因之一，加入另一种不同作用机制的抗血小板药物或许能提高对血小板功能的抑制率。

由北京天坛医院王拥军教授牵头的"氯吡格雷联合阿司匹林与单用阿司匹林相比用于急性非致残性脑血管事件高危患者的疗效比较（CHANCE）"研究[32]表明，氯吡格雷联合阿司匹林在降低非致残性小卒中或高危TIA患者早期卒中复发方面优于单用阿司匹林（90天内卒中发生的相对风险降低了32%），且不增加出血风险。"氯吡格雷联合阿司匹林与单用阿司匹林相比对于减少急性症状性颅内动脉或颈动脉狭窄患者栓子形成疗效的比较（CLAIR）"研究[33]表明，氯吡格雷联合阿司匹林在降低微栓子信号阳性率和微栓子数量方面优于单用阿司匹林。"颅内支架置入与积极药物干预治疗颅内动脉狭窄（SAMMPRIS）"研究[34]显示阿司匹林联合氯吡格雷治疗症状性颅内动脉重度狭窄（70%～99%）患者的卒中或死亡发生率（30天为5.8%，1年为12.2%）明显低于支架组（30天为14.7%，1年为20%）。

双联抗血小板治疗并不总是比单药抗血小板治疗更有效，而且还可能显著增加不良反应发生的风险。"阿司匹林联合氯吡格雷与单用氯吡格雷相比对近期缺血性卒中或短暂性脑缺血发作高危患者的疗效比较（MATCH）"研究[35]提示与氯吡格雷单药治疗相比，阿司匹林与氯吡格雷联合治疗动脉粥样硬化性血栓形成高危患者不能减少心脑血管事件（缺血性卒中以及心肌梗死等）的发生，但显著增加了出血事件。"皮质下小卒中二级预防（SPS3）"试验[36]提示阿司匹林与氯吡格雷联合治疗组和单药阿司匹林治疗组年卒中复发风险没有区别，但联合治疗组发生主要出血事件和死亡的风险加倍。

基于上述研究，下列几种情况，可考虑进行双联抗血小板治疗。①急性非心源性高风险TIA（定义为ABCD2评分≥4，根据年龄、血压、临床特征、TIA持续时间和是否存在糖尿病评估卒中风险；评分范围为0～7分）或轻度缺血性卒中［定义为美国国立卫生研究院卒中量表（National Institutes of Health Stroke Scale，NIHSS）评分≤3分，评分范围为0～42分］：在症状发作后24 h内，患者接受氯吡格雷和阿司匹林联合治疗（氯吡格雷的初始剂量为300 mg，随后每天75 mg，共90天，前

The WASID (Warfarin-Aspirin Symptomatic Intracranial Disease) study[26] showed that aspirin was similar to warfarin in clinical efficacy but safer in patients with symptomatic intracranial arterial stenosis > 70%, thus establishing the clinical status of aspirin in the treatment of intracranial arterial stenosis. Despite the use of aspirin antiplatelet therapy, however, the risk of stroke recurrence remained 18% in the first year. A prospective study of stable cardiovascular disease found that aspirin could reduce the risk of death, myocardial infarction, or stroke more than threefold.[27] Current studies have found that low-dose aspirin (75–150 mg/d) is an effective antiplatelet therapy suitable for long-term use, while blindly increasing the dose of aspirin to increase the preventive effect can offset the net benefit of patients by increased bleeding risk.[28]

1.2.2 Clopidogrel and Ticagrelor

The study of the efficacy and safety of Clopidogrel versus Aspirin in the treatment of ischaemic events (Clopidogrel vs. Aspirin in Patients at Risk of Ischaemic Event, CAPRIE)[29] found that the annual risk of cerebrovascular accident, myocardial infarction, or vascular death was slightly lower in the clopidogrel group than that in the aspirin group (5.32% vs. 5.83%). The patients treated with clopidogrel rarely experience serious adverse effects. Therefore, as an antiplatelet drug, clopidogrel is widely used to prevent cardiovascular and cerebrovascular events. Clopidogrel is a prodrug which is activated by cytochrome P450-3A4 (CYP3A4), and there are significant individual differences in the degree of clopidogrel inhibiting platelets due to different level of CYP3A4 activity.[30] Carriers of CYP2C19 loss-of-function alleles [*2 and/or *3] are strong predictors of clopidogrel ineffectiveness, and patients with symptomatic intracranial atherosclerosis who are resistant to clopidogrel due to genetic variants may have a higher risk of stroke recurrence. Carriers of loss-of-function alleles of CYP2C19 account for up to 58.8% in Asian population,[31] and alternative treatment options need to be sought.

Ticagrelor is not metabolized by CYP2C19 and is not affected by CYP2C19 gene polymorphisms, which is expected to be an effective alternative in patients with clopidogrel resistance. At present, because new antiplatelet drugs (including prasugrel and ticagrelor) increase the risk of bleeding event which might offset the clinical benefits it brings, they are not widely used in the treatment of ischemic stroke. Therefore, more clinical studies are needed to explore the efficacy and safety of novel antiplatelet agents.

1.3 Dual antiplatelet therapy

Activation of alternative pathways during antiplatelet therapy is one of the important causes of antiplatelet insensitivity or resistance, and the addition of another antiplatelet drug with different mechanisms of action may improve the inhibition rate of platelet function.

The CHANCE (Clopidogrel and Aspirin versus Aspirin Alone for the Treatment of High-risk Patients with Acute Non-disabling Cerebrovascular Event) study,[32] led by Professor Yongjun Wang of Beijing Tiantan Hospital, showed that clopidogrel plus aspirin was superior to aspirin alone in reducing early stroke recurrence in patients with non-disabling minor stroke or TIA, with 32% reduction in the relative risk of stroke recurrence in the "dual antiplatelet" treatment group of 90 days without increasing the risk of bleeding. CLAIR (Clopidogrel plus Aspirin versus Aspirin Alone for Reducing Embolisation in Patients with Acute Symptomatic Cerebral or Carotid Artery Stenosis) study[33] indicated that combination of clopidogrel and aspirin was more effective than aspirin alone in reducing microembolic signals in patients with acute symptomatic stenosis. SAMMPRIS (Stenting versus Aggressive Medical Therapy for Intracranial Arterial Stenosis) study[34] indicated that for patients with intracranial arterial severe stenosis (70%–99%), aggressive medical management was superior to percutaneous transluminal angioplasty and stenting (PTAS), because the risk of stroke or death after PTAS was higher (14.7% for 30-day, 20.0% for 1-year) than that of aggressive medical therapy alone (5.8% for 30-day, 12.2% for 1-year).

Dual antiplatelet therapy was not always more effective than single antiplatelet agent and may also significantly increase the risk of adverse events. MATCH (Aspirin and clopidogrel compared with clopidogrel alone after recent ischaemic stroke or transient ischaemic attack in high-risk patients) study[35] revealed that adding aspirin to clopidogrel in high-risk patients with recent ischaemic stroke or TIA was associated with a non-significant difference in reducing major vascular events, however, the risk of life-threatening major bleeding was increased by the addition of aspirin. SPS3 (Secondary Prevention of Small Subcortical Strokes) trial[36] suggested combination of clopidogrel and aspirin in patients with small subcortical strokes was associated with a non-significant difference in reducing risk of recurrent stroke, and an increased risk of major bleeding and death events.

Based on the above studies, dual antiplatelet therapy may be considered in the following situations. (1) Acute non-cardiac high-risk TIA (defined as a score of ≥ 4 on the ABCD2, which assesses the risk of stroke on the basis of age, blood pressure, clinical features, duration of TIA, and presence or absence of diabetes; scores range from 0 to 7), or minor ischemic stroke [defined as a score of ≤ 3 on the National Institutes of Health Stroke Scale (NIHSS), scores range from 0 to 42]: within 24 hours after the symptom onset, the patients receive combination therapy with clopidogrel and aspirin (clopidogrel at an initial dose of 300 mg, followed by 75 mg per day for 90 days, plus aspirin at a dose of 75 mg per day for the

21 天合用阿司匹林，剂量为每天 75 mg）。②发病 7 天内症状性颅内动脉粥样硬化性狭窄伴阳性微栓子信号（其中缺血性卒中定义为 NIHSS 评分≤ 8 分）：患者接受氯吡格雷和阿司匹林联合治疗（氯吡格雷初始剂量为 300 mg，随后每天 75 mg，持续 7 天，联合阿司匹林，剂量为每天 75 ～ 160 mg）。③发病 30 天内的症状性颅内动脉粥样硬化性狭窄（狭窄率 70% ～ 99%）：患者接受氯吡格雷和阿司匹林联合治疗（氯吡格雷 75 mg/d 和阿司匹林 100 mg/d，持续 90 天）。

综上所述，医生应权衡患者特点（狭窄程度、卒中机制、危险因素、出血风险）及抗血小板药物作用机制和特点（是否存在药物抵抗、副作用、费用）来做出合理选择。

二、抗凝药物

抗凝药物包括注射类和口服抗凝药物。注射类抗凝药物包括普通肝素和低分子量肝素。口服抗凝药物包括传统抗凝药物（如维生素 K 拮抗剂华法林）和新型口服抗凝药物（如 X a 因子抑制剂利伐沙班、阿哌沙班等，直接凝血酶抑制剂达比加群、阿加曲班等）。

WASID 研究[26]提示相较于阿司匹林组，华法林治疗发病 90 天内症状性颅内动脉粥样硬化性狭窄（50% ～ 99%）引起的死亡以及严重出血事件发生率明显高于阿司匹林组，而缺血性卒中、轻度脑出血和非卒中相关的血管性死亡事件两组之间无差异。但 WASID 研究的一项事后分析显示对于国际标准化比值（international normalized ratio，INR）维持在理想治疗窗（INR 2.0 ～ 3.0）的患者，卒中风险从每年 24.9% 降低到 5.1%，且每年严重出血事件的发生风险明显低于 INR 在 3.1 ～ 4.4 的患者（3.5% *vs.* 15.2%），而 INR 在 4.5 以上的患者严重出血事件的发生风险更高。这提示如果理想的治疗窗在所有患者中都能得到维持，那么华法林的疗效就会显现出来。

新型口服抗凝药不受治疗窗的限制，且在预防缺血的同时不增加出血风险，为维持最佳治疗效果提供了新的机会。因此，有必要开展临床研究，探讨使用新型口服抗凝药是否较抗血小板药物能更有效地改善症状性颅内动脉狭窄患者的预后。

三、他汀类药物

众多研究显示，他汀类药物的应用可有效降低缺血性卒中的复发风险，已被作为一级推荐写入缺血性卒中二级预防指南。

因此，对于症状性颅内动脉粥样硬化性缺血性卒中患者，强化他汀类药物治疗，使低密度脂蛋白胆固醇（low-density lipoprotein cholesterol，LDL-C）< 1.8 mmol/L 或降幅超过 50%，可降低血管事件再发的风险。

四、危险因素的控制

控制饮食，适度体育锻炼，戒烟、戒酒和其他生活方式的调整，可减少卒中风险。严格控制血糖、血压，其中糖尿病患者的糖化血红蛋白应控制在 7.0% 以下，同时联合他汀类调脂药物，也应用于症状性颅内动脉粥样硬化性狭窄患者的二级预防。

（黄睿）

first 21 days). (2) Symptomatic intracranial atherosclerotic stenosis within 7 days after the symptom onset with positive microembolic signals (ischemic stroke defined as a score of ≤ 8 on the NIHSS): patients receive combination therapy with clopidogrel and aspirin (clopidogrel at an initial dose of 300 mg, followed by 75 mg per day for 7 days, plus aspirin at a dose of 75–160 mg per day for 7 days). (3) Symptomatic intracranial atherosclerotic stenosis (70%–99%) within 30 days after the symptom onset: patients receive combination therapy with clopidogrel and aspirin (clopidogrel 75 mg per day and aspirin 100 mg per day for 90 days).

In summary, physicians should make reasonable choices after weighing patient characteristics (degree of stenosis, stroke mechanism, risk factors, bleeding risk) and action mechanism and characteristics of antiplatelet drug (e.g., presence of drug resistance, side effects, cost).

2. Anticoagulant agents

Anticoagulant agents include injectable and oral anticoagulant drugs. Injectable anticoagulant drugs include unfractionated heparin and low-molecular-weight heparin. Oral anticoagulant drugs include traditional anticoagulant drugs (such as vitamin K antagonist warfarin) and new oral anticoagulant drugs (such as factor Xa inhibitors Rivaroxaban, Apixaban, and direct thrombin inhibitors Dabigatran, Argatroban, etc.).

WASID trial[26] revealed that the incidence of death and major bleeding events due to symptomatic intracranial atherosclerotic stenosis (50%–99%) within 90 days after the symptom onset was significantly higher in the warfarin group than that in the aspirin group, while ischemic stroke, mild cerebral hemorrhage, and non-stroke-related vascular death events were not different between the two groups. However, a post-hoc analysis of the WASID study showed that for patients whose international normalized ratio (INR) were maintained at the ideal therapeutic window (INR 2.0 ~ 3.0), the risk of stroke was reduced from 24.9% to 5.1% per year, and the risk of major bleeding events per year was significantly lower than that for patients with INR between 3.1 and 4.4 (3.5% *vs.* 15.2%), while the risk of major bleeding events was higher in patients with INR above 4.5. It is suggested that if the ideal therapeutic window can be maintained in all patients, then the efficacy of warfarin will be revealed.

Novel oral anticoagulants offer an opportunity to maintain beneficial therapeutic effects within a narrow therapeutic window, preventing ischemia without increasing the risk of bleeding. Clinical studies are necessary to investigate whether new oral anticoagulants are more effective than antiplatelet drugs in improving the prognosis of patients with symptomatic intracranial arterial stenosis.

3. Statin agents

Multiple studies have shown that the statins were effective in reducing the risk of ischemic stroke recurrence, which has been introduced into the guidelines for secondary prevention of ischemic stroke as a primary recommendation.

Hence, for patients with symptomatic intracranial atherosclerotic ischemic stroke, intensive statin therapy, which reduces LDL-C to < 1.8 mmol/L or by more than 50%, could reduce the risk of recurrent vascular events.

4. Control of risk factors

A balanced diet, regular physical activity, smoking cessation, alcohol withdrawal, and other lifestyle modifications may reduce stroke risk. Strictly controlled blood glucose and blood pressure, in which the glycosylated hemoglobin should be controlled below 7.0% for diabetics, combined with the lipid-regulating drugs of statins should also be applied in the secondary prevention of patients with symptomatic ICAS.

(Translated by Rui Huang)

第二节 颅外-颅内血管搭桥手术治疗

1967 年，Yasargil 首先采用颞浅动脉-大脑中动脉（STA-MCA）吻合的方式治疗缺血性脑卒中[37]。然而，1985 年一项比较药物治疗和颅外-颅内动脉搭桥治疗颅内动脉粥样硬化性狭窄的临床研究结果为阴性[38]，文章纳入 1377 例接受手术治疗的症状性颈内动脉或 MCA 动脉粥样硬化性狭窄或闭塞的患者，与内科药物治疗组比较，结果发现 STA-MCA 吻合术未能给卒中患者带来临床获益。随后该研究受到了广泛的讨论，Sundt 等重新调查了参与研究的 62 个研究中心（一些样本量太小的医院以及加拿大研究中心被排除），发现大量接受了手术的患者因为入组及排除标准不合适而没有被纳入研究中，导致研究的随机化出现了问题[39-40]。

为了重新评估颅外-颅内动脉搭桥术能否给缺血性卒中患者带来收益，日本开展了"颅外-颅内动脉搭桥试验（JET）"，其入组标准包含了血流动力学标准，共纳入 192 例患者并进行 2 年的随访，结果显示接受外科手术治疗的患者在主要终点事件（完全卒中和死亡）以及次要终点事件（同侧复发缺血）的发生率方面均有明显降低，并且围术期的卒中发生率< 5%[41]。

2011 年美国开展的"颈动脉闭塞手术研究（COSS）"试验被迫停止。COSS 试验预计纳入的样本量为 372 例，主要终点事件定义为 30 天内卒中或死亡，以及 2 年内发生同侧缺血性卒中。在中期分析时共纳入 195 例患者，包括 97 例手术治疗组和 98 例内科治疗组。试验被叫停主要有两点原因：第一是手术组患者 2 年内同侧卒中复发率 22.7%，这与药物治疗组的 21% 没有显著差异；第二是手术组患者术后 30 天内同侧卒中的发生率为 15%，远高于药物治疗组的 2%[42]。COSS 试验虽然提供了高级别的研究证据以及加入了血流动力学指标氧摄取分数（oxygen extraction fraction，OEF），但是仍然存在一些瑕疵。首先由于患者纳入时机问题[43-44]以及通过正电子发射断层显像（positron emission tomography，PET）检查确定 OEF[45]，导致试验可能并没有筛选出卒中高危患者；其次 Reynolds 等分析了围术期同侧卒中情况，结果发现 14 例术后 30 天内同侧卒中

患者中 12 例发生于术后 2 天内，进一步分析原因发现只有 3 例围术期卒中与搭桥手术技术相关，提示了麻醉、围术期监护、护理等因素的影响超过了手术技术层面[46]。这些可能与该研究纳入了一些不合格的研究中心有关，有些研究中心颅外-颅内搭桥年手术量不足 10 例。最后 COSS 试验设置的主要终点事件并没有包含认知、语言等功能改善指标[47]，也是该试验没有得到广泛认可的原因之一。

2015 年日本公布了 JET-2 试验结果，根据静息状态的脑血流量（cerebral blood flow，CBF）和脑血管反应性（cerebrovascular reactivity，CVR）将患者分为 4 组，然后经过严格的内科药物治疗 2 年，结论为：①经药物治疗的症状性脑血管闭塞并且血流动力学改变轻微的患者预后良好；②颅外-颅内血管搭桥手术对 CBF > 80% 或 CVR > 10% 的患者无明显获益[48]。

基于 COSS 试验的失败、JET 和 JET-2 试验的阳性结果以及近年来颅外-颅内搭桥术在烟雾病治疗中展现的良好效果，2016 年中国宣武医院联合国内多个研究中心开始了"颈动脉和大脑中动脉闭塞手术研究（CMOSS）"试验[49]，研究方案相对于 COSS 试验进行了以下几个方面的改进：①以 CT 灌注成像（CT perfusion，CTP）替代 PET 作为血流动力学评估指标；②建立了更细致的纳入和排除标准，试图挑选出手术适宜人群；③次要结果事件包括了认知、情绪等多种与患者生活质量密切相关的指标，可以更准确地反映病情和疗效。

颅内动脉粥样硬化性狭窄是一种高度异质性疾病，外科手术提供了一种治疗思路，并有其理论依据。虽然 COSS 试验和 JET 试验提供了不同的试验结果、CMOSS 试验还没有得出试验结果，但是颅外-颅内动脉搭桥手术目前仍是治疗缺血性脑卒中的可选手段之一，可能需要我们更严格地筛选合适的患者。未来需要明确手术适宜人群特点、技术规范、手术时机及围术期管理规范等问题。

（王嵘 秦舒森）

Section 2 Extracranial–intracranial bypass surgery

In 1967, Yasargil used superficial temporal artery-middle cerebral artery (STA-MCA) anastomosis to treat ischemic stroke for the first time.[37] However, the clinical study in 1985 comparing drug therapy with bypass surgery for intracranial atherosclerotic stenosis was negative.[38] A total of 1377 patients with symptomatic internal carotid artery or middle cerebral artery stenosis or occlusion due to atherosclerosis treated with bypass surgery were included in the study. STA-MCA bypass surgery did not provide clinical benefit to stroke patients compared with the medical treatment. The study was then widely discussed. Sundt et al. reinvestigated the 62 research centers that participated in the study (hospitals with small sample sizes and Canada research centers were excluded), and found that a large number of patients who had undergone bypass surgery were not included in the study due to inappropriate inclusion and exclusion criteria, leading to the randomization of the study being problematic.[39, 40]

To reassess the benefits of extracranial-intracranial (EC-IC) bypass surgery to patients with atherosclerotic ischemic stroke, the JET (Japanese EC-IC Bypass Trial) study was conducted in Japan. The inclusion criteria included hemodynamic parameter. A total of 192 patients were enrolled and followed up for 2 years. The primary endpoint (complete stroke and death) and secondary endpoint (ipsilateral recurrent ischemia) were significantly reduced in patients undergoing surgical treatment, and the incidence of perioperative stroke was less than 5%.[41]

The COSS (Carotid Occlusion Surgery Study) trial in the United States was halted in 2011. The COSS trial was expected to include a sample size of 372 patients, and the primary end point was defined as stroke or death within 30 days and ipsilateral ischemic stroke within 2 years. A total of 195 patients, 97 in the surgical group and 98 in the drug group, were included in the interim analysis. The trial was stopped for two reasons: first, the 2-year recurrence rate of ipsilateral stroke in the surgery group was 22.7%, which was not significantly different from that of 21% in the drug group; second, the incidence of ipsilateral stroke within the 30 days after surgery was 15%, which was much higher than that of 2% in the drug group.[42] Although the COSS trial provided high-level evidence and added hemodynamic index of oxygen extraction fraction (OEF), it still had some flaws. First, the trial might not screen out patients at high risk of stroke due to the timing of patient inclusion[43, 44] and the determination of OEF by PET examination.[45] Second, Reynolds analyzed the perioperative ipsilateral stroke cases and found that among the 14 cases of ipsilateral stroke patients within 30 days after operation, 12 cases occurred within 2 days

postoperatively. Further analysis showed that only 3 cases of perioperative stroke were associated with bypass surgical technic, suggesting that anesthesia, perioperative monitoring and nursing care may play a more important role than surgical technic.[46] These may be related to the inclusion of several substandard centers in the study, some of which performed less than 10 extracranial-intracranial bypass operations per year. Finally, the main endpoint events set in the COSS trial did not include functional improvement indicators such as cognition and language, which was also one of the reason why the trial was not widely recognized.[47]

The results of the JET-2 study were published in Japan in 2015. According to the resting cerebral blood flow (CBF) and cerebrovascular reactivity (CVR), patients were divided into four groups and received strict drug treatment for 2 years. The conclusions were as follows: (1) After drug treatment, patients with symptomatic cerebral vascular occlusion and slight hemodynamic changes had a good prognosis; (2) For patients of CBF > 80% or CVR > 10%, bypass surgery had no significant benefit.[48]

In the background of the failure of COSS trial, the positive results of JET and JET-2 study, and the good results of EC-IC bypass surgery in Moyamoya disease in recent years, Xuanwu Hospital (China), in collaboration with several other Chinese research centers, started the CMOSS (Carotid or Middle cerebral artery Occlusion Surgery Study) trial in 2016.[49] Compared with the COSS trial, the protocol of the CMOSS trial was improved in the following aspects: (1) CTP was used as hemodynamic evaluation index instead of PET; (2) More detailed inclusion and exclusion criteria were established to select the patients who were suitable for surgery; (3) Secondary outcome events included a variety of indicators closely related to patients' daily life, such as cognition and emotion, which could reflect the state of illness and surgery efficacy more accurately.

Intracranial atherosclerotic stenosis is a highly heterogeneous disease, and the surgical treatment has a theoretical basis. Although the COSS trial and the JET study provided different results, and the CMOSS trial has not been completed, bypass surgery is still one of the possible treatments for ischemic stroke. It requires us to select patients more strictly. In the future, it is necessary to clarify the indications and contraindications of operation, surgical technics, operation time and perioperative management specifications.

(Translated by Shusen Qin)

第三节 血管内介入治疗

颅内动脉粥样硬化性狭窄（ICAS）的介入治疗起源于 20 世纪 80 年代，经过 30 多年的发展，ICAS 介入治疗的材料和技术等都获得长足发展。总结其发展过程，可以归纳为四个阶段。

第一阶段：技术兴起，缺乏材料

1980 年 Sundt 等首次使用球囊扩张血管成形术成功治疗了 2 例难治性基底动脉狭窄[50]。随后的相关研究证实单纯球囊扩张成形术治疗 ICAS 是可行的[51-53]。Hideo Okada 等研究显示单纯球囊扩张成形术治疗 30 天内卒中或死亡的发生率为 6.4%，30 天至 1 年内同侧卒中发生率为 3%[54]。然而，单纯球囊扩张成形术的并发症发生率较高，常见并发症包括血管夹层、继发血栓形成、弹性回缩以及血管破裂等。为了减少单纯球囊扩张成形术并发症，1999 年临床医生首次提出并应用小球囊缓慢扩张技术，这种技术已被神经介入医生广泛接受[55]。

伴随心脏介入技术和材料学的发展，1996 年 Feldman 等使用冠状动脉球囊扩张式支架治疗颈内动脉颅内段狭窄获得成功[56]，随后系列关于冠状动脉支架治疗 ICAS 的支架成形术相关研究被报道[57-60]。同样，球囊扩张式支架治疗 ICAS 也有较高的手术风险。原因在于缺少球囊和支架一体化的设计，使得其整体直径相对较大，限制其通过严重狭窄病变的能力；在迂曲的血管内输送时可能出现支架从球囊上脱落；同时，球囊扩张式支架的命名压高，可能会增加血管破裂的风险或导致血管损伤；此外，这种支架释放后管腔内部的直径一致，尽管这有助于即刻管径的改善、减少再狭窄率，但是由于支架不能顺应血管的自然曲度和形态，可能会导致血管过度扩张而破裂或支架与血管壁贴合不良。

随着研究的深入和技术的积累，颅内动脉狭窄的病变分型研究得到重视，Mori 分型[53] 和 LMA 分型[53] 相继出现。LMA 分型是我国姜卫剑教授等根据颅内动脉狭窄的位置、形态、路径提出了颅内动脉狭窄的分型以预测支架成形术的结果，同时还就并发症发生的相关因素进行了探索[53, 61]。

第二阶段：技术成熟，专用材料相继出现

2004 年全球第一个多中心、前瞻性的应用颅内专用 Neurolink 球囊扩张式支架（Guidant 公司）治疗颅内动脉狭窄的非随机对照研究"症状性椎动脉或颅内动脉粥样硬化性病变的支架术治疗（SSYLVIA）"结果发表[62]。Terada 等报道一项回顾性研究表明对于颈内动脉颅内段狭窄的治疗，支架置入比单纯球囊扩张更有效[63]。球囊扩张式支架治疗 ICAS 的经验和临床效果得到了较为深入的研究。

2004 年中国自主研发一款颅内专用球囊扩张式支架 Apollo 被批准在中国上市。Apollo 支架的输送系统为快速交换球囊导管系统，球囊设计为半顺应性球囊，使支架与血管壁贴合更紧密，同时低压球囊有效降低了血管受损风险。"中国症状性颅内段动脉狭窄 Apollo 支架治疗登记研究（AIRE-CHINA）"在中国 20 家中心开展，入组 159 例患者，手术技术成功率为 98.7%，30 天靶血管事件（包括任何类型卒中、TIA 和死亡）发生率为 4.4%[64]。

在这种背景下，2005 年基于相关研究结果，美国食品和药品监督管理局批准 Gateway-Wingspan 支架系统上市用于治疗症状性 ICAS 患者（狭窄率 ≥50% 且对药物治疗无效）[65]。Wingspan 支架为镍钛合金构成的自膨式支架，被预先安置于一个 3.5F 的非快速交换多腔导管输送系统中。Gateway-Wingspan 支架系统主要有两个操作步骤：亚满意的球囊（Gateway）扩张成形，自膨式支架（Wingspan）置入。该系统临床操作相对复杂，对于技术要求较高。

2016 年中国赛诺医疗科技推出全球首款颅内快速交换型球囊扩张导管 Neuro RX，获得中国国家食品和药品监督管理局的注册认证。该球囊系统与 Gateway 球囊类似，均为半顺应性球囊。

Section 3 Endovascular Therapy

Endovascular treatment of ICAS originated from the 1980s. After more than 30 years of development, the materials and techniques for endovascular treatment of ICAS have experienced a great development, which can be summarized into four stages.

The first stage: the rise of the technology and lack of the materials

In 1980, Thoralf M. Sundt et al successfully treated two cases of refractory basilar artery stenosis using balloon dilatation angioplasty.[50] The subsequent studies demonstrated that simple balloon angioplasty for the treatment of ICAS was feasible.[51-53] Hideo Okada et al revealed that the incidence of stroke or death within 30 days after percutaneous transluminal angioplasty (PTA) treatment was 6.4%, and the incidence of ipsilateral stroke beyond 30 days to 1 year after PTA was 3%.[54] Simple balloon angioplasty has a high incidence of complications, and common complications include vascular dissection, secondary thrombosis, elastic recoil as well as vascular rupture. To reduce the complications of balloon dilatation, slow dilatation technique with the small-size balloon was first proposed and applied by clinicians in 1999, and has been widely accepted by neurointerventionalists.[55]

With the development of cardiac interventional techniques and materials, the use of coronary balloon-expandable stents for the treatment of intracranial internal carotid artery stenosis was successfully performed by Feldman in 1996,[56] followed by a series of studies on coronary stents for ICAS stenting.[57-60] Similarly, balloon-expandable stents have a significant periprocedural risk in the treatment of ICAS, which may be due to the lack of integration design of the balloon and the stent. The large overall diameter limits its ability to pass through severe stenosis lesions. Besides, the stent may be detached from the balloon when passing through a tortuous approach. Moreover, the high nominal pressure of the balloon-expandable stents may increase the risk of vascular rupture or damage to the blood vessel. In addition, the vessel diameter of target segment between proximal and distal end of a stent is consistent after the stent deployment. Although this contributes to the immediate improvement of the vascular diameter and the reduction of the in-stent restenosis (ISR) rate, the failure of stent to comply with the natural curvature and shape of vessel may lead to excessive expansion of vessel and vascular rupture or poor apposition of the stent to vessel wall.

With the deepening of research and the accumulation of technology, attention has been paid to the lesion classification of ICAS. Mori classification[53] and LMA classification[53] have appeared successively. LMA classification is proposed by Professor Jiang Weijian et al in China according to the location, shape, and approach of intracranial artery stenosis to predict the outcome of stenting, and to explore the related factors of complications.[53, 61]

The second stage: mature technology and various special materials

In 2004, the results of the world's first multicenter, prospective non-randomized controlled study SSYLVIA (stenting of symptomatic atherosclerotic lesions in the vertebral or intracranial arteries) using intracranial dedicated Neurolink balloon-expandable stent (Guidant Company) for the treatment of intracranial artery stenosis were published.[62] Terada et al reported a retrospective study showing that stenting for stenosis of the intracranial internal carotid artery is more effective than simple balloon angioplasty.[63] The experience and clinical effects of the balloon-expandable stents used for ICAS have been studied intensively.

In 2004, China independently developed an intracranial special balloon-expandable stent, Apollo, which was approved for marketing in China. The delivery system of the Apollo stent is a fast-exchange balloon catheter system. The semi-compliant balloon design allows for complete stent apposition to the vessel wall, while the balloon with low nominal pressure effectively reduces the risk of vessel damage. A Multicenter Registry Study of Apollo Stenting for Symptomatic Intracranial Artery Stenosis in China (AIRE-CHINA) was performed in 20 sites. A total of 159 patients were recruited. Successful revascularization rate was 98.7%. The incidence of target vascular events (including any stroke, TIA, and death) within 30 days after stenting was 4.4%.[64]

In this context, the Gateway-Wingspan stent system was approved by the US Food and Drug Administration in 2005 for the treatment of patients with symptomatic ICAS (stenosis rate $\geqslant$ 50% and refractory to medical treatment) based on relevant study results.[65] The Wingspan stent is a self-expanding stent constructed of nitinol and is pre-positioned in a 3.5F non-rapid-exchanging multi-lumen catheter delivery system. The Gateway-Wingspan Stent System has two main operation steps: balloon predilatation (Gateway balloon), and placement of self-expanding stent (Wingspan stent). The clinical operation of the system is relatively complicated and requires high technical learning curve.

In 2016, China's Sino-Science Technology launched the world's first intracranial fast-exchange balloon dilatation catheter, called Neuro RX, which was certified by the China National Food and Drug Administration. The semi-compliant balloon system is the same as the Gateway balloon.

第三阶段：临床研究循证时代

随着颅内动脉狭窄血管内介入治疗技术的广泛开展，为验证强化药物治疗与支架成形术治疗预防卒中复发的效果，2008 年美国 Chimowitz 教授启动了 SAMMPRIS 研究[34]。研究首要目标是观察血管成形术联合积极药物治疗预防卒中的效果是否优于单纯积极药物治疗。研究对象为狭窄率 70%～99% 的颅内动脉粥样硬化性病变导致入组前 30 内发生 TIA 或者非致残性卒中［改良 Rankin 量表（modified Rankin scale，mRS）评分 ≤ 3］的患者，并随访 2 年。研究为期 5 年，计划在美国的 50 个中心开展，拟入选患者 764 人。主要研究终点是在入组后 30 天内以及血管内治疗后 30 天内任何卒中和死亡，以及在后来的随访中靶血管相关的缺血性卒中。次要终点是致残性卒中、任何卒中和死亡、心肌梗死以及非卒中相关性出血事件等。最终研究结果显示药物治疗组与支架治疗组 30 天内卒中或死亡发生率分别为 5.8% 和 14.7%，由于支架组出现较高的卒中再发及死亡事件，研究提前终止，提示支架联合积极药物治疗效果并不优于单纯积极药物治疗[66]。但是该研究面临诸多质疑，包括操作者经验不足、病例入组不当、支架治疗组中较多患者给予超大剂量氯吡格雷等。

2015 年 JAMA 杂志发表 "Vitesse 缺血性卒中颅内支架治疗研究（VISSIT）"，该研究比较强化药物治疗和球囊扩张式支架治疗颅内动脉狭窄预防卒中的效果，结果提示支架组术后 30 天内卒中、死亡或颅内出血与严重 TIA 的发生率更高（24.1% *vs.* 9.4%），且 1 年靶血管供应区卒中或严重 TIA 的发生率也更高（36.2% *vs.* 15.1%）[67]。

同时，中国学者也开始关注颅内动脉狭窄的血管内介入治疗，相关登记研究结果相继发表。2015 年，北京天坛医院缪中荣教授牵头的颅内动脉狭窄介入治疗多中心登记研究[64]显示颅内动脉狭窄介入治疗 30 天的卒中、TIA 及死亡的发生率为 4.3%，远低于 SAMMPRIS 研究。2016 年北京宣武医院焦力群教授为首的团队也公布了其颅内动脉狭窄的多中心登记研究结果，共计入组 100 例患者，30 天卒中和死亡发生率为 2%[68]。

2019 年 WEAVE 研究[69]公布，该研究旨在验证 Wingspan 支架系统的安全性，结果发现符合适应证的患者，其接受支架治疗 72 h 内终点事件的发生率仅为 2.6%，远远低于 SAMMPRIS 研究的内科治疗组。此外，WEAVE 研究同时明确了 ICAS 介入治疗的手术时机、规避并发症的相关技术问题及围术期药物使用方法等问题。2021 年 WOVEN 研究[70]也发表，该研究目的是明确 Wingspan 支架系统的远期疗效，结果发现 1 年卒中和死亡率仅为 8.5%，这其中还包括 4 例围术期事件的患者；再狭窄率为 16.8%，再狭窄的 18 例患者中有 7 例出现症状，再狭窄是远期卒中复发的主要原因。

第四阶段：off-label 使用经微导管释放的自膨式支架治疗 ICAS

尽管颅内动脉狭窄的专用支架包括球囊扩张式支架和自膨式支架，但是对复杂的颅内动脉狭窄，仍存在一些困难病例无法得到治疗，也因材料的原因造成并发症。一项德国研究应用 Enterprise 支架治疗 209 例 ICAS 患者，技术成功率为 100%，围术期并发症发生率为 8.1%，平均随访 4.2 个月，症状性再狭窄发生率为 2.3%[71]。另一项研究使用药物涂层球囊预扩张联合 Enterprise 自膨式支架治疗狭窄率 ≥ 50% 的症状性 ICAS 患者，结果显示技术成功率为 81%，并发症发生率为 5%，再狭窄发生率为 3%[72]。一项针对症状性颅内动脉狭窄药物治疗失败的患者应用 Solitaire 支架治疗的安全性及有效性研究中，技术成功率为 100%，30 天并发症发生率为 9.09%，平均随访 9.3 个月支架内再狭窄发生率为 11.36%[73]。此外，还有 Neuform EZ 支架系统用于治疗 ICAS 的小样本研究报道[74]。

总体来说，颅内动脉狭窄的介入治疗效果和安全性均在不断进步，在此过程中也伴随临床医生对疾病认识的加深、技术的成熟和介入材料技术的进步。未来颅内动脉狭窄的介入治疗，一方面要加强对疾病本身的深入研究，另一方面要加强材料技术的研究，以便为临床提供更加安全、便捷和有效的装置。

（徐子奇）

The third stage: evidence based era of clinical research

With the extensive development of endovascular therapy for intracranial artery stenosis, the comparison of the effect of aggressive medical therapy and stent angioplasty in preventing stroke recurrence has become a research hotspot. The SAMMPRIS study was initiated in 2008 by Professor Chimowitz in the United States.[34] SAMMPRIS is the first randomized trial designed to compare percutaneous transluminal angioplasty and stenting (PTAS) plus aggressive medical management with aggressive medical management alone in high-risk patients with intracranial stenosis. The objective population in this trial included patients who had TIA or non-disabling ischemic stroke (modified Rankin scale $\leqslant$ 3) within 30 days before enrollment, due to ICAS with stenosis rate of 70% to 99% confirmed by catheter angiography. The expected mean follow-up duration was 2 years. The expected total study duration was 5 years, and the expected sample size was 764 patients. The trial was planned to be conducted at 50 sites in the United States. Primary endpoints included: (1) any stroke or death within 30 days after enrollment, (2) any stroke or death within 30 days after a revascularization procedure in the culprit lesion, or (3) ischemic stroke in the territory of the culprit artery beyond 30 days. Secondary outcomes included disabling stroke, any stroke or death, myocardial infarction, and major non-stroke hemorrhage, etc. The primary endpoint rate within 30 days after enrollment was 14.7% in the PTAS group and 5.8% in the medical-management group. Enrollment was prematurely stopped, because the rate of stroke or death within 30 days was higher in the PTAS group. This may suggest that PTAS with the use of the medical management was not superior to aggressive medical management alone.[66] However, doubts were cast on the study for the lack of experience of the operator, improper cases enrolled, and the administration of supramaximal clopidogrel to patients in the PTAS group.

In 2015, JAMA published the VISSIT (Vitesse Intracranial Stent Study for Ischemic Stroke Therapy) trial, which compared the effects of aggressive medical therapy and balloon-expandable stent in the treatment of intracranial artery stenosis to prevent stroke recurrence. The results suggested that the incidence of stroke, death or intracranial hemorrhage and severe TIA within 30 days after operation was higher in the stent group (24.1% *vs.* 9.4%), and the 1-year incidence of stroke or severe TIA in the target artery territory was also higher in the stent group (36.2% *vs.* 15.1%).[67]

At the same time, Chinese scholars also started to pay attention to the endovascular treatment of intracranial artery stenosis, and the results of relevant registry studies had been published successively. In 2015, a multicenter prospective registry study of endovascular therapy for intracranial artery stenosis led by Professor Zhongrong Miao from Beijing Tiantan Hospital[64] showed that the incidence of stroke, TIA and death within 30 days after endovascular therapy for intracranial artery stenosis was 4.3%, which was much lower than that in the SAMMPRIS study.[65] In 2016, the team led by Professor Liqun Jiao of Beijing Xuanwu Hospital also published the results of a multi-center registration study on intracranial arterial stenosis. 100 patients were enrolled, and the incidence of stroke and death within 30 days was 2%.[68]

In 2019, the WEAVE study[69] which was designed to verify the safety of the Wingspan stent system, found that patients who met the indications had an incidence of endpoint events of 2.6% within 72 hours after stenting, which was much lower than that in the medical treatment group in the SAMMPIRS study. In addition, the WEAVE study threw light on the timing of endovascular therapy for ICAS, the technique to avoid periprocedural complications, and the periprocedural medicine strategy. The WOVEN study[70] was also published in 2021, aiming to determine the long-term efficacy of the Wingspan stent system. The results showed that one-year incidence of stroke and death was 8.5%, including 4 patients with periprocedural events, while the ISR rate was 16.8%, among which 38.9% (7/18) was symptomatic, and ISR was the main cause of long-term recurrent stroke.

The fourth stage: off-label use of a self-expanding stent released through microcatheter for ICAS

Although stents used for ICAS include balloon-expandable and self-expanding stents, refractory intracranial artery stenosis and material-related complications still exist. A German study used Enterprise stents to treat 209 patients of ICAS. Technical success rate was 100%. Major procedural complications occurred in 16 patients (8.1%). Symptomatic in-stent restenosis was observed in 4 cases (2.3%) during a mean 4.2 months follow-up duration.[71] Another study evaluated safety and efficacy of angioplasty using a drug-eluting balloon (DEB) followed by the implantation of a self-expanding stent (Enterprise) for the treatment of ICAS patients (stenosis rate $\geqslant$ 50%). Technical success rate was 81%. The combined procedure-related permanent neurologic morbidity and mortality in 30 days and beyond was 5%. In-stent restenosis rate was 3%.[72] Another retrospective study evaluated the safety and efficacy of Solitaire stent placement after balloon angioplasty for the treatment of complex symptomatic ICAS. The overall technical success rate was 100%. The overall 30-day incidence of procedure-related complications was 9.09%. In-stent restenosis rate was 11.36% during a mean follow-up period of 9.3 months.[73] In addition, there was an small-sample study of the Neuform EZ stent system for the treatment of ICAS.[74]

Generally speaking, the efficacy and safety of endovascular therapy for ICAS are continuously improving, accompanied by the deepening of clinicians' understanding of the disease, the maturity of technology and the continuous development of endovascular material technology. In the future, the endovascular treatment of ICAS should focus on the following aspects: on the one hand, strengthening the study of the disease mechanism, on the other hand, strengthening the study of material technology to provide a safer, more convenient and effective device for clinical practice.

(Translated by Ziqi Xu)

参考文献（Reference）

［1］Higashida RT，Meyers PM，Connors JJ，3rd，et al. Intracranial angioplasty and stenting for cerebral atherosclerosis：a position statement of the American Society of Interventional and Therapeutic Neuroradiology，Society of Interventional Radiology，and the American Society of Neuroradiology. *Journal of Vascular and Interventional Radiology*，2009，20（7 Suppl）：S312-316. doi：10.1016/j.jvir.2009.04.007［published Online First：2009/07/09］

［2］王伊龙，王拥军，吴敌，等.中国卒中防治研究现状.中国卒中杂志，2007，2（1）：20-37. doi：10.3969/j.issn.1673-5765.2007.01.007

［3］Feigin VL，Lawes CM，Bennett DA，et al. Worldwide stroke incidence and early case fatality reported in 56 population-based studies：a systematic review. *The Lancet Neurology*，2009，8（4）：355-369. doi：10.1016/s1474-4422（09）70025-0［published Online First：2009/02/24］

［4］Bauer R，Sheehan S，Wechsler N，et al. Arteriographic study of sites，incidence，and treatment of arteriosclerotic cerebrovascular lesions. *Neurology*，1962，12：698. doi：10.1212/WNL.12.10.698

［5］Feldmann E，Daneault N，Kwan E，et al. Chinese-white differences in the distribution of occlusive cerebrovascular disease. *Neurology*，1990，40（10）：1541-1545. doi：10.1212/wnl.40.10.1540［published Online First：1990/10/01］

［6］Brust RW，Jr. Patterns of cerebrovascular disease in Japanese and other population groups in Hawaii：an angiographical study. *Stroke*，1975，6（5）：539-542. doi：10.1161/01.str.6.5.539［published Online First：1975/09/11］

［7］黄一宁，高山，王莉鹃，等.闭塞性脑血管病经颅多普勒超声和脑血管造影的比较.中华神经科杂志，1997，2：35-38.

［8］高山，黄家星，黄一宁，等.颅内大动脉狭窄的检查方法和流行病学调查.中国医学科学院学报，2003，1：96-100.

［9］Wong KS，Li H，Chan YL，et al. Use of transcranial Doppler ultrasound to predict outcome in patients with intracranial large-artery occlusive disease. *Stroke*，2000，31（11）：2641-2647. doi：10.1161/01.str.31.11.2641［published Online First：2000/11/04］

［10］王桂红，王拥军，姜卫剑，等.缺血性脑血管病患者脑动脉狭窄的分布及特征.中华老年心脑血管病杂志，2003，5：315-317.

［11］Kasner SE. Natural history of symptomatic intracranial arterial stenosis. *Journal of Neuroimaging*，2009，19（Suppl 1）：20s-21s. doi：10.1111/j.1552-6569.2009.00417.x［published Online First：2009/10/08］

［12］李尧，何晋涛，成冰，等.北京市东城社区40岁以上人群脑动脉狭窄的流行病学调查.中国神经免疫学和神经病学杂志，2009，16（05）：340-343.

［13］Parthasarathy S，Steinberg D，Witztum JL. The role of oxidized low-density lipoproteins in the pathogenesis of atherosclerosis. *Annual Review of Medicine*，1992，43：219-225. doi：10.1146/annurev.me.43.020192.001251［published Online First：1992/01/01］

［14］Masuoka T，Hayashi N，Hori E，et al. Distribution of internal elastic lamina and external elastic lamina in the internal carotid artery：possible relationship with atherosclerosis. *Neurol Med Chir（Tokyo）*，2010，50（3）：179-182. doi：10.2176/nmc.50.179.

［15］Gudiene D，Baltrusaitis K，Rackauskas M. Features of elastic tissue staining and its arrangement in the wall of human basilar artery. *Medicina（Kaunas，Lithuania）*，2003，39（10）：946-950.

［16］Kimura H，Takao M，Suzuki N，et al. Pathologic study of intracranial large artery atherosclerosis in 7260 autopsy cases. *Journal of Stroke and Cerebrovascular Diseases*，2017，26（12）：2821-2827. doi：10.1016/j.jstrokecerebrovasdis.2017.06.056.

［17］Virmani R，Kolodgie FD，Burke AP，et al. Lessons from sudden coronary death：a comprehensive morphological classification scheme for atherosclerotic lesions. *Arterioscler Thromb Vasc Biol*，2000，20（5）：1262-1275.

［18］Yang WJ，Fisher M，Zheng L，et al. Histological characteristics of intracranial atherosclerosis in a Chinese population：a postmortem study. *Front Neurol*，2017，8：488. doi：10.3389/fneur.2017.00488.

［19］Wang Y，Zhao X，Liu L，et al. Prevalence and outcomes of symptomatic intracranial large artery stenoses and occlusions in China：the Chinese Intracranial Atherosclerosis（CICAS）Study. *Stroke*，2014，45（3）：663-669. doi：10.1161/strokeaha.113.003508［published Online First：2014/02/01］

［20］Fontana P，Dupont A，Gandrille S，et al. Adenosine

diphosphate-induced platelet aggregation is associated with P2Y12 gene sequence variations in healthy subjects. *Circulation*, 2003, 108（8）: 989-995. doi: 10.1161/01.Cir.0000085073.69189.88［published Online First: 2003/08/13］

［21］Hollopeter G, Jantzen HM, Vincent D, et al. Identification of the platelet ADP receptor targeted by antithrombotic drugs. *Nature*, 2001, 409（6817）: 202-207. doi: 10.1038/35051599［published Online First: 2001/02/24］

［22］Genton E, Barnett HJ, Fields WS, et al. Cerebral ischemia: the role of thrombosis and of antithrombotic therapy. Study group on antithrombotic therapy. *Stroke*, 1977, 8（1）: 150-175. doi: 10.1161/01.str.8.1.150［published Online First: 1977/01/01］

［23］Antiplatelet Trialists' Collaboration. Secondary prevention of vascular disease by prolonged antiplatelet treatment. *British Medical Journal（Clinical Research ed）*, 1988, 296（6618）: 320-331.［published Online First: 1988/01/30］

［24］Pulcinelli FM, Pignatelli P, Celestini A, et al. Inhibition of platelet aggregation by aspirin progressively decreases in long-term treated patients. *Journal of the American College of Cardiology*, 2004, 43（6）: 979-984. doi: 10.1016/j.jacc.2003.08.062［published Online First: 2004/03/19］

［25］Eikelboom JW, Hirsh J, Weitz JI, et al. Aspirin-resistant thromboxane biosynthesis and the risk of myocardial infarction, stroke, or cardiovascular death in patients at high risk for cardiovascular events. *Circulation*, 2002, 105（14）: 1650-1655. doi: 10.1161/01.cir.0000013777.21160.07［published Online First: 2002/04/10］

［26］Chimowitz MI, Kokkinos J, Strong J, et al. The Warfarin-Aspirin Symptomatic Intracranial Disease Study. *Neurology*, 1995, 45（8）: 1488-1493. doi: 10.1212/wnl.45.8.1488［published Online First: 1995/08/01］

［27］Gum PA, Kottke-Marchant K, Welsh PA, et al. A prospective, blinded determination of the natural history of aspirin resistance among stable patients with cardiovascular disease. *Journal of the American College of Cardiology*, 2003, 41（6）: 961-965. doi: 10.1016/s0735-1097（02）03014-0［published Online First: 2003/03/26］

［28］Antiplatelet Trialists' Collaboration. Collaborative overview of randomised trials of antiplatelet therapy—I: Prevention of death, myocardial infarction, and stroke by prolonged antiplatelet therapy in various categories of patients. *British Medical Journal（Clinical Research ed）*, 1994, 308（6921）: 81-106.［published Online First: 1994/01/08］

［29］CAPRIE Steering Committee. A randomised, blinded, trial of clopidogrel versus aspirin in patients at risk of ischaemic events（CAPRIE）. *Lancet*, 1996, 348（9038）: 1329-1339. doi: 10.1016/s0140-6736（96）09457-3［published Online First: 1996/11/16］

［30］Lau WC, Gurbel PA, Watkins PB, et al. Contribution of hepatic cytochrome P450 3A4 metabolic activity to the phenomenon of clopidogrel resistance. *Circulation*, 2004, 109（2）: 166-171. doi: 10.1161/01.Cir.0000112378.09325.F9［published Online First: 2004/01/07］

［31］Wang Y, Zhao X, Lin J, et al. Association between CYP2C19 loss-of-function allele status and efficacy of clopidogrel for risk reduction among patients with minor stroke or transient ischemic attack. *Journal of the American Medical Association*, 2016, 316（1）: 70-78. doi: 10.1001/jama.2016.8662［published Online First: 2016/06/28］

［32］Wang Y, Wang Y, Zhao X, et al. Clopidogrel with aspirin in acute minor stroke or transient ischemic attack. *The New England Journal of Medicine*, 2013, 369（1）: 11-19. doi: 10.1056/NEJMoa1215340［published Online First: 2013/06/28］

［33］Wong KS, Chen C, Fu J, et al. Clopidogrel plus aspirin versus aspirin alone for reducing embolisation in patients with acute symptomatic cerebral or carotid artery stenosis（CLAIR study）: a randomised, open-label, blinded-endpoint trial. *The Lancet Neurology*, 2010, 9（5）: 489-497. doi: 10.1016/s1474-4422（10）70060-0［published Online First: 2010/03/26］

［34］Chimowitz MI, Lynn MJ, Derdeyn CP, et al. Stenting versus aggressive medical therapy for intracranial arterial stenosis. *The New England Journal of Medicine*, 2011, 365（11）: 993-1003. doi: 10.1056/NEJMoa1105335［published Online First: 2011/09/09］

［35］Diener HC, Bogousslavsky J, Brass LM, et al. Aspirin and clopidogrel compared with clopidogrel alone after recent ischaemic stroke or transient ischaemic attack in high-risk patients（MATCH）: randomised, double-blind, placebo-controlled trial. *Lancet*, 2004, 364（9431）: 331-337. doi: 10.1016/s0140-6736（04）16721-4［published Online First: 2004/07/28］

［36］Benavente OR, White CL, Pearce L, et al. The Secondary Prevention of Small Subcortical Strokes（SPS3）study. *International Journal of Stroke*, 2011, 6（2）: 164-175. doi: 10.1111/j.1747-4949.2010.00573.x［published Online First: 2011/03/05］

［37］Yasargil MG. Microsurgery. Applied to neurosurgery. Stuttgart: Georg Thieme Verlag, 1969.

［38］EC/IC Bypass Study Group. Failure of extracranial-intracranial arterial bypass to reduce the risk of ischemic stroke. Results of an international randomized trial. *The*

New England Journal of Medicine, 1985, 313（19）: 1191-1200. doi: 10.1056/nejm198511073131904 [published Online First: 1985/11/07]

[39] Sundt TM, Jr. Was the international randomized trial of extracranial-intracranial arterial bypass representative of the population at risk? *The New England Journal of Medicine*, 1987, 316（13）: 814-816. doi: 10.1056/nejm198703263161318 [published Online First: 1987/03/26]

[40] Goldring S, Zervas N, Langfitt T. The Extracranial-Intracranial Bypass Study. A report of the committee appointed by the American Association of Neurological Surgeons to examine the study. *The New England Journal of Medicine*, 1987, 316（13）: 817-820. doi: 10.1056/nejm198703263161319

[41] Ogasawara K, Ogawa A. JET study（Japanese EC-IC Bypass Trial）. *Nihon Rinsho*, 2006, 64（Suppl 7）: 524-527.

[42] Powers WJ, Clarke WR, Grubb RL, Jr., et al. Extracranial-intracranial bypass surgery for stroke prevention in hemodynamic cerebral ischemia: the Carotid Occlusion Surgery Study randomized trial. *Journal of the American Medical Association*, 2011, 306（18）: 1983-1992. doi: 10.1001/jama.2011.1610 [published Online First: 2011/11/10]

[43] Rothwell PM, Eliasziw M, Gutnikov SA, et al. Endarterectomy for symptomatic carotid stenosis in relation to clinical subgroups and timing of surgery. *Lancet*, 2004, 363（9413）: 915-924. doi: 10.1016/s0140-6736（04）15785-1 [published Online First: 2004/03/27]

[44] Kasner SE, Chimowitz MI, Lynn MJ, et al. Predictors of ischemic stroke in the territory of a symptomatic intracranial arterial stenosis. *Circulation*, 2006, 113（4）: 555-563. doi: 10.1161/circulationaha.105.578229 [published Online First: 2006/01/25]

[45] Carlson AP, Yonas H, Chang YF, et al. Failure of cerebral hemodynamic selection in general or of specific positron emission tomography methodology: Carotid Occlusion Surgery Study（COSS）. *Stroke*, 2011, 42（12）: 3637-3639. doi: 10.1161/strokeaha.111.627745 [published Online First: 2011/10/01]

[46] Reynolds MR, Grubb RL, Jr., Clarke WR, et al. Investigating the mechanisms of perioperative ischemic stroke in the Carotid Occlusion Surgery Study. *Journal of Neurosurgery*, 2013, 119（4）: 988-995. doi: 10.3171/2013.6.Jns13312 [published Online First: 2013/08/06]

[47] Marshall RS, Festa JR, Cheung YK, et al. Randomized Evaluation of Carotid Occlusion and Neurocognition（RECON）trial: main results. *Neurology*, 2014, 82（9）:

744-751. doi: 10.1212/wnl.0000000000000167 [published Online First: 2014/01/31]

[48] Kataoka H, Miyamoto S, Ogasawara K, et al. Results of prospective cohort study on symptomatic cerebrovascular occlusive disease showing mild hemodynamic compromise [Japanese Extracranial-Intracranial Bypass Trial（JET）-2 Study]. *Neurologia Medico-chirurgica*, 2015, 55（6）: 460-468. doi: 10.2176/nmc.oa.2014-0424 [published Online First: 2015/06/05]

[49] Ma Y, Gu Y, Tong X, et al. The Carotid and Middle cerebral artery Occlusion Surgery Study（CMOSS）: a study protocol for a randomised controlled trial. *Trials*, 2016, 17（1）: 544. doi: 10.1186/s13063-016-1600-1 [published Online First: 2016/11/18]

[50] Sundt TM, Jr., Smith HC, Campbell JK, et al. Transluminal angioplasty for basilar artery stenosis. *Mayo Clinic Proceedings*, 1980, 55（11）: 673-680. [published Online First: 1980/11/01]

[51] Higashida RT, Tsai FY, Halbach VV, et al. Transluminal angioplasty for atherosclerotic disease of the vertebral and basilar arteries. *Journal of Neurosurgery*, 1993, 78（2）: 192-198.

[52] Yokote H, Terada T, Ryujin K, et al. Percutaneous transluminal angioplasty for intracranial arteriosclerotic lesions. *Neuroradiology*, 1998, 40（9）: 590-596. doi: 10.1007/s002340050651 [published Online First: 1998/11/10]

[53] Mori T, Fukuoka M, Kazita K, et al. Follow-up study after intracranial percutaneous transluminal cerebral balloon angioplasty. *American Journal of Neuroradiology*, 1998, 19（8）: 1525-1533. [published Online First: 1998/10/08]

[54] Okada H, Terada T, Tanaka Y, et al. Reappraisal of primary balloon angioplasty without stenting for patients with symptomatic middle cerebral artery stenosis. *Neurologia Medico-chirurgica*, 2015, 55（2）: 133-140. doi: 10.2176/nmc.oa.2014-0156 [published Online First: 2015/03/10]

[55] Marks MP, Wojak JC, Al-Ali F, et al. Angioplasty for symptomatic intracranial stenosis: clinical outcome. *Stroke*, 2006, 37（4）: 1016-1020. doi: 10.1161/01.STR.0000206142.03677.c2 [published Online First: 2006/02/25]

[56] Feldman RL, Trigg L, Gaudier J, et al. Use of coronary Palmaz-Schatz stent in the percutaneous treatment of an intracranial carotid artery stenosis. *Catheterization and Cardiovascular Diagnosis*, 1996, 38（3）: 316-319. doi: 10.1002/（sici）1097-0304（199607）38:3＜316::Aid-ccd23＞3.0.Co; 2-d [published Online First: 1996/07/01]

［57］Gomez CR，Misra VK，Liu MW，et al. Elective stenting of symptomatic basilar artery stenosis. *Stroke*，2000，31（1）：95-99. doi：10.1161/01.str.31.1.95［published Online First：2000/01/08］

［58］Mori T，Kazita K，Chokyu K，et al. Short-term arteriographic and clinical outcome after cerebral angioplasty and stenting for intracranial vertebrobasilar and carotid atherosclerotic occlusive disease. *American Journal of Neuroradiology*，2000，21（2）：249-254.［published Online First：2000/03/01］

［59］Levy EI，Horowitz MB，Koebbe CJ，et al. Transluminal stent-assisted angiplasty of the intracranial vertebrobasilar system for medically refractory，posterior circulation ischemia：early results. *Neurosurgery*，2001，48（6）：1215-1221；discussion 1521-1523. doi：10.1097/00006123-200106000-00002［published Online First：2001/06/01］

［60］Lylyk P，Cohen JE，Ceratto R，et al. Angioplasty and stent placement in intracranial atherosclerotic stenoses and dissections. *American Journal of Neuroradiology*，2002，23（3）：430-436.［published Online First：2002/03/20］

［61］Jiang WJ，Du B，Leung TW，et al. Symptomatic intracranial stenosis：cerebrovascular complications from elective stent placement. *Radiology*，2007，243（1）：188-197. doi：10.1148/radiol.2431060139［published Online First：2007/03/30］

［62］Lutsep HL，Barnwell SL，Mawad M，et al. Stenting of Symptomatic Atherosclerotic Lesions in the Vertebral or Intracranial Arteries（SSYLVIA）：study results. *Stroke*，2004，35（6）：1388-1392. doi：10.1161/01.STR.0000128708.86762.d6［published Online First：2004/04/24］

［63］Terada T，Tsuura M，Matsumoto H，et al. Endovascular therapy for stenosis of the petrous or cavernous portion of the internal carotid artery：percutaneous transluminal angioplasty compared with stent placement. *Journal of Neurosurgery*，2003，98（3）：491-497. doi：10.3171/jns.2003.98.3.0491［published Online First：2003/03/26］

［64］Miao Z，Zhang Y，Shuai J，et al. Thirty-day outcome of a Multicenter Registry Study of Stenting for Symptomatic Intracranial Artery Stenosis in China. *Stroke*，2015，46（10）：2822-2829. doi：10.1161/strokeaha.115.010549［published Online First：2015/08/20］

［65］Bose A，Hartmann M，Henkes H，et al. A novel，self-expanding，nitinol stent in medically refractory intracranial atherosclerotic stenoses：the Wingspan study. *Stroke*，2007，38（5）：1531-1537. doi：10.1161/strokeaha.106.477711［published Online First：2007/03/31］

［66］Derdeyn CP，Chimowitz MI，Lynn MJ，et al. Aggressive medical treatment with or without stenting in high-risk patients with intracranial artery stenosis（SAMMPRIS）：the final results of a randomised trial. *Lancet*，2014，383（9914）：333-341. doi：10.1016/s0140-6736（13）62038-3［published Online First：2013/10/31］

［67］Zaidat OO，Fitzsimmons BF，Woodward BK，et al. Effect of a balloon-expandable intracranial stent vs medical therapy on risk of stroke in patients with symptomatic intracranial stenosis：the VISSIT randomized clinical trial. *Journal of the American Medical Association*，2015，313（12）：1240-1248. doi：10.1001/jama.2015.1693［published Online First：2015/03/25］

［68］Gao P，Wang D，Zhao Z，et al. Multicenter prospective trial of stent placement in patients with symptomatic high-grade intracranial stenosis. *American Journal of Neuroradiology*，2016，37（7）：1275-1280. doi：10.3174/ajnr.A4698［published Online First：2016/02/13］

［69］Alexander MJ，Zauner A，Chaloupka JC，et al. WEAVE trial：final results in 152 on-label patients. *Stroke*，2019，50（4）：889-894.

［70］Alexander MJ，Zauner A，Gupta R，et al. The WOVEN trial：Wingspan One-year Vascular Events and Neurologic Outcomes. *J Neurointerv Surg*，2021，13（4）：307-310. doi：10.1136/neurintsurg-2020-016208.

［71］Vajda Z，Schmid E，Güthe T，et al. The modified Bose method for the endovascular treatment of intracranial atherosclerotic arterial stenoses using the Enterprise stent. *Neurosurgery*，2012，70（1）：91-101；discussion 101. doi：10.1227/NEU.0b013e31822dff0f［published Online First：2011/07/23］

［72］Vajda Z，Güthe T，Perez MA，et al. Prevention of intracranial in-stent restenoses：predilatation with a drug eluting balloon，followed by the deployment of a self-expanding stent. *Cardiovascular and Interventional Radiology*，2013，36（2）：346-352. doi：10.1007/s00270-012-0450-9［published Online First：2012/08/08］

［73］Duan G，Feng Z，Zhang L，et al. Solitaire stents for the treatment of complex symptomatic intracranial stenosis after antithrombotic failure：safety and efficacy evaluation. *Journal of Neurointerventional Surgery*，2016，8（7）：680-684. doi：10.1136/neurintsurg-2015-011734［published Online First：2015/06/05］

［74］Hähnel S，Ringleb P，Hartmann M. Treatment of intracranial stenoses using the Neuroform stent system：initial experience in five cases. *Neuroradiology*，2006，48（7）：479-485. doi：10.1007/s00234-006-0081-4［published Online First：2006/05/25］

第二部分

颅内动脉粥样硬化性狭窄的血管内介入治疗

Part Ⅱ

Endovascular Therapy for Intracranial Atherosclerotic Stenosis

第四章

常规颅内动脉粥样硬化性狭窄的血管内介入治疗

第一节　颈内动脉颅内段

病例 1　右颈内动脉 C7 段重度狭窄

（一）临床病史及影像分析

患者，男性，53 岁，主因"言语不利伴口角歪斜 2 个月"入院。

当地医院头部 MRI 示右侧额叶急性梗死病灶（图 4.1.1 A），MRA 示右颈内动脉交通段管腔狭窄（图 4.1.1 B）。予内科药物治疗后仍有症状反复，为进一步治疗收入我院。

既往史：高血压、2 型糖尿病、脂蛋白代谢紊乱。

查体：神经系统查体未见明显异常。

CTP：右侧大脑半球异常灌注区，CBF 下降，CBV 基本正常，MTT 及 TTP 延长（图 4.1.1 C）。

术前 DSA：右颈内动脉交通段（C7 段）偏心性狭窄，狭窄处发出胚胎型右大脑后动脉（图 4.1.2 A～C）。未见明显同侧大脑前动脉及大脑后动脉向右大脑中动脉供血区域代偿（图 4.1.2 D～F）。

血栓弹力图：花生四烯酸（AA）抑制率 93.1%，腺苷二磷酸（ADP）抑制率 10.5%。

入院后给予双联抗血小板（阿司匹林 100 mg 1 次 / 日＋西洛他唑 100 mg 2 次 / 日）、降脂（阿托伐他汀 20 mg 1 次 / 日）等治疗。

（二）诊断

症状性右颈内动脉 C7 段重度狭窄。

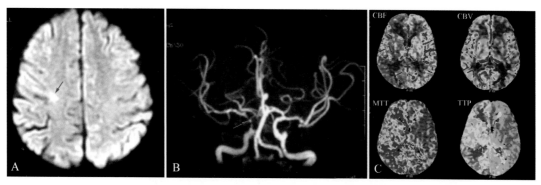

图 4.1.1　**A**. MRI 示右侧额叶急性梗死病灶（箭头示）；**B**. MRA 示右颈内动脉交通段管腔狭窄（箭头示）；**C**. CTP 示右侧大脑半球异常灌注区

Chapter 4

Endovascular Therapy for Common Intracranial Atherosclerotic Stenosis

Section 1　Intracranial Segments of the Internal Carotid Artery

Case 1　Severe stenosis of the C7 segment of the right internal carotid artery

1. Clinical presentation and radiological studies

A 53-year-old male patient presented with slurred speech and left facial droop for two months.

The MRI revealed an acute infarct in the right frontal lobe (Fig. 4.1.1 A). The MRA showed severe stenosis in the C7 segment of the right internal carotid artery (ICA) (Fig. 4.1.1 B). Despite medical treatment, the patient continued to experience recurrent symptoms.

The patient's medical history includes hypertension, type 2 diabetes mellitus, and dyslipidemia.

He was neurologically intact on admission.

The CT perfusion (CTP) demonstrated the prolongation of MTT and TTP with normal CBV and decreased CBF in the right ICA territory (Fig. 4.1.1 C).

The DSA showed severe eccentric stenosis in the C7 segment of the right ICA and a persistent fetal-type right posterior cerebral artery originating from the stenotic segment (Fig. 4.1.2 A–C). Poor pial collaterals were observed from both the right anterior and posterior cerebral arteries to the right middle cerebral artery (MCA) (Fig. 4.1.2 D–F).

Thromboelastography showed 93.1% inhibition of arachidonic acid (AA) and 10.5% inhibition of adenosine diphosphate (ADP).

Upon admission, he was prescribed dual antiplatelet therapy consisting of daily Aspirin (100 mg) and twice daily Cilostazol (100 mg), as well as daily Atorvastatin (20 mg).

2. Diagnosis

Symptomatic severe stenosis of the C7 segment of the right internal carotid artery.

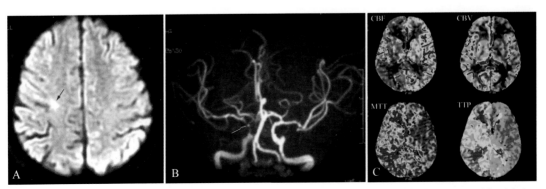

Fig. 4.1.1　MRI showed a new infarct in the right frontal lobe (arrow) (**A**). MRA showed severe stenosis of the C7 segment of the right internal carotid artery (arrow) (**B**). CTP perfusion demonstrated hypoperfusion in the right internal carotid artery territory (**C**)

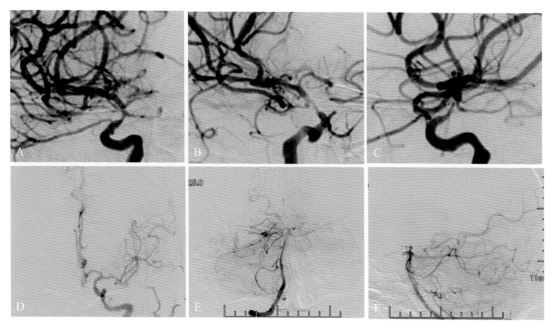

图 4.1.2　术前 DSA 提示右颈内动脉 C7 段狭窄，狭窄处发出胚胎型右大脑后动脉（**A ～ C**）。未见明显同侧大脑前动脉及大脑后动脉向右大脑中动脉供血区域代偿（**D ～ F**）

（三）术前讨论

　　患者右颈内动脉 C7 段重度狭窄，CTP 示右侧大脑半球低灌注，双联抗血小板聚集治疗后症状仍发作，有介入治疗指征。

　　治疗策略：患者右颈内动脉交通段重度狭窄，拟微导丝通过后球囊预扩张基础上再放置球囊扩张式支架。

　　相关风险：医源性夹层或血管破裂、急性或亚急性血栓形成等。

（四）治疗过程

　　全麻下右股动脉入路，6F 导引导管放至右颈内动脉 C1 段远端，造影显示右颈内动脉 C7 段重度狭窄，狭窄处管壁不光滑（图 4.1.3 A 和 B）。Transend 微导丝（0.014 in，300 cm）（1 in = 2.54 cm）通

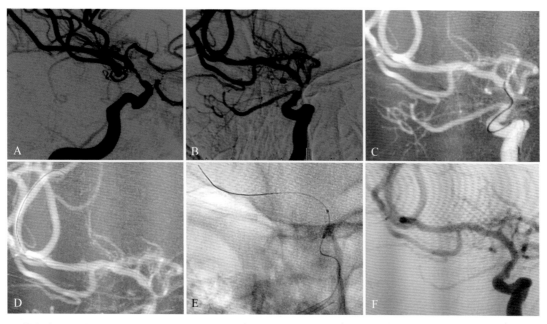

图 4.1.3　血管内介入治疗过程。**A 和 B**. 术前造影显示右颈内动脉 C7 段重度狭窄，狭窄处管壁不光滑；**C 和 D**. Transend 微导丝通过右颈内动脉 C7 狭窄段，至右大脑中动脉 M2 段；**E**. Gateway 球囊扩张狭窄病变 2 次；**F**. 释放支架后造影显示支架贴壁良好，残余狭窄率约 10%

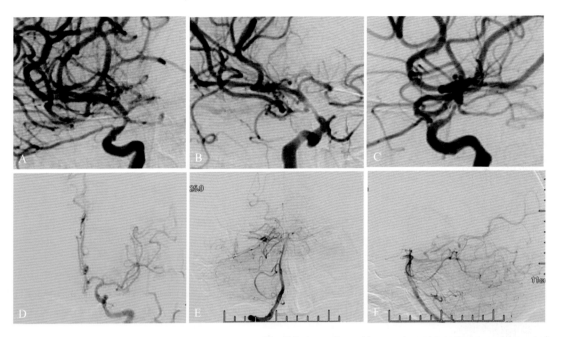

Fig. 4.1.2   DSA showed severe eccentric stenosis of the C7 segment of the right internal carotid artery. A persistent fetal-type right posterior cerebral artery arose from the stenotic segment (**A**–**C**). The pial collaterals from the right anterior and posterior cerebral artery to the right middle cerebral artery were poor (**D**–**F**)

3. Treatment schedule

The patient had a severe stenosis in the C7 segment of the right ICA. CTP suggested hypoperfusion in its target territory. Endovascular therapy was indicated because the patient failed medical treatment.

Treatment approach: Primary balloon dilatation plus balloon-expandable stent was considered for the lesion.

Potential risks of the procedure included iatrogenic dissection, vessel perforation, and acute in-stent thrombosis.

4. Treatment

Under general anesthesia, a 6F guide catheterwas positioned at the distal C1 segment of the right internal carotid artery. The angiogram confirmed a severe stenosis in the C7 segment with an irregular surface (Fig. 4.1.3 A, B). A Transend microwire (0.014 in, 300 cm) was navigated into

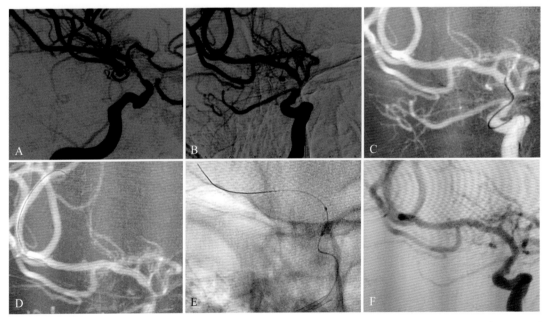

Fig. 4.1.3   The angiogram before stenting revealed severe stenosis of the C7 segment with an irregular surface (**A**, **B**). The Transend microwire was navigated into the M2 segment of the right middle cerebral artery (**C**, **D**). The lesion was dilated twice with a Gateway balloon (**E**). After stent implantation, the angiogram showed excellent stent apposition with residual stenosis of 10% (**F**)

过右颈内动脉 C7 狭窄段，至右大脑中动脉 M2 段（图 4.1.3 C 和 D）。沿微导丝送入 Gateway 球囊（2.5 mm×15 mm）预扩张 2 次后（图 4.1.3 E），放置 Apollo 支架（2.5 mm×8 mm）。球囊扩张后支架贴壁良好，残余狭窄率约为 10%，前向血流分级（mTICI 分级）3 级（图 4.1.3 F）。

术后查体同前。术后第二天复查头颅 CTA 示右颈内动脉 C7 段支架内血流通畅（图 4.1.4 A）。CTP 示右侧大脑半球灌注较术前改善（图 4.1.4 B）。

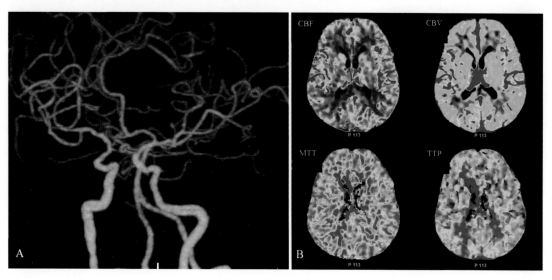

图 4.1.4　**A**. 术后 CTA 示右颈内动脉 C7 段支架内血流通畅；**B**. 术后 CTP 示右侧大脑半球灌注较术前改善

（五）讨论

本例右颈内动脉 C7 段病变略有成角，但病变直径较短（5 mm 左右），故选择球囊扩张式支架。对于颅内动脉狭窄病变，放置球囊扩张式支架前，使用球囊预扩张有助于后续支架定位及防止长度较短的支架释放过程中出现移位现象。本例患者术前血栓弹力图提示 ADP 抑制率为 10.5%，我们经验性将氯吡格雷更换为西洛他唑，但此临床抉择尚无循证医学证据支持。

（吴岩峰　王现旺　李红闪　韩明　李强
杨海华　霍晓川　李晓青）

4.1　手术操作视频
（病例 1）

the M2 segment of the right MCA (Fig. 4.1.3 C, D). The lesion was dilated twice with a 2.5 mm×15 mm Gateway balloon (Fig. 4.1.3 E). After balloon pre-dilation, a 2.5 mm× 8 mm Apollo stent was used to cover the lesion fully. After stent implantation, the angiogram showed excellent stent

apposition with residual stenosis of 10% (Fig. 4.1.3 F).

Postprocedural CT angiography demonstrated the patency of the C7 segment of the right ICA (Fig.4.1.4 A). The CTP results showed improved perfusion parameters (Fig.4.1.4 B).

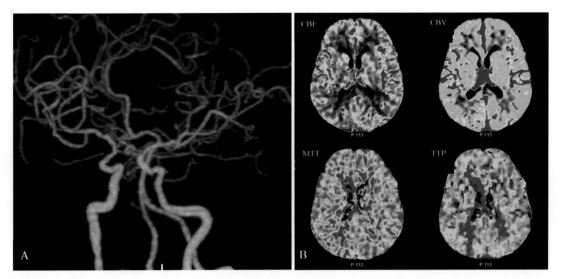

Fig. 4.1.4   Postprocedural CT angiography demonstrated the patency of the C7 segment of the right internal carotid artery (**A**). The CTP result showed improved perfusion parameters (**B**)

5. Comments

Although the lesion had a mild bend, it was less than 5 mm in length, so a balloon-mounted stent was preferred. The pre-dilation before balloon-mounted stent placement would prevent stent migration during stent placement. In this case, we empirically substituted Cilostazol for Clopidogrel

since the ADP inhibition was 10.5% in thromboelastography, although there is no strong clinical evidence to support this practice.

(Translated by Ning Ma, revised by Zhikai Hou and Lei Feng)

4.1   Video of endovascular therapy (Case 1)

第二节　大脑中动脉 M1 段

病例 2　右大脑中动脉 M1 段重度狭窄

（一）临床病史及影像分析

患者，男性，47 岁，主因"言语不利，左侧肢体活动不利 2 月余"入院。

病后就诊当地医院，行头部 CT 及头部 MRI 提示右侧半卵圆中心多发脑梗死（图 4.2.1 A ～ F）。头颅 CTA 示右大脑中动脉 M1 段近端重度狭窄（图 4.2.2 A 和 B）。CTP 示右侧大脑半球低灌注，右顶叶和内侧分水岭区 MTT 和 TTP 延长（图 4.2.2 C）。予以内科药物保守治疗，临床症状缓解。患者

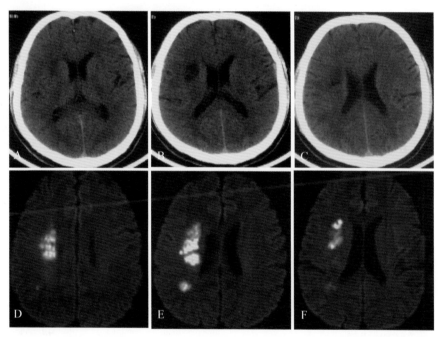

图 4.2.1　头颅 CT（**A ～ C**）及头部 MRI（**D ～ F**）提示右侧半卵圆中心多发脑梗死

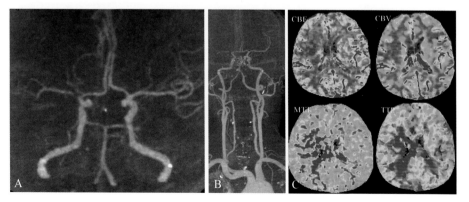

图 4.2.2　头颅 CTA 提示右大脑中动脉 M1 段近端重度狭窄（**A 和 B**），头颅 CTP 提示右侧大脑半球低灌注（**C**）

Section 2 The M1 Segment of the Middle Cerebral Artery

Case 2 Severe stenosis of the M1 segment of the right middle cerebral artery

1. Clinical presentation and radiological studies

A 47-year-old man presented with dysarthria and left hemiparesis for 2 months.

The results of both the CT scan and MRI indicated multiple acute infarcts in the right centrum semiovale (Fig. 4.2.1 A–F). CT angiography (CTA) revealed severe stenosis at the proximal segment of the right middle cerebral artery (MCA) (Fig. 4.2.2 A, B). The CT perfusion (CTP) demonstrated prolongation of MTT and TTP in the right parietal lobe and deep watershed areas (Fig. 4.2.2 C). His symptoms were only partially alleviated with medical

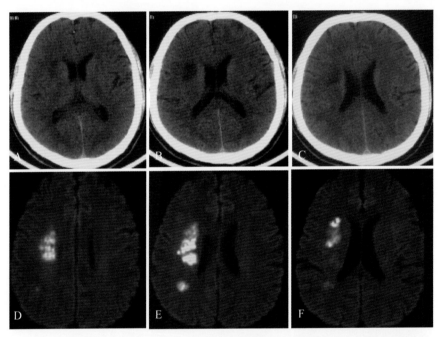

Fig. 4.2.1 The CT scan (**A**–**C**) and MRI (**D**–**F**) showed acute infarcts in the right centrum semiovale

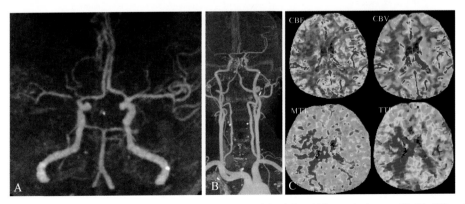

Fig. 4.2.2 CT angiography revealed a severe stenosis at the proximal segment of the right middle cerebral artery (**A**, **B**). CT perfusion demonstrated hypoperfusion in the right cerebral hemisphere (**C**)

为进一步治疗就诊于我院。

既往史：高血压病史。

查体：左侧中枢性面舌瘫。

血栓弹力图：ADP 抑制率 90.8%，AA 抑制率 100%。

DSA：右大脑中动脉 M1 段近端重度狭窄，狭窄处有豆纹动脉发出；未见明显后循环向前循环代偿（图 4.2.3 A～F）。

高分辨率磁共振管壁成像：右大脑中动脉管壁偏心增厚，管腔上壁强化明显（图 4.2.4 A 和 B）。

入院后给予双联抗血小板（阿司匹林 100 mg 1 次 / 日＋氯吡格雷 75 mg 1 次 / 日）、降脂（阿托伐他汀钙片 20 mg 1 次 / 日）治疗。

（二）诊断

症状性右大脑中动脉 M1 段近端重度狭窄。

（三）术前讨论

患者 CT 和 MRI 提示右半卵圆中心梗死，梗死病灶呈串珠样改变，结合 CT 灌注成像所示的低灌注，考虑右大脑中动脉 M1 段近端重度狭窄是本次发病的责任病变，有血管内介入治疗指征。

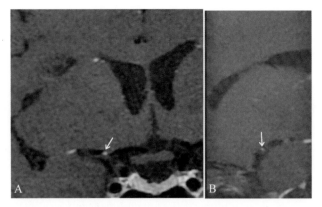

图 4.2.4　**A**. 高分辨率磁共振管壁成像提示右大脑中动脉管壁偏心增厚；**B**. 管腔上壁强化明显（箭头示）

治疗策略：鉴于病变长度较短，拟先球囊扩张，如无明显弹性回缩或夹层形成，不准备放置支架。

相关风险：穿支卒中、急性血栓形成等。

（四）治疗过程及随访

全麻下右股动脉入路，将 6F 导引导管放置在右颈内动脉 C1 段。造影显示右大脑中动脉 M1 段近端重度狭窄（图 4.2.5 A）。将 Transend 微导丝（0.014 in，300 cm）放置在右大脑中动脉上干。经

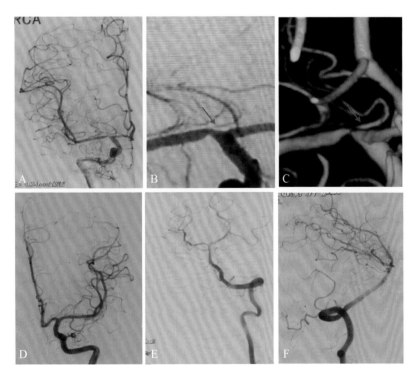

图 4.2.3　DSA 提示右大脑中动脉 M1 段近端重度狭窄，狭窄处有豆纹动脉发出（箭头示），未见明显后循环向前循环代偿（A～F）

treatments.

The patient had a medical history of hypertension.

Physical examination showed left central facial and lingual paralysis.

Thromboelastography revealed 90.8% inhibition of ADP and 100% inhibition of AA.

The digital subtraction angiography (DSA) showed severe stenosis at the proximal segment of the right MCA, with lenticulostriate arteries arising from the opposite wall of the eccentric plaque, and poor collateral circulation from the posterior circulation to the anterior circulation (Fig. 4.2.3 A–F).

High-resolution MRI showed eccentric vessel wall thickening and an enhancement of the superior wall of the right middle cerebral artery (Fig. 4.2.4 A, B).

He was on a dual antiplatelet regimen (Aspirin 100 mg daily and Clopidogrel 75 mg daily) and Atorvastatin (20 mg daily) at admission.

2. Diagnosis

Symptomatic severe stenosis of the proximal segment of the right middle cerebral artery.

3. Treatment schedule

The distribution of cerebral infarcts and CTP suggested hypoperfusion from severe right MCA stenosis was the culprit of strokes. Endovascular therapy was indicated as the physical limitation of flow could not be removed with medical therapy.

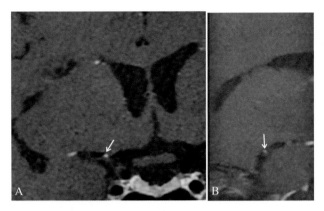

Fig. 4.2.4 High-resolution MRI showed an eccentric thickening vessel wall (**A**) with strong enhancement on the superior wall of the right middle cerebral artery (arrow) (**B**)

Treatment approach: primary balloon dilation would be used for the short stenosis lesion. Stenting would be reserved for severe recoil or dissection after angioplasty. Potential complications included perforator stroke and acute in-stent thrombosis.

4. Treatment and follow-up

Under general anesthesia, a 6F guide catheter was placed at the C1 segment of the right internal carotid artery. Angiogram confirmed severe stenosis at the proximal segment of the right MCA(Fig. 4.2.5 A). A Transend microwire (0.014 in, 300 cm) was navigated into the superior

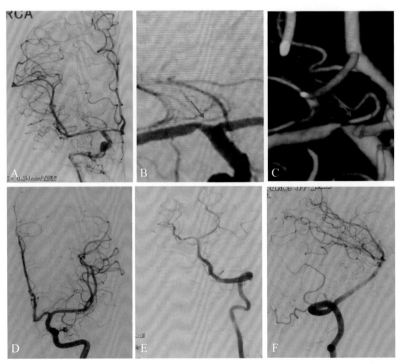

Fig. 4.2.3 DSA demonstrated severe stenosis at the proximal segment of the right cerebral middle artery, lenticulostriate arteries arising from the opposite wall of the eccentric plaque (arrow) (**A–C**). There was poor collateral compensation to the right cerebral hemisphere from the contralateral anterior circulation and posterior circulation (**D–F**)

微导丝送入 Gateway 球囊（2.0 mm×9 mm）扩张狭窄段，扩张后残余狭窄率约为 30%，局部对比剂滞留，不除外夹层（图 4.2.5 B）。置入 Wingspan 支架（3.0 mm×15 mm），完全覆盖狭窄段（图 4.2.5 C）。支架释放后造影提示夹层消失，残余狭窄率约 15%（图 4.2.5 D）。观察 10 min 无改变结束治疗。

术后 7 个月 CTA 和 CTP：右大脑中动脉 M1 段支架内通畅（图 4.2.6 A），右侧大脑半球低灌注较术前明显改善（图 4.2.6 B）。

（五）讨论

本例右大脑中动脉 M1 段近端狭窄，因病变长度较短，拟单纯球囊扩张，但因扩张后局部夹层，故予以支架贴合。狭窄处有穿支动脉发出，干预过程未造成其损伤，与以下两个因素有关：①开口位于斑块对侧；②选择稍小直径的球囊扩张病变。

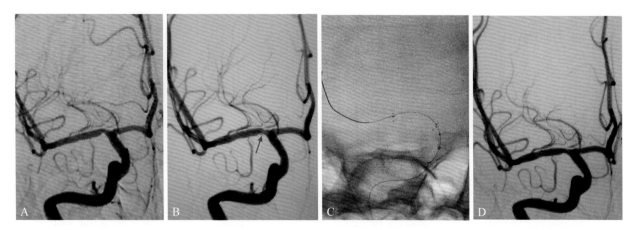

图 4.2.5　血管内介入治疗过程如下：术前造影显示右大脑中动脉 M1 段近端重度狭窄（**A**）；球囊扩张后造影显示残余狭窄率约为 30%，局部夹层形成（箭头）（**B**）；释放 Wingspan 支架（**C**）；支架释放后造影提示夹层消失，残余狭窄率约 15%（**D**）

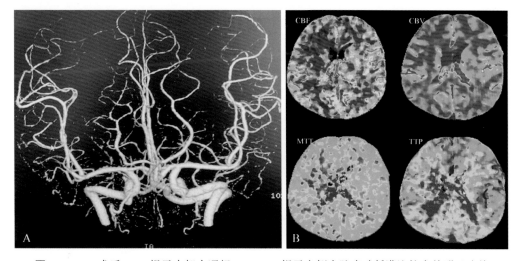

图 4.2.6　**A.** 术后 CTA 提示支架内通畅；**B.** CTP 提示右侧大脑半球低灌注较术前明显改善

（苗春芝　杨连琦　王坤）

4.2　手术操作视频
（病例 2）

division of the right MCA. The lesion was dilated with a 2.0 mm×9 mm Gateway balloon. Angiogram after the balloon angioplasty showed a residual stenosis of 30% with contrast stasis in the inferior wall, suggesting a dissection (Fig. 4.2.5 B). A 3.0 mm×15 mm Wingspan self-expanding stent was used to cover the lesion (Fig. 4.2.5 C). After stent implantation, the degree of residual stenosis rate was 15%, and dissection disappeared (Fig. 4.2.5 D). Ten minutes later, a final angiogram showed no changes in the stented vessel.

Seven months later, repeated CTA demonstrated the patency of the right MCA (Fig. 4.2.6 A), and the CTP result showed improved perfusion in the right deep watershed areas (Fig. 4.2.6 B).

5. Comments

The lesion location and short stenotic length in the proximal right MCA led to the decision of choosing balloon angioplasty as the primary treatment. A stent was later deployed to cover the dissection from balloon angioplasty. To note, lenticulostriate arteries arising from the stenotic segment were not compromised by either angioplasty or stenting. The origin of the lenticulostriate arteries arising from the opposite wall of the plaque and the use of an undersized balloon may contribute to the preservation of this artery.

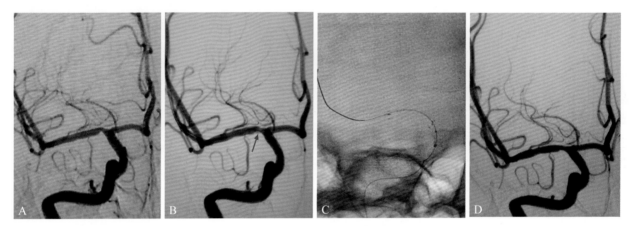

Fig. 4.2.5   Angiogram confirmed severe stenosis of the proximal segment of the right middle cerebral artery (**A**). Angiogram after the balloon dilation showed a residual stenosis of 30% with contrast stasis in the inferior wall (arrow) (**B**). A 3.0 mm×15 mm Wingspan self-expanding stentwas used to coverthe lesion (**C**). After the stent implantation, an angiogram showed the degree of residual stenosis was 15%, and arterial dissection disappeared. (**D**)

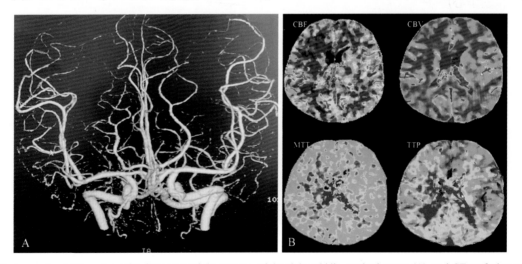

Fig. 4.2.6   Post-procedural CT angiography demonstrated the patency of the right middle cerebral artery (**A**), and CT perfusion result showed improved perfusion in the right deep watershed areas (**B**)

(Translated by Ning Ma, revised by Zhikal Hou and Lei Feng)

4.2   Video of endovascular therapy (Case 2)

第三节　基底动脉

病例 3　快速进展的基底动脉粥样硬化性狭窄

（一）临床病史及影像分析

患者，男性，53 岁，主因"发作性耳鸣 7 个月，加重伴头晕及行走不稳 5 个月"入院。

7 个月前患者于当地医院行头颅 MRA 未见明显血管狭窄（图 4.3.1）。5 个月前患者突然出现头晕、昏沉感，伴行走不稳，似醉酒感。3 天后突发左侧肢体无力，口角歪斜，同时伴有构音障碍，行 MRI 示右侧脑桥体梗死，MRA 示基底动脉中段重度狭窄（图 4.3.2）。

行血管炎免疫检查未见特殊异常，行 CTA 检查仍提示基底动脉狭窄（图 4.3.3）。行高分辨率磁共振成像（high-resolution MRI，HRMRI）检查提示基底动脉管壁偏心增厚（图 4.3.4）。病后一直口服阿司匹林、氯吡格雷、瑞舒伐他汀治疗。20 天前再次出现头晕症状，为行介入治疗就诊于我院。

既往史：类风湿关节炎病史 20 余年，高血压及糖尿病史；本次发病前 2 个月，患者每天坚持健身运动，且运动量较大。

入院后 HRMRI：基底动脉中远段管壁明显不规则、粗细不均，局部管壁不均匀增厚，中段局部管壁环状不均匀增厚，右侧稍明显，远段局部管壁以左侧增厚明显，呈长 T1 信号，MP-RAGE 序列未见明显异常高信号。增强扫描示，基底动脉局部管壁环形强化，局部右后壁明显点状强化（图

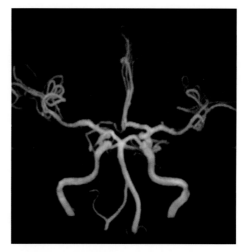

图 4.3.1　MRA 示颅内大血管未见明显狭窄

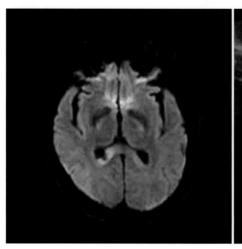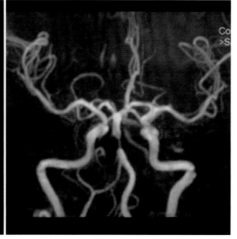

图 4.3.2　MRI 示右侧脑桥体梗死，MRA 示基底动脉中段重度狭窄

Section 3 The Basilar Artery

Case 3 Rapidly progressing atherosclerotic stenosis of the basilar artery

1. Clinical presentation and radiological studies

A 53-year-old man was admitted to the hospital due to paroxysmal tinnitus for seven months. His symptoms gradually worsened, accompanied by dizziness and unstable walking in the past five months.

The MRA seven months ago showed no obvious abnormality in the intracranial segments of the cerebral artery. (Fig. 4.3.1). Five months ago, he felt dizzy and drowsy, accompanied by unstable walking. Three days later, he suffered from weakness in the left limbs, deviated mouth, and dysarthria. The MRI result showed new cerebral infarcts in the right corpus callosum. The MRA result showed severe stenosis of the middle segment of the basilar artery (BA) (Fig. 4.3.2).

There was no abnormal autoimmune antibody or inflammation factors related to cerebral vasculitis. CT angiography revealed severe stenosis at the middle segment of the BA (Fig. 4.3.3). The high-resolution MRI (HRMRI) showed an eccentric thickened lesion located at the BA (Fig. 4.3.4). The patient had recurrent dizziness under the aggressive medical treatment, including dual-antiplatelet and intensive risk factor control.

The patient had a medical history of rheumatoid arthritis for more than 20 years. And he was complicated with hypertension and diabetes mellitus.

High-resolution MRI showed the focal vessel wall, especially the left vessel wall, of the middle and distal segments of the basilar artery unevenly thickened. The MPRAGE sequence didn't show the hyperintense lesions of the vessel wall. The contrast-enhanced sequence showed the circumferential wall enhancement of the basilar artery and strong spot-like enhancement on the right posterior wall

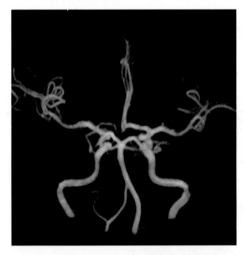

Fig. 4.3.1 The MRA seven months ago showed no obvious abnormality in the intracranial segments of the cerebral artery

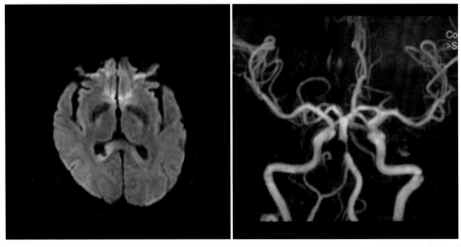

Fig. 4.3.2 The MRI result showed acute cerebral infarct in the corpus callosum, and the MRA indicated severe stenosis of the middle segment of the basilar artery

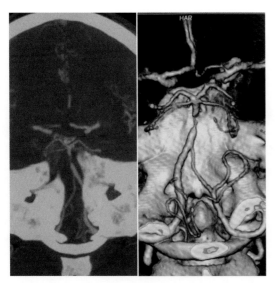

图 4.3.3 CTA 示基底动脉重度狭窄

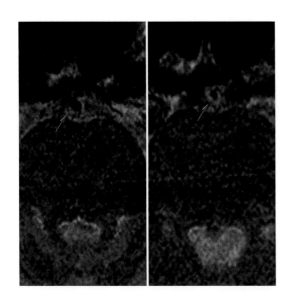

图 4.3.4 HRMRI 示基底动脉管壁偏心增厚，管壁未见高信号

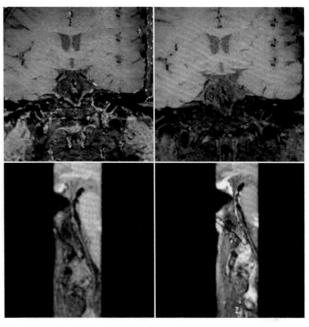

图 4.3.5 入院后 HRMRI 示基底动脉中远段局部管壁不均匀增厚，中段管壁右侧增厚明显，远段管壁左侧增厚明显。增强扫描示基底动脉管壁环形强化，右后壁点状强化

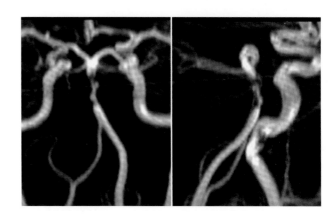

图 4.3.6 入院后 MRA 示基底动脉重度狭窄

4.3.5）。MRA 提示基底动脉重度狭窄（图 4.3.6）。

TCD：基底动脉收缩期峰值速度大于 200 cm/s，伴有湍流频谱，乐性杂音。

术前 DSA：基底动脉中段重度狭窄，狭窄段存在 2 个充盈缺损，并可见双侧小脑前下动脉及多个细小穿支动脉起于狭窄段（图 4.3.7）。

血栓弹力图：ADP 抑制率 19.3%，AA 抑制率 46.6%。

类风湿因子：10.6 IU/ml（正常值 0～15.9 IU/ml）。

红细胞沉降率：54 mm/h（正常值 0～15 mm/h）。

超敏 C 反应蛋白：12.2 mg/L（正常值 0～3.0 mg/L）

入院后给予双联抗血小板（阿司匹林 100 mg 1 次/日＋氯吡格雷 75 mg 1 次/日）及降脂（阿托伐他汀 20 mg 1 次/日）治疗。

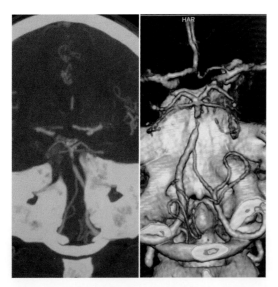

Fig. 4.3.3 CT angiography showed severe stenosis of the basilar artery

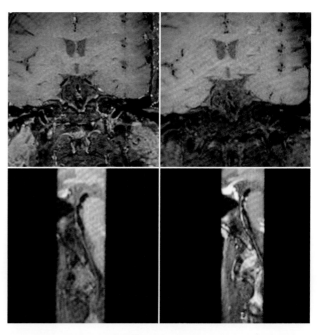

Fig. 4.3.5 HRMRI showed the focal vessel wall, especially the left vessel wall, of the middle and distal segments of the basilar artery unevenly thickened. The contrast-enhanced sequence showed the circumferential wall enhancement of the basilar artery and strong spot-like enhancement on the right posterior wall of the basilar artery

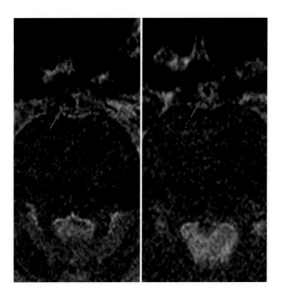

Fig. 4.3.4 HRMRI showed an eccentric thickening wall of the basilar artery

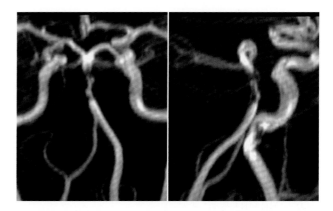

Fig. 4.3.6 MRA after admission showed severe stenosis of the basilar artery

of the basilar artery (Fig. 4.3.5). The MRA result revealed severe stenosis of the basilar artery (Fig. 4.3.6).

TCD showed that the peak systolic velocity of the basilar artery was more than 200 cm/s, accompanied by a turbulent frequency spectrum and musical noise.

Preprocedural DSA demonstrated severe stenosis of the middle segment of the basilar artery along with two filling defects. Bilateral anterior inferior cerebellar arteries and multiple perforator arteries arose from the stenosis segment (Fig. 4.3.7).

Thromboelastography revealed 19.3% inhibition of ADP and 46.6% inhibition of AA.

Rheumatoid factor: 10.6 IU/ml (0–15.9 IU/ml).

Erythrocyte sedimentation rate: 54 mm/h (0–15 mm/h).

High-sensitivity C-reactive protein: 12.2 mg/L (0–3.0 mg/L).

He was on a dual antiplatelet regimen (Aspirin 100 mg daily and Clopidogrel 75 mg daily) and Atorvastatin (20 mg daily) at admission.

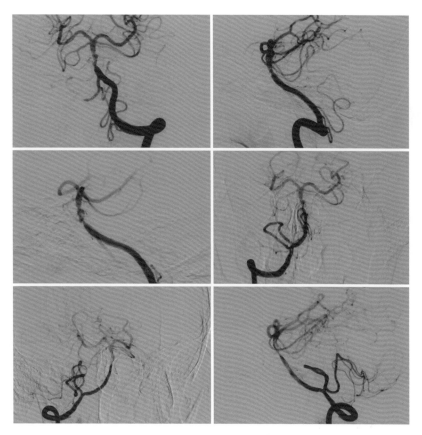

图 4.3.7　术前 DSA 示基底动脉中段重度狭窄

（二）诊断

症状性基底动脉重度狭窄。

（三）术前讨论

第一，患者基底动脉狭窄进展迅速并出现临床症状，HRMRI 提示系动脉粥样硬化斑块所致。予以抗血小板治疗后仍有症状反复，可以考虑血管内介入治疗。第二，HRMRI 提示斑块负荷较重，血管造影提示局部充盈缺损，狭窄段毗邻双侧小脑前下动脉及多个细小穿支动脉，其治疗风险主要是术后穿支卒中，对应策略为球囊扩张时应避免压力过大。第三，红细胞沉降率增快及超敏 C 反应蛋白增高考虑与患者类风湿关节炎相关。

（四）治疗过程及随访

全麻下右股动脉入路，6F Envy 导引导管置于左椎动脉 V2 段，造影示基底动脉中段重度狭窄。

Traxcess 微导丝与 Echelon-10 微导管同轴越过病变，撤出微导丝经微导管造影证实位于真腔。交换技术后经 Docking 微导丝送入 Trek 球囊（2.5 mm×8 mm），先后扩张球囊 2 次（扩张压力 6 atm），然后送入 Apollo 支架（2.5 mm×13 mm）至狭窄段，6 atm 扩张球囊释放支架，其后显示狭窄明显改善，残余狭窄率 30%，前向血流 mTICI 分级 3 级（图4.3.8）。

术后 TCD：基底动脉收缩期峰值流速 102 cm/s，频谱正常。

术后 44 个月 DSA：基底动脉支架内通畅（图4.3.9）。

（五）讨论

颅内动脉粥样硬化性狭窄能在较短时间（2 个月）内进展迅速，并引发临床症状。本例选择直径稍小的球囊及支架，采用低扩张压力主要是预防术后穿支卒中。本例支架也可选择自膨式支架。

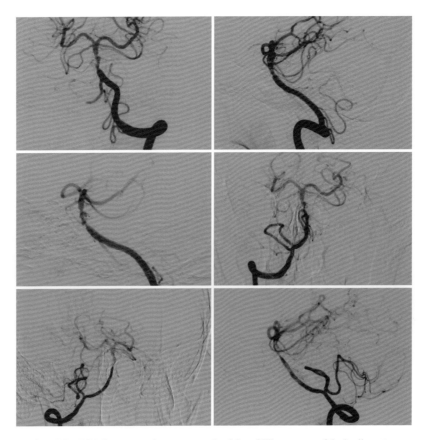

Fig. 4.3.7   DSA demonstrated severe stenosis of the middle segment of the basilar artery

2. Diagnosis

Symptomatic severe stenosis of the basilar artery.

3. Treatment schedule

The patient exhibited a stenosis located at the middle segment of the basilar artery that advanced rapidly and developed into severe stenosis within a brief period. High-resolution MRI suggested the presence of advanced atherosclerotic plaque, which carried a heavy plaque burden in the stenosis. Endovascular therapy was indicated because the patient had a recurrent stroke despite dual anti-platelet therapy and intensive control of vascular risk factors. The heavy plaque burden and anatomical characteristics of the culprit lesions, adjacent to the bilateral anterior inferior cerebellar arteries and multiple perforator arteries of the basilar artery, presented a high risk of perforator stroke as the major complication. The endovascular approach was to avoid excessive pressure when expanding the balloon. The elevated erythrocyte sedimentation rate and high-sensitivity C-reactive protein may be associated with rheumatoid arthritis.

4. Treatment and follow-up

Under general anesthesia, a 6 F guide catheter was placed at the V2 segment of the left vertebral artery. The angiogram confirmed severe stenosis of the middle segment of the basilar artery. An Echelon-10 microcatheter was coaxially advanced through the lesion using a Traxcess microwire. A transcatheter angiogram confirmed the microcatheter was situated in the true lumen of the basilar artery. Following the exchange technique, a 2.5 mm × 8 mm Trek balloon was delivered using a Docking microwire. The stenosis lesion was dilated twice with a pressure of 6 atm. Then a 2.5 mm × 13 mm Apollo stent was used to cover the lesion fully. After the stent implantation, the final angiogram showed the degree of residual stenosis was 30%, and the antegrade blood flow was grade Ⅲ (Fig. 4.3.8).

TCD showed the peak systolic velocity of the basilar artery was 102 cm/s with a regular frequency spectrum.

DSA performed 44 months after stent placement demonstrated the basilar artery stent remained patent. (Fig. 4.3.9).

5. Comments

Intracranial stenosis caused by atherosclerosis can rapidly progress, even within a short period of two months. In this case, a small-size balloon and balloon-mounted stent were selected with a low dilation pressure to prevent perforator occlusion after the procedure. Alternatively, A self-expanding stent could also be chosen for the basilar artery stenting in this case.

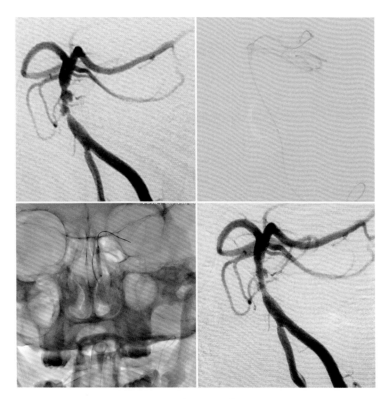

图 4.3.8　支架置入后造影显示狭窄明显改善，前向血流 mTICI 分级 3 级

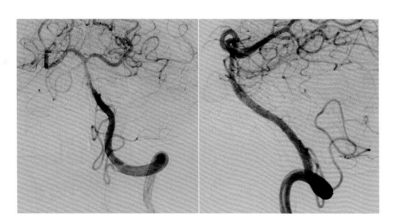

图 4.3.9　术后 44 个月 DSA 提示基底动脉支架内通畅

（马宁）

4.3　手术操作视频
（病例 3）

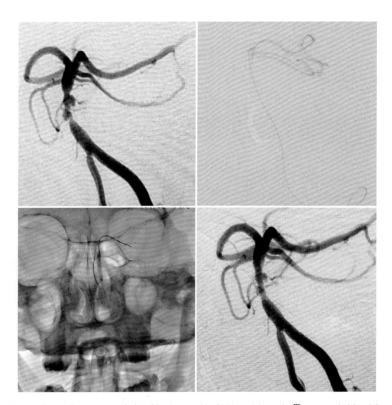

Fig. 4.3.8   The angiogram revealed residual stenosis of 30%, with grade Ⅲ antegrade blood flow

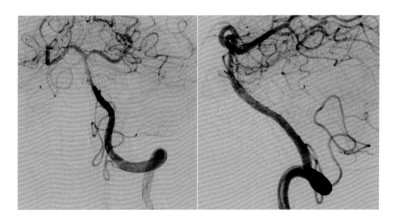

Fig. 4.3.9   DSA performed 44 months after stent placement demonstrated the basilar artery stent remained patent

4.3   **Video of endovascular therapy (Case 3)**

(Translated by Rongrong Cui, Revised by Zhikai Hou)

病例 4　基底动脉中段重度狭窄

（一）临床病史及影像分析

患者，男性，主因"突发头晕、呕吐伴意识障碍 4 天"入院。

既往史：糖尿病史。

查体：神经系统查体未见明显异常。

入院后完善头部 MRI：显示脑桥、小脑半球、枕叶多发梗死灶（图 4.3.10 A 和 B）。

头部 MRA：右椎动脉颅内段严重迂曲，基底动脉中段重度狭窄，双侧大脑后动脉狭窄（图 4.3.11 A 和 B）。

DSA：右颈内动脉 C6 段中度狭窄，右颈内动脉 C1 段迂曲（图 4.3.12 A 和 B），左颈内动脉 C1 段迂曲，无明显血管狭窄（图 4.3.12 C 和 D），基底动脉中段重度狭窄，双侧大脑后动脉狭窄（图 4.3.12 E 和 F）。

入院后给予双联抗血小板（阿司匹林 100 mg 1 次 / 日＋氯吡格雷 75 mg 1 次 / 日）以及强化降脂（阿托伐他汀 40 mg 1 次 / 日）等治疗。

（二）诊断

症状性基底动脉中段重度狭窄。

（三）术前讨论

结合患者病史及相关影像学检查，患者基底动脉供血区域多发梗死，考虑基底动脉中段重度狭窄系责任病变，拟对其进行血管内介入治疗。

相关风险：基底动脉中段富含穿支，穿支卒中概率大，此外还有动脉破裂、急性血栓形成以及栓子脱落等风险。

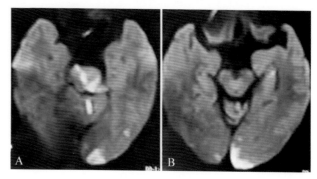

图 4.3.10　头颅磁共振 DWI 提示脑桥、小脑半球、枕叶多发梗死灶（**A** 和 **B**）

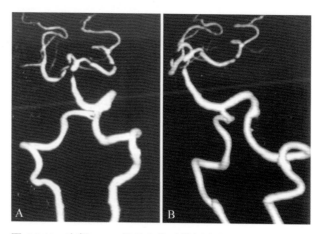

图 4.3.11　头部 MRA 提示右椎动脉颅内段严重迂曲，基底动脉中段重度狭窄，双侧大脑后动脉狭窄（**A** 和 **B**）

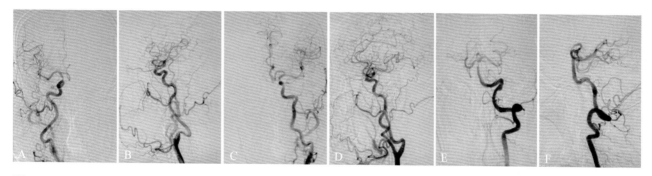

图 4.3.12　DSA。**A** 和 **B**. 右颈内动脉 C6 段中度狭窄，右颈内动脉 C1 段迂曲；**C** 和 **D**. 左颈内动脉 C1 段迂曲，无明显血管狭窄；**E** 和 **F**. 基底动脉中段重度狭窄，双侧大脑后动脉狭窄

Case 4　Severe stenosis of the mid-basilar artery

1. Clinical presentation and radiological studies

A man was admitted to the hospital due to sudden dizziness, vomiting, and alteration of consciousness for 4 days.

He had a history of diabetes mellitus.

He was neurologically intact on admission.

MRI showed multiple infarcts in the pons, cerebellar hemispheres, and bilateral occipital lobes (Fig. 4.3.10 A, B).

MRA revealed severe tortuosity of the intracranial segment of the right vertebral artery, severe stenosis of the mid-basilar artery, and stenosis of the bilateral posterior cerebral arteries (Fig. 4.3.11 A, B).

DSA revealed moderate stenosis of the C6 segment of the right internal carotid artery, severe tortuosity of the C1 segment of the right internal carotid artery (Fig. 4.3.12 A, B), severe twisting of the C1 segment of the left internal carotid artery (Fig. 4.3.12 C, D), severe stenosis of the mid-basilar artery, and stenosis of the bilateral posterior cerebral arteries (Fig. 4.3.12 E, F).

At the time of admission, he was receiving a dual antiplatelet regimen consisting of daily doses of Aspirin (100 mg) and Clopidogrel (75 mg), as well as Atorvastatin (40 mg) daily.

2. Diagnosis

Symptomatic severe stenosis of the mid-basilar artery.

3. Treatment schedule

The multiple cerebral infarcts involved in the territory of the basilar artery suggested severe basilar artery stenosis as the culprit lesions of strokes. Therefore, endovascular therapy was recommended for this patient. Related risks included perforating artery occlusion, arterial rupture, and in-stent thrombosis.

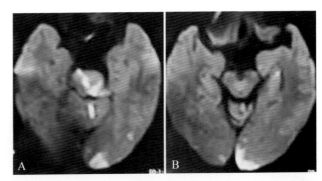

Fig. 4.3.10　MRI showed multiple infarcts in the pons, cerebellar hemispheres, and bilateral occipital lobes (**A, B**)

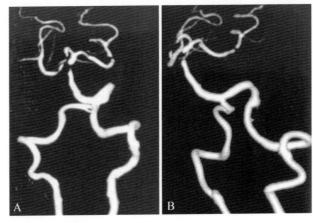

Fig. 4.3.11　MRA showed severe tortuosity of the intracranial segment of the right vertebral artery, severe stenosis of the mid-basilar artery, and stenosis of the bilateral posterior cerebral arteries (**A, B**)

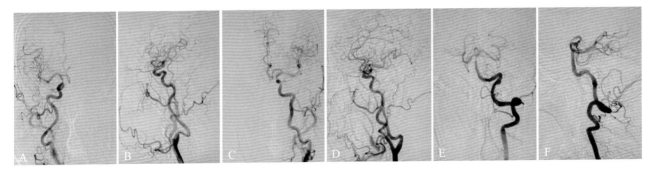

Fig. 4.3.12　DSA showed moderate stenosis of the C6 segment of the right internal carotid artery, severe tortuosity of the C1 segment of the right internal carotid artery (**A, B**), severe twisting of the C1 segment of the left internal carotid artery (**C, D**), severe stenosis of the mid-basilar artery, and stenosis of the bilateral posterior cerebral arteries (**E, F**)

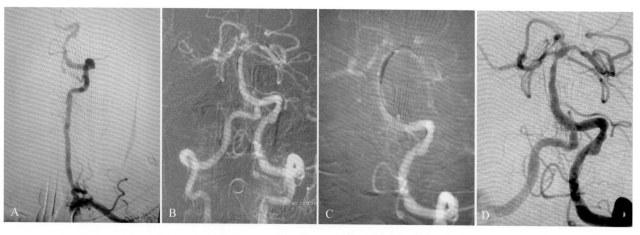

图 4.3.13　**A**. 术前造影；**B**. 微导丝到位；**C**. 球囊扩张；**D**. 术后造影

（四）治疗过程

全麻下右股动脉穿刺入路，置入 6F 鞘，造影见左椎动脉起始部迂曲（图 4.3.13 A），将 6F 导引导管送至左椎动脉 V2 段，沿导引导管送入 Synchro 微导丝（0.014 in，300 cm），小心通过狭窄段至左大脑后动脉（图 4.3.13 B），沿微导丝送入 Ultra Soft 球囊（2.0 mm×15 mm），加压至 6 atm 扩张（图 4.3.13 C），造影见狭窄明显改善，撤出球囊，沿微导丝送入 XT-27 微导管，撤出微导丝，沿微导管送入 Neuroform EZ 支架（3.0 mm×15 mm），准确对位后成功释放支架，造影见前向血流较前明显改善（mTICI 分级 3 级），分支显影良好，支架贴壁良好。观察 10 min 后造影，血流通畅，无急性血栓形成（图 4.3.13 D），撤出导管，结束手术。患者术后无新发神经功能缺损征象。

（五）讨论

本例患者基底动脉中段重度狭窄，结合病史有血管内介入治疗指征。因穿支卒中风险大，故选择稍小直径球囊预扩张并放置自膨式支架，以在改善供血的同时最大程度降低手术风险。

（李郁芳　陈湘　雒东江）

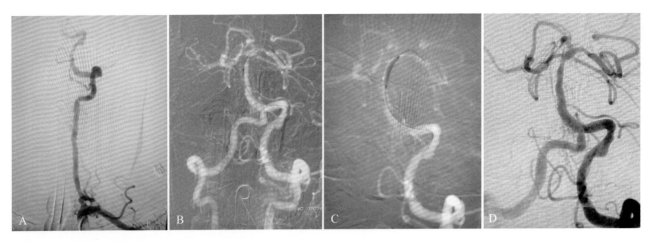

Fig. 4.3.13 (**A**) An angiogram before stenting. (**B**) The Synchro microwire was navigated into the left posterior cerebral artery. (**C**) The lesion was pre-dilated with an Ultra Soft balloon. (**D**) An angiogram after stent implantation

4. Treatment

Under general anesthesia, an angiogram showed the tortuous access of the V1 segment of the left vertebral artery (Fig. 4.3.13 A). A 6F guide catheter was placed at the V2 segment of the left vertebral artery. A Synchro microwire (0.014 in, 300 cm) was navigated into the P2 segment of the left posterior cerebral artery (Fig. 4.3.13 B). The lesion was pre-dilated with a 2.0 mm×15 mm Ultra Soft balloon (Fig. 4.3.13 C). The angiogram showed the degree of stenosis was significantly improved. Then a Neuroform EZ stent (3.0 mm×15 mm) was delivered along the XT-27 microcatheter to cover the lesion. Ten minutes later, the angiogram after stent implantation showed excellent stent apposition with the grade Ⅲ of antegrade blood flow (Fig. 4.3.13 D).

5. Comments

Based on the medical history and radiological findings, the patient was indicated to perform balloon angioplasty and stenting. To reduce the risk of perforator stroke after stenting, a small-size balloon was chosen for pre-dilatation before inserting a self-expanding stent.

(Translated by Rongrong Cui, Revised by Zhikai Hou)

第四节　椎基底动脉交界区

病例 5　双侧椎基底动脉交界区重度狭窄

（一）临床病史及影像分析

患者，女性，61 岁，主因"反复头晕 5 月余"入院。每次头晕发作持续 0.5 h 左右，无其他伴随症状和体征。

在当地医院就诊行头部 MRI 未见新发脑梗死（图 4.4.1）。头部 MRA 及 CTA 示右椎动脉优势，双侧椎基底动脉交界区狭窄（图 4.4.2 和图 4.4.3）。

给予双联抗血小板、他汀类药物等治疗仍有反复发作。入院前 10 天曾晕倒一次，伴短暂意识不清，家人诉持续 3～4 min 后清醒，无肢体抽搐等不适，未行相关影像检查。现为行血管内介入治疗而入我院。

既往史：高血压病史 30 年，高脂血症病史 4 年，糖尿病病史 2 年；3 个月前行冠状动脉旁路移植术。

查体：神经系统查体未见阳性定位体征。

实验室检查：低密度脂蛋白胆固醇（LDL-C）2.13 mmol/L。

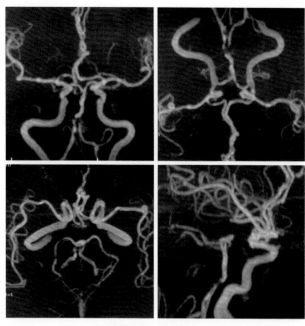

图 4.4.2　头部 MRA 示右椎动脉优势，双侧椎基底动脉交界区狭窄

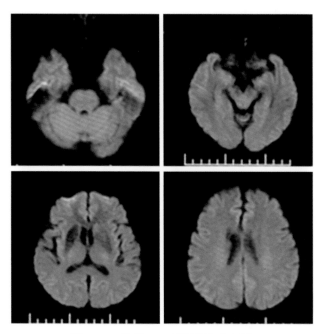

图 4.4.1　头部 MRI 示无新发脑梗死

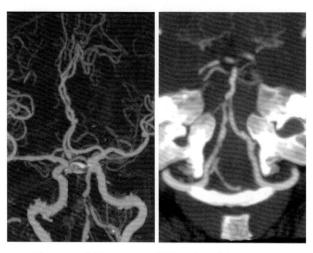

图 4.4.3　头部 CTA 示双侧椎基底动脉交界区狭窄

Section 4 The Vertebro–basilar Artery Junction

Case 5 Severe stenosis of the bilateral vertebro-basilar artery junction

1. Clinical presentation and radiological studies

A 61-year-old woman presented with paroxysmal dizziness for over 5 months. Each episode of the dizziness symptom lasted for around 0.5 hours.

MRI did not show any new cerebral infarction (Fig. 4.4. 1). MRA and CTA revealed a dominant right vertebral artery and severe stenosis at the junction of bilateral vertebro-basilar arteries (Fig. 4.4.2 and Fig. 4.4.3).

Despite aggressive medical treatment, including dual antiplatelet therapy and excellent control of risk factors, she experienced recurrent dizziness. Ten days prior to admission, the patient had a sudden episode of transient unconsciousness lasting 3–4 minutes. She was subsequently transferred to our hospital for endovascular treatment.

The patient had been living with hypertension for 30 years, hyperlipidemia for 4 years, and diabetes mellitus for 2 years. Additionally, she underwent coronary artery bypass grafting 3 months prior to admission.

The patient presented with no neurological deficits at the time of admission. Laboratory results showed that the low-density lipoprotein cholesterol level was 2.13 mmol/L.

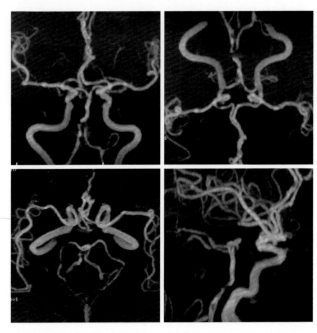

Fig. 4.4.2 MRA showed a dominant right vertebral artery and severe stenosis at the junction of bilateral vertebro-basilar arteries

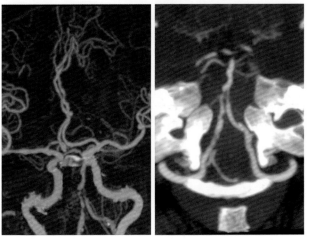

Fig. 4.4.3 CTA showed severe stenosis of the bilateral vertebro-basilar artery junction

Fig. 4.4.1 MRI showed no cerebral infarct

血栓弹力图：AA 抑制率 100%，ADP 抑制率86.6%。

DSA：右椎动脉 V4 段及基底动脉近端串联重度狭窄（图 4.4.4），左椎动脉开口迂曲，左椎动脉V4 段重度狭窄，发出小脑后下动脉（PICA）后以远显影浅淡（图 4.4.5），右侧颈内动脉系统未见明显异常（图 4.4.6），左颈内动脉交通段动脉瘤（2 mm×2.5 mm）（图 4.4.7）。

入院后给予双联抗血小板（阿司匹林 100 mg 1 次 / 日＋替格瑞洛 90 mg 2 次 / 日）、降脂（阿托伐他汀 20 mg 1 次 / 日）等治疗。

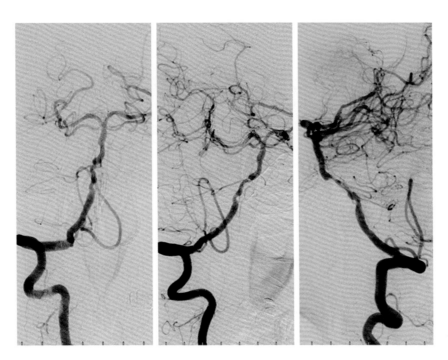

图 4.4.4　DSA 示右椎动脉 V4 段及基底动脉近端串联重度狭窄

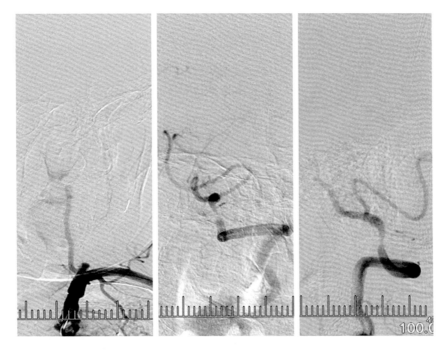

图 4.4.5　DSA 示左椎动脉开口迂曲，左椎动脉 V4 段重度狭窄

Thromboelastography revealed 100% inhibition of AA and 86.6% inhibition of ADP.

After conducting a DSA, it was revealed that the patient had a tandem stenosis of the V4 segment of the right vertebral artery and proximal basilar artery (Fig. 4.4.4). Additionally, there was a tortuous opening of the left vertebral artery, severe stenosis of the V4 segment of the left vertebral artery (Fig. 4.4.5), and no significant stenosis of the right internal carotid artery (Fig. 4.4.6). Furthermore, there was also an aneurysm (2 mm×2.5 mm) in the communicating segment of the left internal carotid artery (Fig. 4.4.7).

Upon admission, the patient was prescribed a dual antiplatelet regimen consisting of daily Aspirin at 100 mg and twice-daily Ticagrelor at 90 mg, as well as Atorvastatin at 20 mg daily.

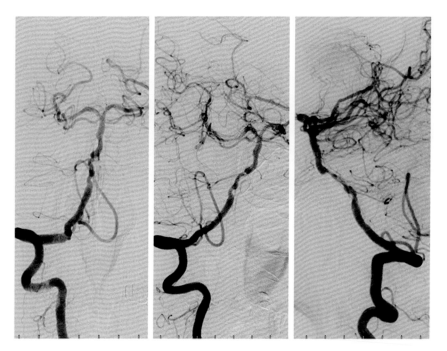

Fig. 4.4.4 DSA showed tandem stenosis of the V4 segment of the right vertebral artery and the proximal basilar artery

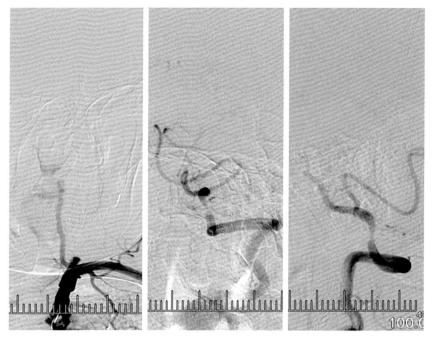

Fig. 4.4.5 DSA showed a tortuous opening of the left vertebral artery and severe stenosis of the V4 segment of the left vertebral artery

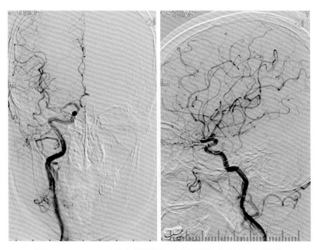

图 4.4.6　DSA 示右侧颈内动脉系统未见明显异常

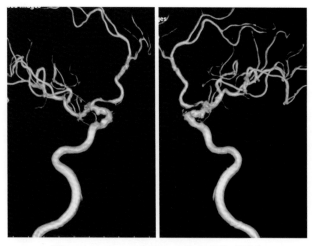

图 4.4.7　DSA 示左颈内动脉交通段动脉瘤

（二）诊断

双侧椎基底动脉交界区重度狭窄。

（三）术前讨论

患者近期有反复头晕等表现，药物治疗效果不佳。DSA 提示双侧椎基底动脉交界区重度狭窄，侧支代偿差，有血管内介入治疗指征。

治疗策略：右椎动脉优势，拟选择右椎动脉入路，但右椎动脉 V4 段-基底动脉病变较长，拟先用球囊预扩张，再放置长度匹配的自膨式支架。左颈内动脉交通段动脉瘤暂时予以保守治疗。

相关风险：穿支闭塞、支架内血栓形成。

（四）治疗过程

全麻下右股动脉入路，6F 导引导管至右椎动脉 V2 段远端，术前造影示右椎基底动脉交界区重度狭窄，局部可见充盈缺损，考虑斑块掀起（图 4.4.8）。

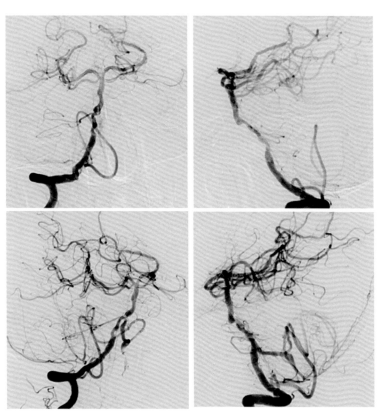

图 4.4.8　术前 DSA 示右椎基底动脉交界区重度狭窄

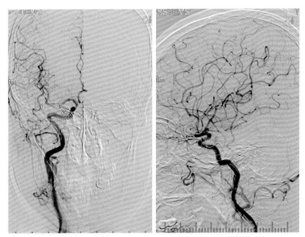

Fig. 4.4.6 DSA showed no significant stenosis of the right internal carotid artery

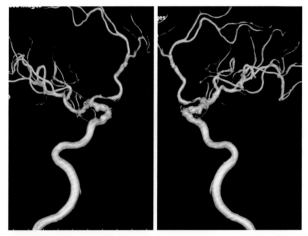

Fig. 4.4.7 DSA showed a communicating segment aneurysm of the left internal carotid artery

2. Diagnosis

Symptomatic severe stenosis of the bilateral vertebrobasilar artery junction.

3. Treatment schedule

Despite receiving aggressive medical treatment, the patient experienced recurrent dizziness. Angiogram results showed severe stenosis at the junction of the bilateral vertebrobasilar arteries with poor collateral compensation. Consequently, endovascular treatment was deemed appropriate.

Endovascular treatment approach: The dominant right vertebral artery was selected as the access approach for the procedure. In the present case, the stenotic lesion located at the junction of the right vertebral and basilar arteries was found to be of considerable length. Consequently, balloon pre-dilation was performed prior to the deployment of a self-expanding stent. As for the smallsized aneurysm at the communicating segment of the left internal carotid artery, routine radiological follow-up was advised.

Potential procedural complications include occlusion of the perforating arteries and in-stent thrombosis.

4. Treatment

Under general anesthesia, a 6 F guide catheter was placed at the distal end of the V2 segment of the right vertebral artery. The angiography confirmed severe stenosis in the junction of the right vertebral-basilar artery, with a locally visible filling defect that was considered to be caused by plaque uplift (Fig. 4.4.8). Under the roadmap, the Synchro

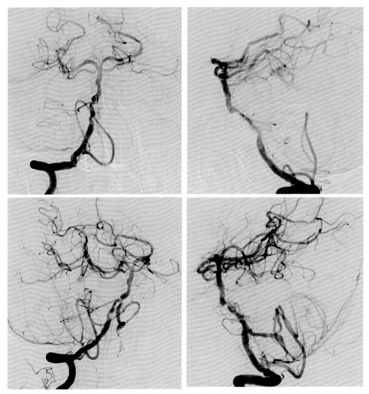

Fig. 4.4.8 DSA showed severe stenosis at the junction of the right vertebral-basilar artery

路径图下沿导引导管送入 Synchro 微导丝（0.014 in，200 cm）及 Echelon-10 微导管通过狭窄段，至左大脑后动脉 P2 段，交换送入 Transend 微导丝（0.014 in，300 cm），撤出微导管，沿微导丝送入 Gateway 球囊（2.25 mm×20 mm）于狭窄处预扩张（图 4.4.9），撤出球囊导管，沿微导丝送入 Wingspan 自膨式支架（3 mm×20 mm），造影提示支架释放后贴壁良好，前向血流 mTICI 分级 3 级（图 4.4.10）。

术后查体同前。

术后头部 CT：未见出血（图 4.4.11）。

术后头部 CTA：右椎动脉 V4 段及基底动脉支架内通畅（图 4.4.12）。

（五）讨论

本例系双侧椎基底动脉交界区狭窄，处理上一般选择优势侧。该病例的病变稍长，不适合放置球囊扩张式支架。此外，因考虑穿支闭塞的风险，球囊直径的选择也略有保守。

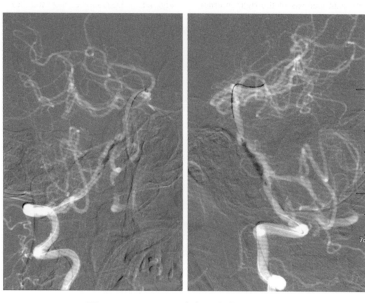

图 4.4.9　Gateway 球囊于狭窄处预扩张

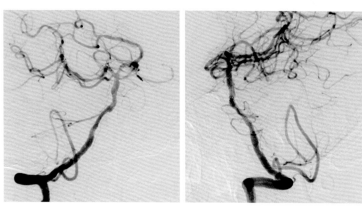

图 4.4.10　术后 DSA 示支架释放后贴壁良好，前向血流 mTICI 分级 3 级

microwire (0.014 in, 200 cm) and Echelon-10 microcatheter were navigated through the stenosis lesion and advanced towards the P2 segment of the left posterior cerebral artery. Following the exchange technique, a Transend microwire (0.014 in, 300 cm) was navigated through the target lesion. A 2.25 mm×20 mm Gateway balloon was used to pre-dilate the lesion. (Fig. 4.4.9). Subsequently, a 3 mm×20 mm Wingspan stent was deployed to cover the lesion totally. Post-stent implantation angiogram showed excellent stent wall apposition, and the antegrade blood flow of the right vertebral artery achieved grade 3 (Fig. 4.4.10).

The non-contrast CT scan conducted after the procedure displayed no evidence of cerebral hemorrhage. (Fig. 4.4. 11).

The postprocedural CTA revealed that the stent at the vertebro-basilar artery junction was patent. (Fig. 4.4. 12).

5. Comments

In the aforesaid case featuring stenosis at the junction of the bilateral vertebro-basilar arteries, the dominant artery was usually subjected to treatment. However, due to the lesion's length, deployment of a balloon-expandable stent was contraindicant. What's more, the conservative selection of balloon diameter was based on the concern over potential occlusion of perforating arteries.

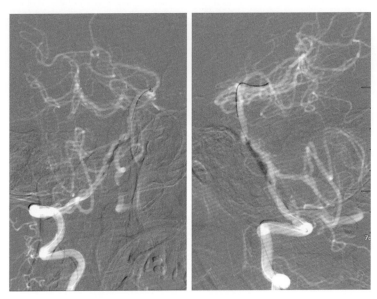

Fig. 4.4.9   The stenosis lesion at the right vertebro-basilar artery junction was pre-dilated using a Gateway balloon

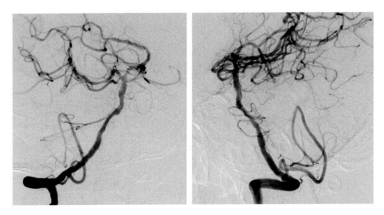

Fig. 4.4.10   Post-stent implantation angiogram showed excellent stent wall apposition, and the antegrade blood flow of the right vertebral artery achieved a grade 3

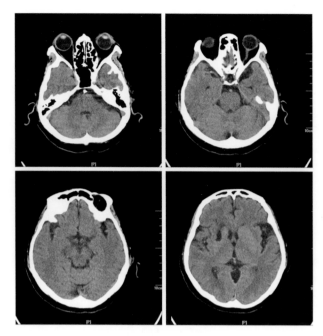

图 4.4.11　头部 CT 未见出血

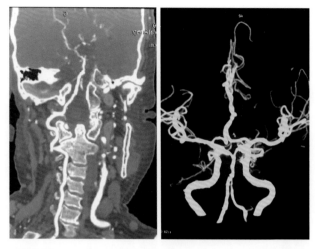

图 4.4.12　头部 CTA 示右椎基底动脉交界区支架内通畅

（王天保　宋立刚　马宁）

4.4　手术操作视频
（病例 5）

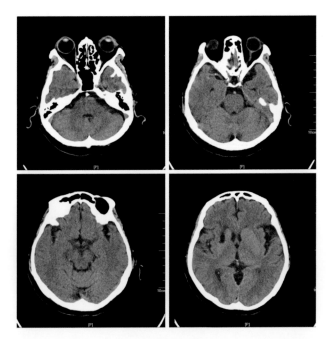

Fig. 4.4.11   Postprocedural CT scan revealed the absence of cerebral hemorrhage

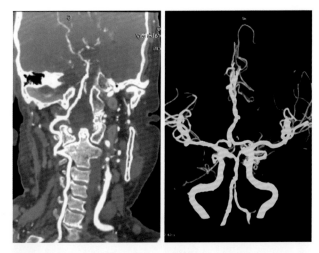

Fig. 4.4.12   Postprocedural CTA revealed that the stent at the vertebro-basilar artery junction was patent

(Translated by Rongrong Cui, Revised by Zhikai Hou)

4.4   Video of endovascular therapy (Case 5)

第五节 大脑中动脉分叉部

病例 6 右大脑中动脉分叉部重度狭窄

（一）临床病史及影像分析

患者，男性，主因"突发言语不能伴左侧肢体无力3周"入院。

既往史：既往体健，无高血压、糖尿病、脑梗死等病史。

查体：运动性失语，左侧肢体针刺觉减退。

入院后完善头部MRI：右侧大脑半球多发急性梗死灶（图4.5.1A和B）。

头部MRA：右大脑中动脉分叉部重度狭窄（图4.5.2A和B）。

头部CTP：右侧大脑半球低灌注（图4.5.3A～D）。

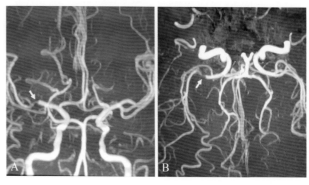

图4.5.2 头部MRA提示右大脑中动脉分叉部重度狭窄（箭头）（**A**和**B**）

入院后给予双联抗血小板（阿司匹林100 mg 1次/日＋氯吡格雷75 mg 1次/日）以及强化降脂（阿托伐他汀40 mg 1次/日）等治疗。

（二）诊断

症状性右大脑中动脉分叉部重度狭窄。

（三）术前讨论

结合患者病史及相关影像学检查，考虑右大脑中动脉为责任动脉，且右侧大脑半球低灌注，有血管内治疗指征。

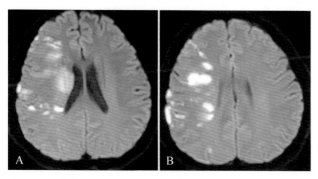

图4.5.1 头部MRI提示右侧大脑半球多发急性梗死灶（**A**和**B**）

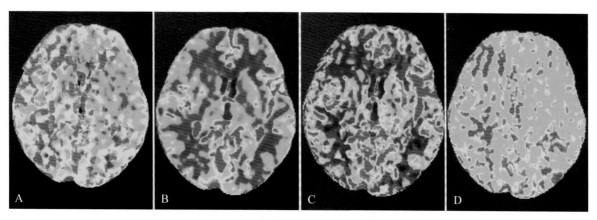

图4.5.3 头部CTP提示右侧大脑半球低灌注（**A**～**D**）

Section 5　The Middle Cerebral Artery Bifurcation

Case 6　Severe stenosis of the right middle cerebral artery bifurcation

1. Clinical presentation and radiological studies

A male patient was hospitalized with a history of sudden speech impairment and hemiplegia on the left side for three weeks.

The patient had no known medical history of hypertension, diabetes, cerebral infarction, or any other relevant conditions. Upon physical examination, the patient displayed evident motor aphasia and decreased pinprick sensation in the left limb.

MRI showed multiple acute infarcts in the right cerebral hemisphere (Fig. 4.5.1 A, B).

MRA indicates significant stenosis at the right middle cerebral artery bifurcation. (Fig. 4.5.2 A, B).

The CTP results indicated a noteworthy hypoperfusion in the region supplied by the right middle cerebral artery. (Fig. 4.5.3 A–D).

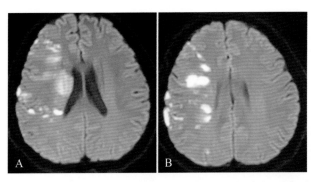

Fig. 4.5.1　MRI showed multiple acute infarcts in the right cerebral hemisphere (**A**, **B**)

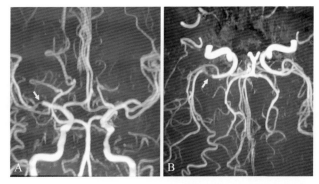

Fig. 4.5.2　MRA showed severe stenosis at the right middle cerebral artery bifurcation (arrow) (**A**, **B**)

Upon admission, he initiated dual antiplatelet therapy consisting of daily doses of 100 mg of Aspirin and 75 mg of Clopidogrel, as well as intensive statin therapy with a daily dose of 40 mg of Atorvastatin.

2. Diagnosis

Symptomatic severe stenosis of the right middle cerebral artery bifurcation.

3. Treatment schedule

Considering the patient's medical history and radiological findings, the right middle cerebral artery was identified as the culprit vessel, with notable hypoperfusion within the distal territory of the stenotic lesion. Consequently, the patient was deemed a candidate for endovascular treatment.

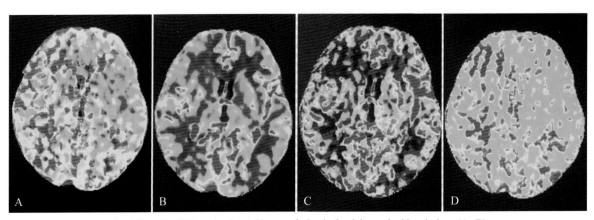

Fig. 4.5.3　The CTP results showed hypoperfusion in the right cerebral hemisphere (**A**–**D**)

相关风险：医源性夹层、动脉破裂、穿支事件以及急性血栓形成等。

（四）治疗过程

全麻下右股动脉穿刺入路，置入 6F 鞘，术前造影示右大脑中动脉分叉部重度狭窄（图 4.5.4 A 和 B），左颈动脉造影未见明显异常（图 4.5.4 C 和 D），后循环造影未见明显异常（图 4.5.4 E 和 F）。将 6F 导引导管送至右颈内动脉 C2 段，沿导引导管送入 Transend 微导丝，小心通过狭窄段至 M2 段（图 4.5.5 A），沿微导丝送入 Gateway 球囊（1.5 mm× 9 mm），加压扩张（图 4.5.5 B），造影见残余狭窄率约为 50%（图 4.5.5 C），撤出球囊，沿微导丝送入 XT-27 微导管，撤出微导丝，沿微导管送入 Neuroform EZ 支架（2.5 mm×20 mm），准确对位后成功释放支架，造影见前向血流较前明显改善，mTICI 分级 3 级，分支均显影良好，支架贴壁良好。于动脉内缓慢推注替罗非班 0.25 mg，观察 10 min 后造影，血流通畅，无急性血栓形成（图 4.5.5 D），撤出导管，结束手术。

（五）讨论

本例患者右大脑中动脉分叉部重度狭窄，手术风险大，球囊扩张后残余狭窄较重，故给予支架置入。

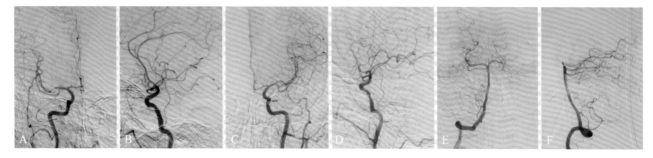

图 4.5.4　术前造影提示右大脑中动脉分叉部重度狭窄（**A** 和 **B**），左侧颈动脉未见明显异常（**C** 和 **D**），后循环未见明显异常（**E** 和 **F**）

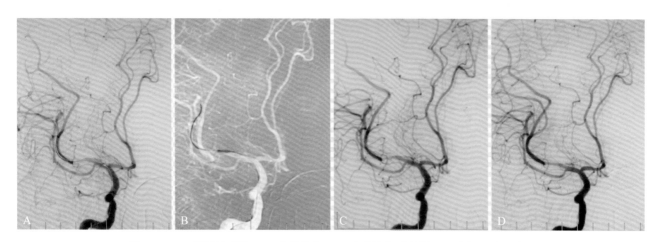

图 4.5.5　**A**. 微导丝到位；**B**. 球囊扩张；**C**. 球囊扩张后造影；**D**. 支架释放后造影

（阎龙）

4.5　手术操作视频
（病例 6）

Potential procedural risks included iatrogenic dissection, arterial rupture, perforating artery occlusion and, acute in-stent thrombosis.

4. Treatment

Following induction of general anesthesia, access to the right femoral artery was achieved, and a 6 French guide catheter sheath was subsequently inserted with precision. The angiogram revealed a severe stenosis at the bifurcation of the right middle cerebral artery (Fig. 4.5.4 A, B), while no significant abnormalities were detected in the left carotid artery (Fig. 4.5.4 C, D) or posterior circulation systems (Fig. 4.5.4 E, F). The 6F guide catheter was placed at the C2 segment of the right internal carotid artery. A Transend microwire was advanced into the M2 segment of the right middle cerebral artery (Fig. 4.5.5 A). After the pre-dilatation with a 1.5 mm×9 mm Gateway balloon (Fig.

4.5.5 B), the angiogram showed residual stenosis at an estimated degree of 50% (Fig. 4.5.5 C). Subsequently, a 2.5 mm×20 mm Neuroform EZ stent was employed to cover the lesion. Follow-up angiogram revealed excellent wall appostion of stent, with a grade 3 of antegrade blood flow. A dosage of 0.25 mg Tirofiban was administered intra-arterially to prevent acute in-stent thrombosis. After an observation period of ten minutes, the final angiogram showed an unobstructed stent. (Fig. 4.5.5 D).

5. Comments

Our report describes a patient with severe stenosis at the bifurcation of the right middle cerebral artery. Given the lesion's location at the bifurcation of trunk, the procedure carried a high potential risk. A stent was implanted due to considerable residual stenosis following balloon angioplasty.

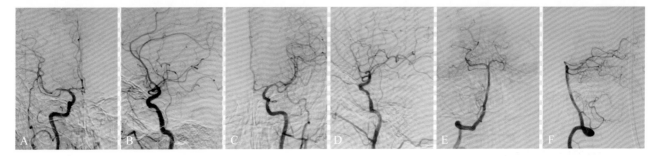

Fig. 4.5.4   The angiogram before the procedure showed severe stenosis at the right middle cerebral artery bifurcation (**A, B**), no significant abnormalities in the left carotid artery (**C, D**) and posterior circulation systems (**E, F**)

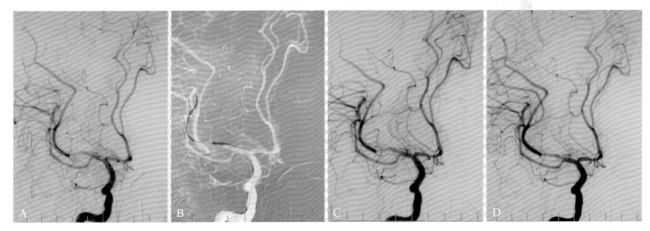

Fig. 4.5.5   (**A**) A Transend microwire was navigated to the M2 segment of the right middle cerebral artery. (**B**) The lesion was dilated using a Gateway balloon. (**C**) The angiogram following the balloon angioplasty. (**D**) The angiogram following the stent implantation

(Translated by Rongrong Cui, Revised by Zhikai Hou)

4.5   Video of endovascular therapy (Case 6)

第六节 椎动脉颅内段

病例 7 左椎动脉 V4 段重度狭窄

（一）临床病史及影像分析

患者，女性，72 岁，主因"头晕 1 月余"入院。

既往史：高血压、糖尿病病史。

查体：神经系统查体未见明显异常。

头颅 MRI 示左侧小脑半球多发新近梗死（图 4.6.1 A 和 B）。MRA 示双椎动脉 V4 段重度狭窄，

基底动脉顶端略显扩张（图 4.6.1 C）。

头颅 CTA 示双椎动脉均衡型，右椎动脉 V4 段远端重度狭窄，左椎动脉 V4 段长段狭窄，狭窄近端可见管壁钙化，基底动脉尖可见扩张，累及双侧大脑后动脉开口（图 4.6.2 A 和 B）。CTP 提示后循环供血区域低灌注（图 4.6.2 C）。

入院后予以双联抗血小板（阿司匹林 100 mg

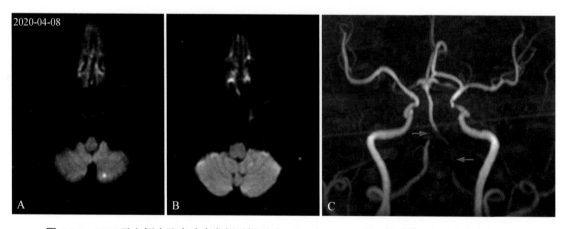

图 4.6.1 DWI 示左侧小脑半球多发新近梗死（**A** 和 **B**），MRA 示双椎动脉 V4 段重度狭窄（**C**）

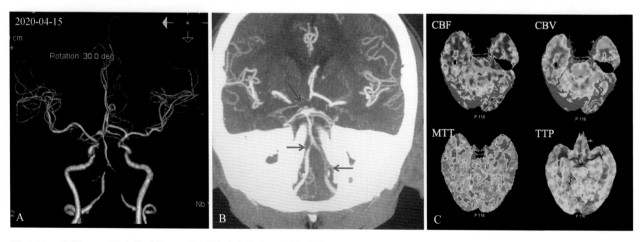

图 4.6.2 头颅 CTA 示右椎动脉 V4 段远端重度狭窄，左椎动脉 V4 段长段狭窄，基底动脉尖扩张，累及双侧大脑后动脉开口（**A** 和 **B**）。CTP 示后循环供血区域低灌注（**C**）

Section 6 The Intracranial Vertebral Artery

Case 7 Severe stenosis of the V4 segment of the left vertebral artery

1. Clinical presentation and radiological studies

A 72-year-old woman presented with dizziness lasting for over one month.

She had a history of hypertension and diabetes mellitus.

She was neurologically intact on admission.

MRI showed multiple infarcts in the left cerebellar hemisphere (Fig. 4.6.1 A, B). The MRA displayed significant stenosis at the V4 segment of both vertebral arteries, along with ectasia of the vessel at the apex of the basilar artery. (Fig. 4.6.1 C).

Upon review of the CTA results, it was found that both vertebral arteries had equal diameters, but with the addition of severe stenosis at the distal V4 segment in the right vertebral artery and an extensive stenotic lesion along the V4 segment at the left vertebral artery. Furthermore, there was vessel ectasia at the apex of the basilar artery, which affected the opening of both posterior cerebral arteries (Fig. 4.6.2 A, B). CTP indicated hypoperfusion in the territory of posterior circulation (Fig. 4.6.2 C).

Following admission, she was prescribed a dual antiplatelet regimen consisting of daily doses of aspirin at 100 mg and clopidogrel at 75 mg, as well as atorvastatin at a

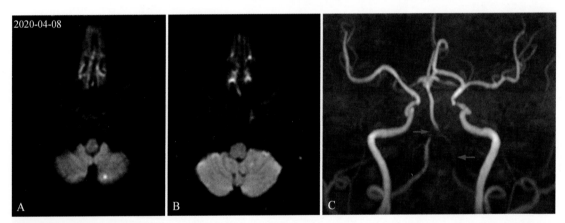

Fig. 4.6.1 The MRI showed multiple infarcts in the left cerebellar hemisphere (**A, B**), the MRA showed severe stenosis at the V4 segment of the bilateral vertebral arteries (**C**)

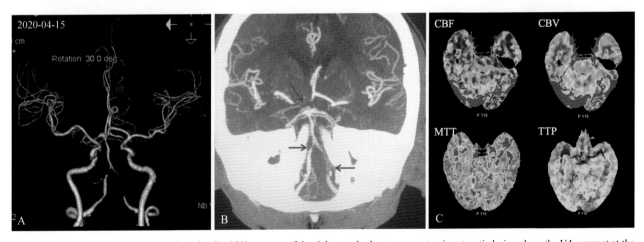

Fig. 4.6.2 CTA revealed severe stenosis at the distal V4 segment of the right vertebral artery, an extensive stenotic lesion along the V4 segment at the left vertebral artery, and vessel ectasia at the top of the basilar artery with the opening of both posterior cerebral arteries being involved (**A, B**). CTP indicated hypoperfusion within the posterior circulation territory (**C**)

1 次 / 日＋氯吡格雷 75 mg 1 次 / 日）及阿托伐他汀（20 mg 1 次 / 日）等治疗。

（二）诊断

双椎动脉 V4 段狭窄。

（三）术前讨论

患者存在双椎动脉 V4 段狭窄，结合患者左侧小脑半球多发梗死，考虑左椎动脉 V4 段系本次发病责任血管，拟行干预治疗。MRA 和 CTA 提示左椎动脉病变较长，拟球囊扩张后放置自膨式支架。病变近端管壁存在钙化，治疗过程中有扩张困难的可能。患者基底动脉顶端扩张，需要血管造影以进一步明确诊断。术中和术后需要控制好血压，预防高灌注。其他治疗风险包括穿支卒中、支架内急性血栓形成等。

（四）治疗过程

全麻下右股动脉穿刺入路。治疗前 DSA 显示右后交通动脉开放，但基底动脉未见逆行显影（图 4.6.3 A ～ D）。左椎动脉 V4 段重度狭窄，狭窄长度

较 MRA 和 CTA 所示短，mTICI 分级 1 级（图 4.6.3 E 和 F）。右椎动脉 V4 段狭窄，狭窄程度较 MRA 和 CTA 所示狭窄程度轻，基底动脉顶端扩张（图 4.6.3 G 和 H）。

路径图下将 6F 导引导管置于左椎动脉 V2 段远端（图 4.6.4 A），将 Synchro 微导丝（0.014 in，300 cm）结合 Gateway 球囊（2.75 mm×15 mm）扩张病变一次（图 4.6.4 B ～ D）。扩张后病变局部管壁掀起。其后于狭窄处释放 Wingspan 支架（3.5 mm×15 mm）。支架释放后造影显示，支架完全张开并贴壁，残余狭窄率约为 10%，mTICI 分级 3 级（图 4.6.4 E 和 F）。观察 10 min，重复造影局部无变化。其后三维血管造影显示基底动脉顶端扩张，正位呈倒三角形，侧位呈球形，累及双侧大脑后动脉开口（图 4.6.4 G），对此改变，未予以处理。

（五）讨论

本例显示对于颅内血管重度狭窄，因前向血流减慢，CTA 或者 MRA 都可能对病变长度有不同程度夸大。颅内偏心钙化病变较环形钙化更容易扩张，本例较为顺利的扩张过程也佐证了这一点。扩

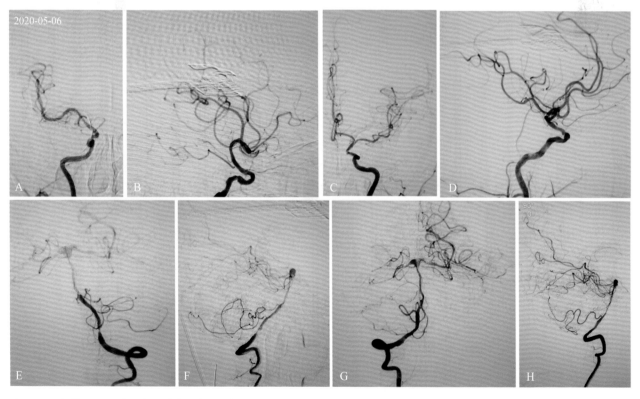

图 4.6.3　术前 DSA 示右后交通动脉开放，基底动脉未见逆行显影（**A ～ D**），左椎动脉 V4 段重度狭窄，狭窄长度较 MRA 和 CTA 所示短，mTICI 分级 1 级（**E 和 F**），右椎动脉 V4 段狭窄，狭窄程度较 MRA 和 CTA 所示轻，基底动脉顶端扩张（**G 和 H**）

daily dosage of 20 mg.

2. Diagnosis

Symptomatic stenosis of the V4 segment of the bilateral vertebral artery.

3. Treatment schedule

The patient was diagnosed with significant stenosis at the V4 segment of both vertebral arteries. Given the presence of multiple infarctions in the left cerebellar hemisphere, it was believed that the left vertebral artery V4 segment is the main responsible vessel for this condition. In light of this, endovascular treatment of the V4 segment of the left vertebral artery had been advised for the patient. The results of both the MRA and CTA revealed the stenosis lesion at the V4 segment of the left vertebral artery was extensive. The lesion was treated with the implantation of a self-expanding stent after balloon angioplasty. However, the presence of calcification along the vessel wall at the V4 segment of the left vertebral artery may pose some challenges during the process of balloon dilatation. Angiography is required to confirm the presence of vessel ectasia at the apex of the basilar artery. Potential complications included hyperperfusion syndrome, perforating artery occlusion, and acute/subacute in-stent thrombosis.

4. Treatment

Under general anesthesia, the endovascular procedure was performed through right femoral artery access. The angiogram displayed a patent right posterior communicating artery (Fig. 4.6.3 A–D), and a marked stenosis at the V4 segment of the left vertebral artery with a length of stenosis shorter than that observed on MRA and CTA. (Fig. 4.6.3 E, F). The angiogram also detected a slight stenosis at the distal V4 segment of the right vertebral artery and ectasia of the vessel at the apex of the basilar artery. (Fig. 4.6.3 G, H).

The 6F guide catheter was positioned at the distal V2 segment of the left vertebral artery (Fig. 4.6.4 A). Subsequently, the lesion was pre-dilated with a 2.75 mm×15 mm Gateway balloon (Fig. 4.6.4 B–D). A 3.5 mm×15 mm Wingspan self-expanding stent was used to cover the lesion completely. After stent implantation, the angiogram exhibited excellent stent attachment to the vessel wall, with the residual stenosis of only 10% (Fig. 4.6.4 E, F). Additionally, A three-dimensional angiogram depicted a vessel ectasia at the top of the basilar artery, forming an inverted triangle when viewed anteriorly, and a spherical shape under lateral observation. The ectasia involved both posterior cerebral arteries (Fig. 4.6.4 G). We did not treat the vessel ectasia of the basilar artery.

5. Comments

The imaging modalities of CTA or MRA may overestimate the length of intracranial artery stenosis, attributable to the slow antegrade flow at the stenotic region. This case indicates that intracranial artery stenosis that exhibits an eccentric calcification is more amenable to

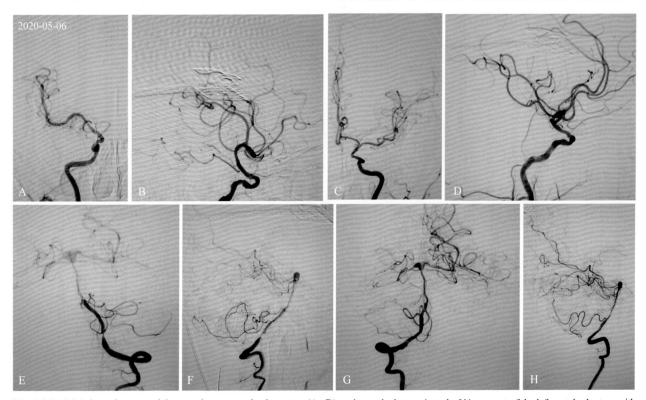

Fig. 4.6.3　DSA showed a patent right posterior communicating artery (**A–D**), and a marked stenosis at the V4 segment of the left vertebral artery with a length of stenosis shorter than that observed on MRA and CTA. (**E, F**). The angiogram also detected a slight stenosis at the distal V4 segment of the right vertebral artery and ectasia of the vessel at the apex of the basilar artery (**G, H**)

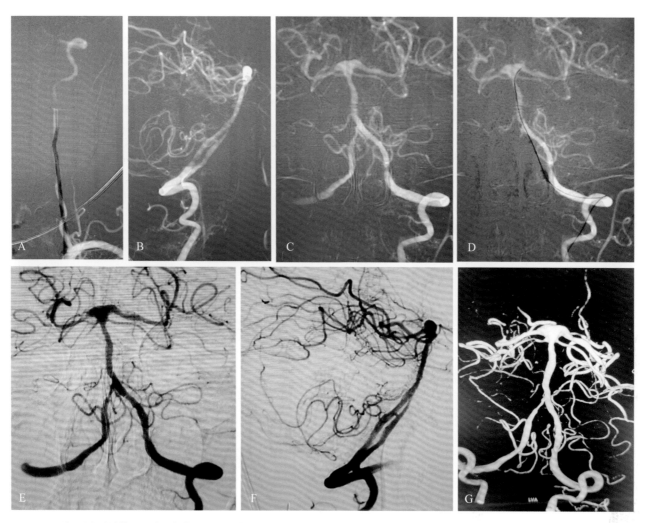

图 4.6.4　放置导引导管于左椎动脉 V2 段远端（**A**），Gateway 球囊扩张病变（**B ～ D**），支架释放后造影示支架贴壁良好，残余狭窄率约为 10%，mTICI 分级 3 级（**E 和 F**）。三维血管造影示基底动脉顶端扩张，正位呈倒三角形，侧位呈球形，累及双侧大脑后动脉开口（**G**）

张后局部管壁掀起，未见明显血流分层现象，考虑系局部斑块被挤压移位。对于基底动脉顶端扩张，不除外动脉瘤可能，未来会密切随访观察，如有增大趋势或发生形态学变化，再考虑进一步干预治疗。

（尤吉栋　杨冬旭　贾白雪　孙立倩　马宁）

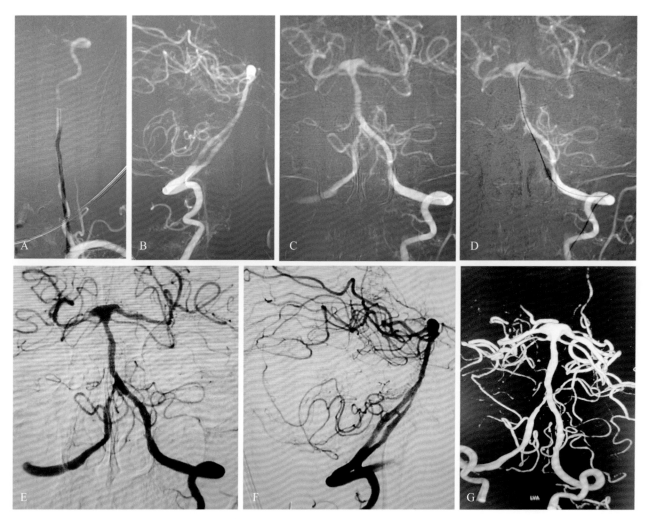

Fig. 4.6.4   The 6F guide catheter was placed at the distal V2 segment of the left vertebral artery (**A**). The lesion was pre-dilated with a Gateway balloon (**B–D**). After stent implantation, the angiogram exhibited excellent stent attachment to the vessel wall, with the residual stenosis of only 10% (**E**, **F**). A three-dimensional angiogram depicted a vessel ectasia at the top of the basilar artery, forming an inverted triangle when viewed anteriorly, and a spherical shape under lateral observation. (**G**)

expansion, as opposed to that circular calcifications. After the balloon dilation, the focal vessel wall was uplifted without any discernible blood flow stratification, which could be attributed to plaque compaction and displacement. The ectasia of the vessel at the basilar artery apex could be a precursor of an aneurysm. Regular monitoring is essential to identify any increase in size and morphological changes of the lesion.

(Translated by Rongrong Cui, Revised by Zhikai Hou)

第七节　大脑前动脉 A1 段

病例 8　左大脑前动脉 A1 段重度狭窄

（一）临床病史及影像分析

患者，女性，60 岁，主因"右侧肢体无力伴言语不利 1 个月"入院。

当地医院头部 MRI 提示左侧额颞顶叶急性梗死灶（图 4.7.1），头部 CTA 提示双侧大脑前动脉 A1 段重度狭窄以及左侧大脑中动脉闭塞（图 4.7.2），为求血管内治疗转入我院。

既往史：高血压 21 年，糖尿病 8 年，脑梗死 8 年。

查体：运动性失语，右侧肢体肌力 4 级。

入院后头部 CTA ＋ CTP：CTA 示左侧大脑中动脉闭塞，左侧颈内动脉 C5 ～ C7 段以及双侧大脑前动脉 A1 段重度狭窄（图 4.7.3）；CTP 示左侧额颞顶叶大片状低灌注区域（图 4.7.4）。

入院后 DSA：左侧大脑中动脉闭塞，左侧颈内动脉 C5 ～ C7 段以及双侧大脑前动脉 A1 段重度狭窄（图 4.7.5）。

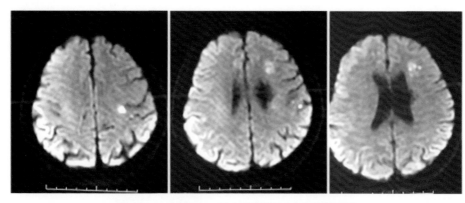

图 4.7.1　头部 MRI 示左侧额颞顶叶急性梗死灶

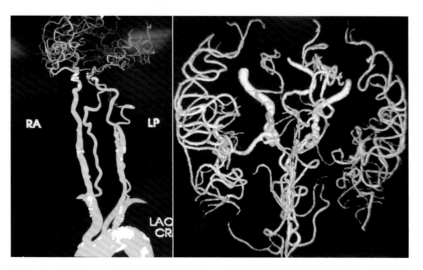

图 4.7.2　头部 CTA 示双侧大脑前动脉 A1 段重度狭窄以及左侧大脑中动脉闭塞

Section 7   The A1 Segment of the Anterior Cerebral Artery

Case 8   Severe stenosis of the A1 segment of the left anterior cerebral artery

1. Clinical presentation and radiological studies

A woman, aged 60, was admitted to the hospital for right hemiplegia and dysphasia for a month.

The MRI conducted at a nearby hospital revealed multiple infarctions in the left frontal, temporal, and parietal lobes. (Fig. 4.7.1). The CTA revealed a significant stenosis of the A1 segment of the bilateral anterior cerebral arteries and occlusion of the left middle cerebral artery (Fig. 4.7.2). She was referred to our hospital for endovascular therapy.

She had a medical history of hypertension for 21 years, diabetes mellitus for 8 years, and ischemic stroke for 8 years.

Neurological evaluation indicated motor aphasia and grade 4 weakness in the right limbs.

Upon admission, the CTA results revealed critical stenosis of the A1 segment in both anterior cerebral arteries, as well as the C5–C7 segments of the left internal carotid artery, and total occlusion of the left middle cerebral artery (Fig. 4.7.3). The CTP scan exhibited hypoperfusion in the region of the left frontal, temporal, and parietal lobes (Fig. 4.7.4).

Subsequent to admission, DSA confirmed severe stenosis in the A1 segment of both anterior cerebral arteries, as well as in the C5–C7 segments of the left internal carotid artery, and complete occlusion of the left middle cerebral artery (Fig. 4.7.5).

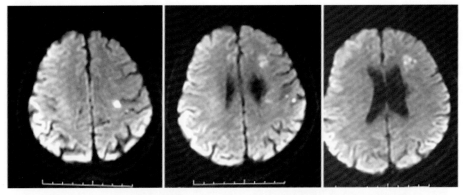

Fig. 4.7.1   MRI showed multiple infarcts in the left frontal, temporal, and parietal lobes

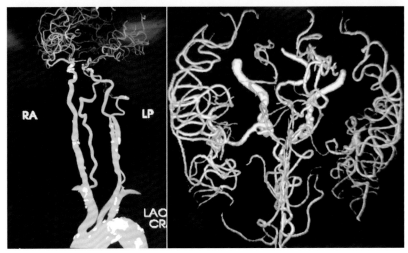

Fig. 4.7.2   The CTA revealed a significant stenosis of the A1 segment of the bilateral anterior cerebral arteries and occlusion of the left middle cerebral artery

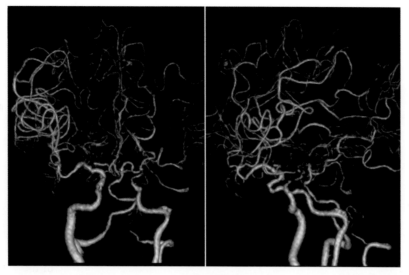

图 4.7.3 入院后头部 CTA 示左侧大脑中动脉闭塞，左侧颈内动脉 C5～C7 段以及双侧大脑前动脉 A1 段重度狭窄

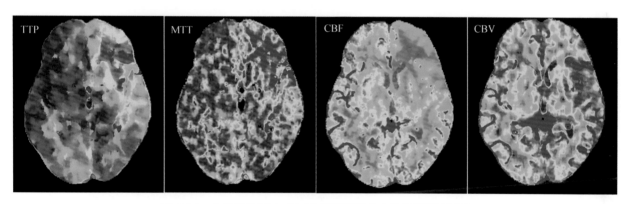

图 4.7.4 入院后头部 CTP 示左侧额颞顶叶大片状低灌注区域

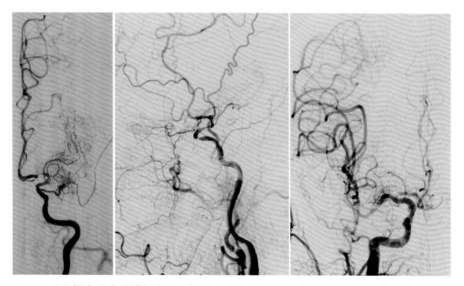

图 4.7.5 DSA 示左侧大脑中动脉闭塞，左侧颈内动脉 C5～C7 段以及双侧大脑前动脉 A1 段重度狭窄

病后一直口服阿司匹林（100 mg 1 次 / 日）、氯吡格雷（75 mg 1 次 / 日）进行双联抗血小板治疗，以及阿托伐他汀（40 mg 1 次 / 日）降脂治疗。

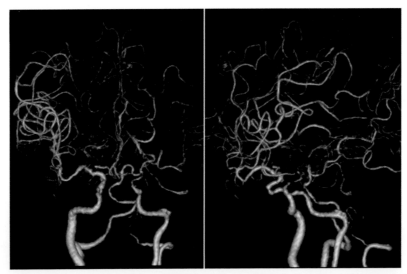

Fig. 4.7.3   The CTA results revealed critical stenosis of the A1 segment in both anterior cerebral arteries, as well as the C5–C7 segments of the left internal carotid artery, and total occlusion of the left middle cerebral artery

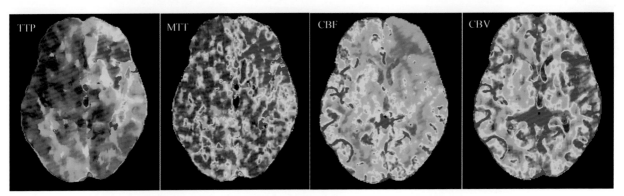

Fig. 4.7.4   The CTP scan exhibited hypoperfusion in the region of the left frontal, temporal, and parietal lobes

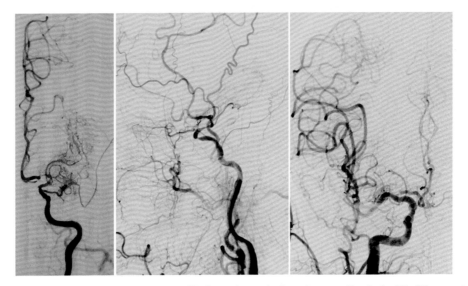

Fig. 4.7.5   DSA confirmed severe stenosis in the A1 segment of both anterior cerebral arteries, as well as in the C5–C7 segments of the left internal carotid artery, and total occlusion of the left middle cerebral artery

Following the onset of symptoms, she was prescribed a dual antiplatelet regimen, comprising of a daily dose of 100 mg of aspirin and 75 mg of clopidogrel, in addition to a daily dose of 40 mg of atorvastatin.

（二）诊断

症状性左大脑前动脉 A1 段以及左颈内动脉 C5 ～ C7 段重度狭窄。

（三）术前讨论

结合患者病史及相关影像学检查，考虑左颈内动脉系统为本次发病责任血管，且头部 CTP 提示左侧额叶低灌注明显，拟同期处理左大脑前动脉 A1 段以及左颈内动脉 C5 ～ C7 段狭窄段。相关风险包括医源性夹层、急性血栓形成、动脉破裂等。

（四）治疗过程

全麻下右股动脉穿刺入路，置入 6F 导引导管送至左颈内动脉 C1 段，造影显示左颈内动脉 C5 ～ C7 段局限性重度狭窄，左大脑中动脉闭塞，左大脑前动脉 A1 段重度狭窄（图 4.7.6）。Synchro 微导丝（0.014 in，300 cm）带 Echelon-10 微导管同轴通过左大脑前动脉 A1 段狭窄病变至左大脑前动脉 A2 段（图 4.7.7 A），因血管迂曲，退出 Synchro 微导丝，更换为 Transend 微导丝（0.014 in，300 cm）送至大脑前动脉 A2 段。沿微导丝将 Gateway 球囊（1.5 mm×15 mm）送至左大脑前动脉 A1 段及左颈内动脉 C5 ～ C7 段狭窄段，准确定位后将球囊缓慢加压至 6 atm，持续 20 s（图 4.7.7 B），造影示左大脑前动脉 A1 段残余狭窄率约为 20%，左颈内动脉 C5 ～ C7 段残余狭窄率约为 30%（图 4.7.7 C 和 D）。观察 10 min 后，造影显示左颈内动脉及左大脑前动脉前向血流良好，无急性血栓形成，远端分支血管无急性闭塞征象（图 4.7.8），撤出导管，结束手术。

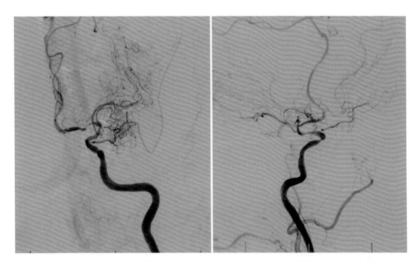

图 4.7.6　术前 DSA 示左颈内动脉 C5 ～ C7 段局限性重度狭窄，左大脑中动脉闭塞，左大脑前动脉 A1 段重度狭窄

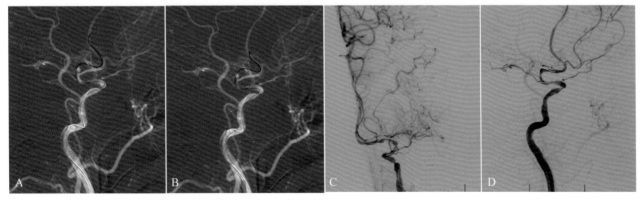

图 4.7.7　**A**. Synchro 微导丝带 Echelon-10 微导管同轴通过左大脑前动脉 A1 段狭窄病变至左大脑前动脉 A2 段；**B**. Gateway 球囊依次扩张左大脑前动脉 A1 段及左颈内动脉 C5 ～ C7 段狭窄段；**C** 和 **D**. 球囊扩张后造影显示左大脑前动脉 A1 段残余狭窄率约为 20%，左颈内动脉 C5 ～ C7 段残余狭窄率约为 30%

2. Diagnosis

Symptomatic severe stenosis of the A1 segment of left anterior cerebral artery and C5–C7 segments of the left internal carotid artery.

3. Treatment schedule

Based on a review of the patient's medical history and radiological studies, it has been determined that the patient has suffered from multiple infarctions within the territory of the left internal carotid artery, leading to significant hypoperfusion in this area. In light of this, it has been recommended that the patient undergo endovascular treatment to address the stenosis of the A1 segment of the left anterior cerebral artery and the C5–C7 segments of the left internal carotid artery. Possible risks associated with the procedure include but are not limited to iatrogenic dissection, in-stent thrombosis, and arterial rupture.

4. Treatment

Under general anesthesia, a 6 F guide catheter was inserted into the C1 segment of the left internal carotid artery. Upon angiography, severe stenosis was revealed in A1 segment of the left anterior cerebral artery and the C5–C7 segments of the left internal carotid artery, as well as complete occlusion of the left middle cerebral artery (Fig.4.7.6). The Synchro microwire (0.014 in, 300 cm) and the Echelon-10 microcatheter coaxially advanced through the stenosis segment of the left anterior cerebral artery to reach the A2 segment (Fig. 4.7.7 A). Due to the tortuous approach, the Synchro microwire was substituted with the Transend microwire. A 1.5 mm×15 mm Gateway balloon was utilized to sequentially dilate the stenosis lesions of the A1 segment of the left anterior cerebral artery and the C5–C7 segments of the left internal carotid artery (Fig. 4.7.7 B). The post-balloon dilatation angiogram revealed a residual stenosis of 20% in the A1 segment of the left anterior cerebral artery, as well as a residual stenosis of 30% in the C5–C7 segments of the left internal carotid artery (Fig. 4.7.7 C, D). After a ten-minute observation, the angiogram indicated that there was no evidence of elastic recoil in the treated vessel wall, and there was no signs of acute thrombosis or occlusion in the distal branches (Fig. 4.7.8).

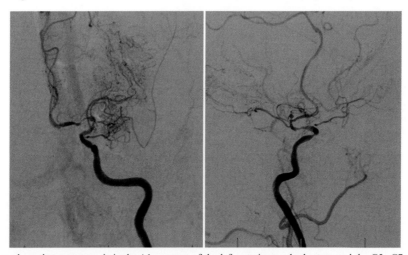

Fig. 4.7.6   The angiogram showed severe stenosis in the A1 segment of the left anterior cerebral artery and the C5–C7 segments of the left internal carotid artery, as well as total occlusion of left middle cerebral artery

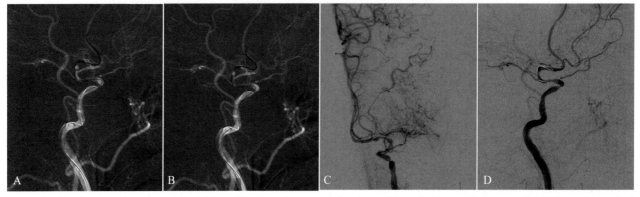

Fig. 4.7.7   The Synchro microwire and the Echelon- 10 microcatheter coaxially advanced through the stenosis segment of the left anterior cerebral artery to reach the A2 segment (**A**). A 1.5 mm×15 mm Gateway balloon was utilized to sequentially dilated the stenosis lesions of the A1 segment of the left anterior cerebral artery and the C5–C7 segments of the left internal carotid artery (**B**). The post-balloon dilatation angiogram revealed a residual stenosis of 20% in the A1 segment of the left anterior cerebral artery, as well as a residual stenosis of 30% in the C5–C7 segments of the left internal carotid artery. (**C, D**)

术后第 1 天患者右侧肢体无力较前加重，右上肢肌力 3 级，右下肢肌力 4 级，考虑穿支梗死。术后第 3 天肢体无力较前明显好转，右侧肢体肌力均为 4 级。

术后第 3 天头部 CTA ＋ CTP：左颈内动脉 C5 ～ C7 段以及左大脑前动脉 A1 段血管通畅（图 4.7.9），左大脑半球低灌注情况较术前改善（图 4.7.10）。

（五）讨论

本例患者脑梗死，责任血管为左颈内动脉系统，造影显示左颈内动脉 C5 ～ C7 段以及左大脑前动脉 A1 段重度狭窄，且对应的左侧额颞顶叶大片状低灌注，故同期处理左颈内动脉以及左大脑前动脉的狭窄病变。

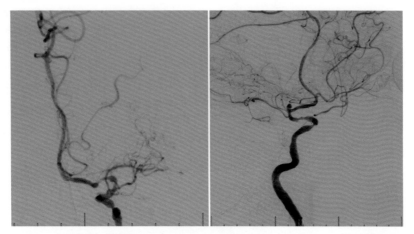

图 4.7.8　术后造影示左颈内动脉及左大脑前动脉前向血流良好，无急性血栓形成

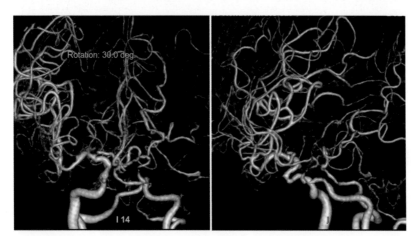

图 4.7.9　术后第 3 天头部 CTA 示左颈内动脉 C5 ～ C7 段以及左大脑前动脉 A1 段血管通畅

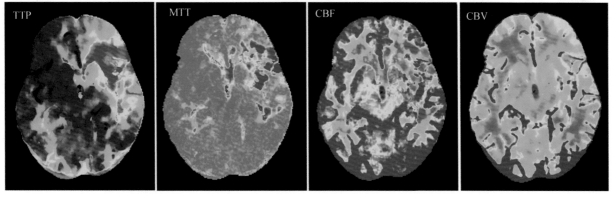

图 4.7.10　术后第 3 天头部 CTP 示左大脑半球低灌注情况较术前改善

（阎龙）

The day following the procedure, weakness in the right upper limb worsened with the muscle strength declining to grade 3. However, two days later, there was an improvement in muscle weakness, with the right upper limb now at grade 4 strength.

The third day after the procedure, a follow-up CTA revealed patency in the C5–C7 segments of the left internal carotid artery as well as the A1 segment of the left anterior cerebral artery (Fig. 4.7.11). Additionally, the CTP results showed an improvement in hypoperfusion in the territory of the left internal carotid artery, in comparison to pre-procedure results (Fig. 4.7.12).

5. Comments

This case concerns a patient with multiple infarctions within the left internal carotid artery's territory. The angiogram indicated severe stenosis in the C5–C7 segments of the left internal carotid artery, as well as the A1 segment of the left anterior cerebral artery. Additionally, there was critical hypoperfusion in the regions of the left frontal, temporal, and parietal lobes. As a result, it has been recommended that the patient undergo endovascular treatment to address the stenosis in the C5–C7 segments of the left internal carotid artery and the A1 segment of the left anterior cerebral artery.

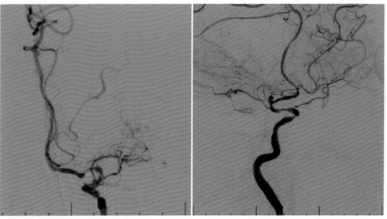

Fig. 4.7.8   The final angiogram indicates that there is no evidence of elastic recoil in the treated vessel wall, and there are no signs of acute thrombosis or occlusion in the distal branches

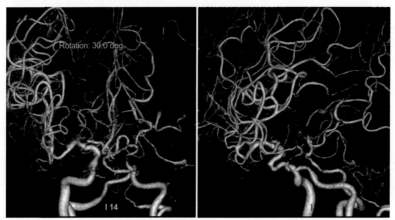

Fig. 4.7.9   Follow-up CTA revealed patency in the C5–C7 segments of the left internal carotid artery as well as the A1 segment of the left anterior cerebral artery

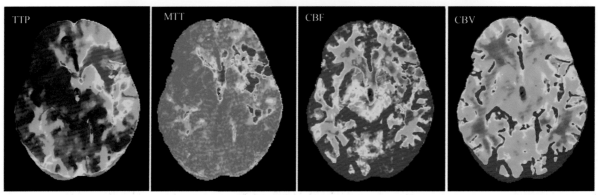

Fig. 4.7.10   CTP results showed an improvement in hypoperfusion in the territory of the left internal carotid artery

(Translated by Rongrong Cui, Revised by Zhikai Hou)

第五章

特殊病变的血管内介入治疗

第一节　长节段病变

病例 9　右颈内动脉 C7 段长节段狭窄

（一）临床病史及影像分析

患者，女性，62 岁，主因"左侧肢体无力伴言语含糊 1 月余"入院。

当地医院头部 MRI 示右侧放射冠多发脑梗死（图 5.1.1 A 和 B）。头颈部 CTA 示右颈内动脉 C7 段狭窄（图 5.1.1 C 和 D）。患者经内科药物治疗，症状仍有反复。为进一步治疗，就诊于我院。

既往史：患高血压及 2 型糖尿病十余年。

查体：神经系统查体未见明显异常。

糖化血红蛋白：10.1%。

血栓弹力图：AA 抑制率 100%，ADP 抑制率 26.2%。

术前 DSA：右颈内动脉 C7 段长节段重度狭窄，右颈内动脉系孤立颈动脉系统，右大脑前动脉 A1 段发育不良或者缺如（图 5.1.2 A）。前交通动脉开放，右大脑前动脉经软脑膜动脉向右大脑中动脉供血区域代偿（图 5.1.2 B 和 C）。未见明显后循环参与代偿（图 5.1.2 D）。

入院后给予双联抗血小板（阿司匹林 100 mg 1 次 / 日 ＋ 氯吡格雷 75 mg 1 次 / 日）、降脂（阿托伐他汀 20 mg 1 次 / 日）治疗，以及控制血压、降糖等治疗。

（二）诊断

症状性右颈内动脉 C7 段长节段重度狭窄。

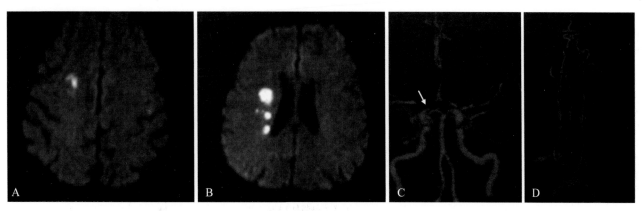

图 5.1.1　**A** 和 **B**. 头部 MRI 提示右侧放射冠多发脑梗死；**C** 和 **D**. 头颈部 CTA 提示右颈内动脉 C7 段狭窄

79

Chapter 5

Advanced Endovascular Therapy for ICAS

Section 1 Long–segment stenoses

Case 9 Long-segment stenosis in the C7 segment of the right internal carotid artery

1. Clinical presentation and radiological studies

A 62-year-old woman was hospitalized due to leftsided weakness and dysarthria persisting for over a month.

MRI revealed multiple infarctions in the right corona radiata (Fig. 5.1.1 A, B). CT angiography demonstrated a severe, long-segment stenosis in the C7 segment of the right internal carotid artery (Fig. 5.1.1 C, D). Her symptoms recurred despite the aggressive medical treatment, prompting her transfer to our hospital for endovascular treatment.

She had a past medical history of hypertension and diabetes mellitus, which had been present for over a decade.

Upon admission, her neurological examination revealed no abnormalities.

The glycated hemoglobin level was recorded at 10.1%.

Thromboelastography results indicated 100% inhibition of AA and 26.2% inhibition of ADP.

The DSA revealed a significant, long-segment narrowing affecting the C7 segment of the right internal carotid artery, along with a hypoplastic or absent A1 segment of the right anterior cerebral artery (Fig. 5.1.2 A). The anterior communicating artery was found to be patent, and collateral blood flow through pial arteries from the right anterior cerebral artery was observed compensating the territories of the right middle cerebral artery (Fig. 5.1.2 B, C). The collateral perfusion from the posterior circulation to the right carotid artery territory was determined to be inadequate (Fig. 5.1.2 D).

Upon admission, a dual antiplatelet regimen was prescribed for her, consisting of a daily dose of 100mg aspirin and 75 mg clopidogrel, alongside a daily dose of 20 mg atorvastatin.

2. Diagnosis

Symptomatic severe long-segment stenosis in the C7 segment of the right internal carotid artery.

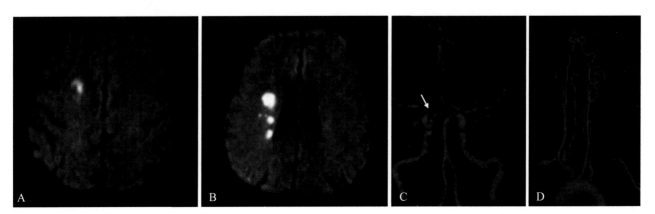

Fig. 5.1.1　MRI showed multiple infarcts in the right corona radiata (**A, B**). The CTA revealed a severe stenosis in the C7 segment of the right internal carotid artery (**C, D**)

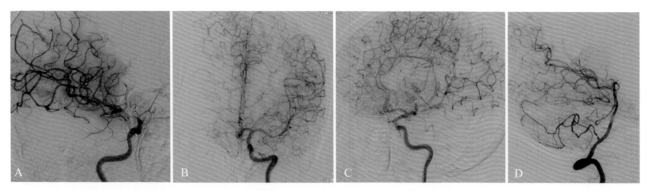

图 5.1.2 **A**. DSA 示右颈内动脉 C7 段长节段重度狭窄，右颈内动脉系孤立颈动脉系统，右大脑前动脉 A1 段发育不良或者缺如；**B** 和 **C**. 前交通动脉开放，右大脑前动脉经软脑膜动脉向右大脑中动脉供血区域代偿；**D**. 未见明显后循环参与代偿

（三）术前讨论

本例患者右颈内动脉 C7 段重度狭窄，为本次发病责任血管。因内科药物治疗症状仍有反复，血管造影显示侧支代偿较差，准备予以血管内介入治疗。

治疗策略：右颈内动脉 C7 段狭窄段病变长度约为 10 mm，拟选择长度 15 mm 的球囊扩张。狭窄段有脉络膜前动脉发出，拟稍小直径球囊预扩张以避免损伤脉络膜前动脉。

相关风险：脉络膜前动脉闭塞、高灌注综合征、急性血栓形成、动脉夹层等。

（四）治疗过程

全麻下右股动脉入路，将 6F 导引导管放至右颈内动脉 C1 段远端，造影示右颈内动脉 C7 段长节段重度狭窄（图 5.1.3 A 和 B）。路径图下将 Transend 微

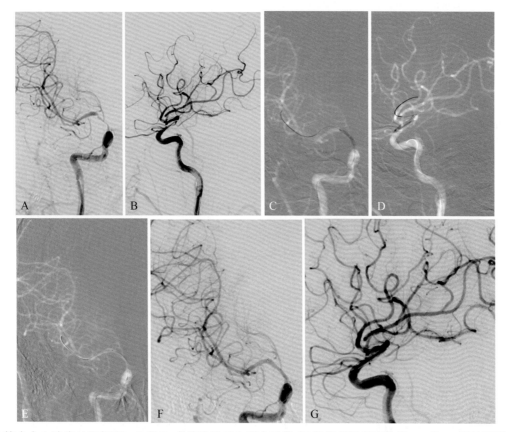

图 5.1.3 血管内介入治疗过程如下：**A** 和 **B**. 术前造影示右颈内动脉 C7 段长节段重度狭窄；**C** 和 **D**. 微导丝到位，Gateway 球囊扩张；**E**. 放置导引导管于右颈内动脉 C3 段以增加系统支撑力；**F** 和 **G**. 释放支架，术后造影显示支架贴壁良好，前向血流 mTICI 分级 3 级，脉络膜前动脉完好

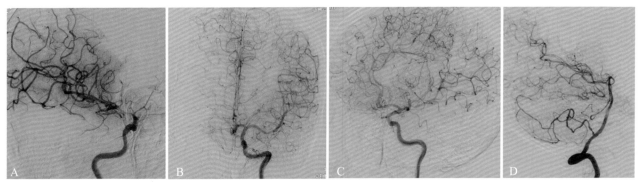

Fig. 5.1.2 DSA revealed a significant, long-segment narrowing affecting the C7 segment of the right internal carotid artery, along with a hypoplastic or absent A1 segment of the right anterior cerebral artery (**A**). The anterior communicating artery was found to be patent, and collateral blood flow through pial arteries from the right anterior cerebral artery was observed compensating the territories of the right middle cerebral artery (**B, C**). The collateral perfusion from the posterior circulation to the right carotid artery territory was determined to be inadequate (**D**)

3. Treatment schedule

This case reported a patient with a long-segment stenosis in the C7 segment of the right internal carotid artery. Despite receiving aggressive medical treatment, she experienced a recurrent ischemic event. Furthermore, angiography revealed inadequate collateral circulation to the territory supplied by the diseased artery. She had an indication for endovascular intervention to enhance distal blood perfusion.

Treatment approach: To treat a stenosis exceeding 10mm in the C7 segment of the right internal carotid artery, a 15 mm balloon was utilized to dilate the stenotic lesion. However, as the anterior choroidal artery arose from the stenotic segment, a

smaller balloon was selected (with a diameter less than that of the target artery) to minimize potential vascular injury.

Possible complications included occlusion of the anterior choroidal artery, hyperperfusion syndrome, artery dissection, as well as acute and subacute in-stent thrombosis.

4. Treatment

Under general anesthesia, a 6F guide catheter was positioned at the C1 segment of the right internal carotid artery. An angiogram confirmed a critical and long-segment stenosis in the C7 segment of the right internal carotid artery. (Fig. 5.1.3 A, B). A Transend microwire (0.014 in, 300 cm) was advanced into

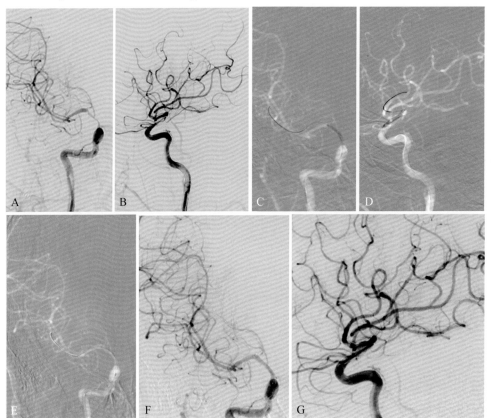

Fig. 5.1.3 An angiogram confirmed a critical and long-segment stenosis in the C7 segment of the right internal carotid artery. (**A, B**). The guide catheter was navigated to the C3 segment of the right internal carotid artery to provide enhanced radial support force during the implanation of the stent (**E**). The final angiogram demonstrated excellent stent wall apposition, and a grade 3 antegrade blood flow in the right internal carotid artery, and the anterior choroidal artery remained intact (**F, G**)

导丝（0.014 in，300 cm）送至右大脑中动脉 M2 段，沿微导丝送入 Gateway 球囊（2.0 mm×15 mm）于狭窄处扩张（图 5.1.3 C 和 D），撤出球囊导管。后沿微导丝送入 Wingspan 自膨式支架（3.0 mm×15 mm），期间将导引导管送至右颈内动脉 C3 段，以增加系统支撑力（图 5.1.3 E）。支架于病变处释放后造影提示支架贴壁良好，前向血流 mTICI 分级 3 级，脉络膜前动脉未受影响（图 5.1.3 F 和 G）。

术后立即复查头部 CT 未见出血，查体同前。

（五）讨论

本例治疗难度在于如何保护脉络膜前动脉，在实施边支保护技术困难的情况下，采用稍小直径球囊扩张后放置自膨式支架，以避免损伤重要边支血管。此外，患者右颈内动脉系孤立颈动脉系统，避免大直径球囊扩张，也会减少术后高灌注综合征发生的概率。

（姚丽娜　宋立刚）

病例 10　右椎动脉 V4 段长节段重度狭窄

（一）临床病史及影像分析

患者，男，46 岁，主因"头晕 3 个月，眩晕伴恶心、呕吐 2 个月"入院。

当地医院头颅 MRI 和 MRA 提示左侧小脑较小梗死灶（图 5.1.4），右椎动脉 V4 段狭窄，基底动脉远段显影欠佳，左椎动脉 V4 段未见显影（图 5.1.5）。

当地医院 DSA 示右椎动脉 V4 段次全闭塞，基底动脉有顺向显影，前向血流减慢（图 5.1.6），左椎动脉 V3 段闭塞，见基底动脉经脊髓前动脉代偿显影（图 5.1.7）。予以双联抗血小板及降脂药物治疗后，患者症状缓解，为进一步治疗收入我院。

既往史：高血压病史，吸烟。

查体：神经系统查体未见明显异常。

血栓弹力图：AA 抑制率 97.1%，ADP 抑制率 70.1%。

头部 CTA＋CTP：右椎动脉 V4 段长节段重度狭窄，左椎动脉 V3 段闭塞，基底动脉近端见开窗（图 5.1.8）；后循环分布区低灌注（图 5.1.9）。

高分辨率磁共振成像：左椎动脉闭塞，管腔可见高信号血栓，负荷量较大；右椎动脉管壁增厚，管腔狭窄（图 5.1.10）。

入院后继续给予双联抗血小板（阿司匹林 100 mg 1 次 / 日＋氯吡格雷 75 mg 1 次 / 日）、降脂（瑞舒伐他汀 10 mg 1 次 / 日）等治疗。

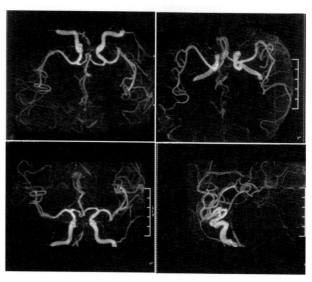

图 5.1.5　MRA 示右椎动脉 V4 段狭窄，基底动脉远段显影欠佳，左椎动脉 V4 段未见显影

图 5.1.4　MRI 示左侧小脑较小梗死灶

the M2 segment of the right middle cerebral artery. The lesion was pre-dilated using a 2.0 mm×15 mm Gateway balloon (Fig. 5.1.3 C, D). And a 3.0 mm×15 mm Wingspan stent was employed to cover the lesion totally. The guide catheter was navigated to the C3 segment of the right internal carotid artery to provide supporting force during the implanation of the stent (Fig. 5.1.3 E). The final angiogram demonstrated excellent stent wall apposition, and a grade 3 antegrade blood flow in the right internal carotid artery. Furthermore, the anterior choroidal artery remained intact (Fig. 5.1.3 F, G).

The post-procedural CT scan revealed complete absence of any cerebral hemorrhage.

5. Comments

The main challenge in this case was to avoid damage to the anterior choroidal artery during the endovascular procedure. As application of side branch protection was restricted, practical approaches such as the use of sub-maximal balloon angioplasty and implantation of self-expanding stents were employed to protect the vital size branch originating from the lesion. To prevent the occurrence of postoperative hyperperfusion syndrome, we performed a submaximal angioplasty on the patient's right internal carotid artery, which was an isolated carotid system.

(Translated by Rongrong Cui, Revised by Zhikai Hou)

Case 10   Severe long-segment stenosis in the V4 segment of the right vertebral artery

1. Clinical presentation and radiological studies

A 46-year-old male was hospitalized for experiencing dizziness for 3 months, accompanied by nausea and vomiting for the last 2 months.

MRI revealed a small infarction located in the left cerebellar hemisphere (Fig. 5.1.4). MRA indicated severe stenosis in the V4 segment of the right vertebral artery, with poor visualization of the distal part of the basilar artery and absence of visualization of the V4 segment of the left vertebral artery (Fig. 5.1.5).

DSA revealed a subtotal occlusion in the V4 segment of the right vertebral artery (Fig. 5.1.6), as well as an occlusion in the V3 segment of the left vertebral artery. The basilar artery was indirectly visualized via compensatory blood flow from the anterior spinal artery (Fig. 5.1.7).

He had a medical background of hypertension and a personal history of cigarette smoking.

He was neurologically intact on admission.

Thromboelastography test revealed 97.1% inhibition of AA and 70. 1% inhibition of ADP.

CT angiography demonstrated a severe long-segment

stenosis in the V4 segment of the right vertebral artery, occlusion in the V3 segment of the left vertebral artery, as well as a fenestration at the proximal segment of the basilar artery (Fig. 5.1.8). Furthermore, CTP indicated critical hypoperfusion in the posterior circulation territory (Fig. 5.1.9).

High- resolution MRI showed a complete occlusion of the left vertebral artery, attributed to the formation of a high-intensity thrombus within its lumen. Additionally, the right vertebral artery displayed a thickened wall, leading to a restricted lumen (Fig. 5.1.10).

Following admission, a dual antiplatelet regimen consisting of daily administration of 100 mg Aspirin and 75 mg Clopidogrel as well as daily dose of 10 mg Rosuvastatin were initiated.

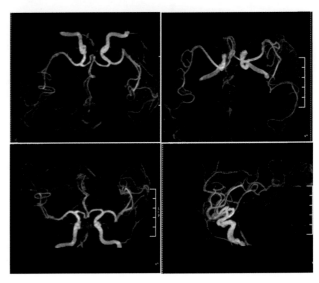

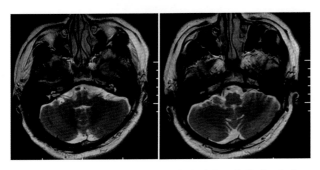

Fig. 5.1.4 MRI showed a small infarct in the left cerebellar hemisphere

Fig. 5.1.5 MRA indicated severe stenosis in the V4 segment of the right vertebral artery, with poor visualization of the distal part of the basilar artery and absence of visualization of the V4 segment of the left vertebral artery

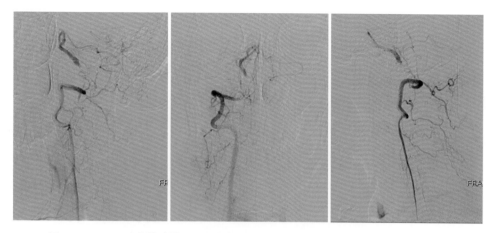

图 5.1.6 DSA 示右椎动脉 V4 段次全闭塞，基底动脉有顺向显影，前向血流减慢

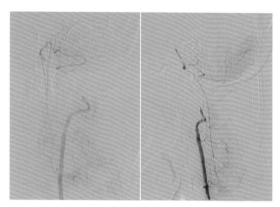

图 5.1.7 DSA 示左椎动脉 V3 段闭塞，见基底动脉经脊髓前动脉代偿显影

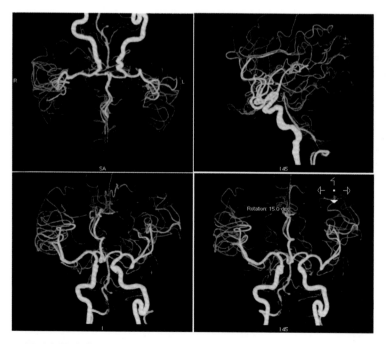

图 5.1.8 CTA 提示右椎动脉 V4 段长节段重度狭窄，左椎动脉 V3 段闭塞，基底动脉近端见开窗

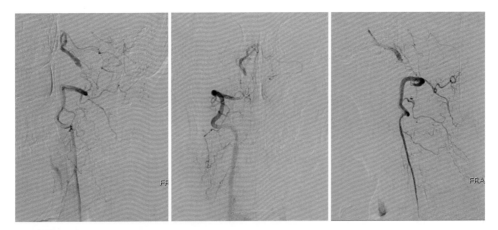

Fig. 5.1.6 DSA revealed a subtotal occlusion in the V4 segment of the right vertebral artery and an antegrade opacification of the basilar artery

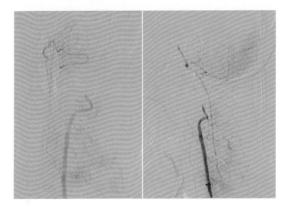

Fig. 5.1.7 DSA indicated an occlusion in the V3 segment of the left vertebral artery, while visualization of the basilar artery was indirectly achieved through compensatory blood flow from the anterior spinal artery

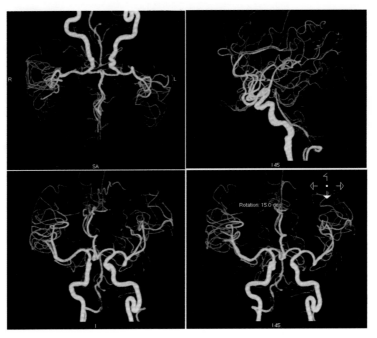

Fig. 5.1.8 CTA showed a severe long-segment stenosis in the V4 segment of the right vertebral artery, occlusion in the V3 segment of the left vertebral artery, as well as a fenestration at the proximal segment of the basilar artery

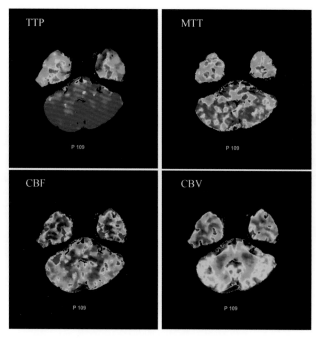

图 5.1.9　CTP 见后循环低灌注

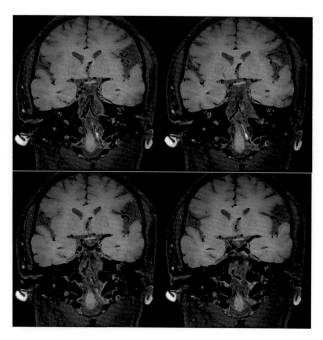

图 5.1.10　高分辨率 MRI 提示左椎动脉闭塞，管腔可见高信号血栓，负荷量较大；右椎动脉管壁增厚，管腔狭窄

（二）诊断

症状性右椎动脉 V4 段狭窄。

（三）术前讨论

患者表现为后循环缺血症状，左椎动脉 V3 段及右椎动脉 V4 段考虑系本次发病责任血管。左椎动脉血栓负荷量大，闭塞长度长，开通困难。而右椎动脉病变经过抗栓治疗后病变严重程度有所改善，拟处理右椎动脉 V4 段病变。

治疗策略：小直径长球囊扩张，再放置自膨式支架。

相关风险：穿支闭塞事件及后循环区域术后高灌注。

（四）治疗过程

全麻下右股动脉入路，将 6F 导引导管放至右椎动脉 V2 段远端，造影示右椎动脉 V4 段重度狭窄，狭窄率约为 95%，狭窄长度 13 mm（图 5.1.11）。路径图下沿导引导管送入 Transend 微导丝（0.014 in，300 cm）越过病变至基底动脉中段，沿微导丝送入 Gateway 球囊（2.75 mm×15 mm）于狭窄处预扩张（图 5.1.12），其后送入 XT-27 微导管，释放

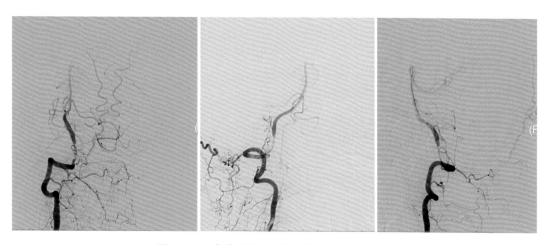

图 5.1.11　术前造影示右椎动脉 V4 段重度狭窄

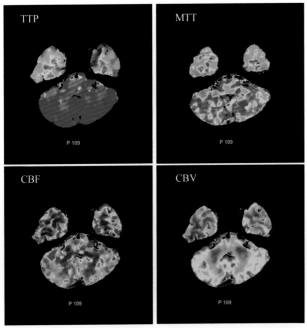

Fig. 5.1.9 CTP showed critical hypoperfusion in the posterior circulation territory

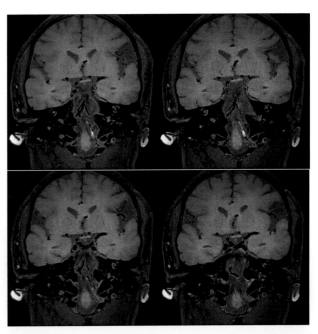

Fig. 5.1.10 High-resolution MRI showed a complete occlusion of the left vertebral artery, attributed to the formation of a high-intensity thrombus within its lumen. Additionally, the right vertebral artery displayed a thickened wall, leading to a restricted lumen

2. Diagnosis

Symptomatic severe stenosis of the V4 segment of the right vertebral artery.

3. Treatment schedule

This case involved an ischemic event in the posterior circulation, with both the V3 segment of the left vertebral artery and the V4 segment of the right vertebral artery being considered as the culprit arteries. Due to both the long-segment occlusion and the presence of a heavy-load thrombus, recanalization of the left vertebral artery was a challenge. After aggressive medical therapy, there was improvement in the degree of stenosis in the right vertebral artery, leading us to decide to perform a stent procedure in the V4 segment of the same artery.

Treatment approach: in the management of the stenotic lesion, we employed an elongated and small-diameter balloon for initial pre-dilatation, following a self-expanding stent to cover the stenosis lesion.

Potential complications included occlusion of the perforating artery and hyperperfusion syndrome.

4. Treatment

Under general anesthesia, a 6F guide catheter was positioned at the V2 segment of the right vertebral artery. The angiogram indicated a 95% stenosis and a 13 mm lesion located in the V4 segment of the same artery (Fig.5.1.11). A Transend microwire (0.014 in, 300 cm) was navigated into the middle segment of the basilar artery. The stenotic lesion was dilated using a 2.75 mm×15 mm Gateway balloon (Fig. 5.1.12). A 4.0 mm×20 mm Neuroform EZ

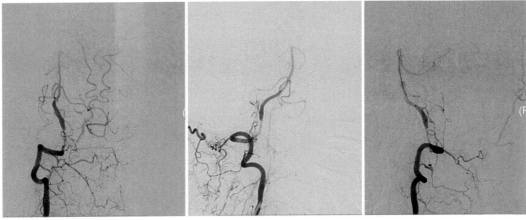

Fig. 5.1.11 Angiogram showed severe stenosis in the V4 segment of the right vertebral artery

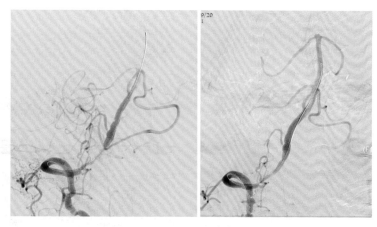

图 5.1.12　Gateway 球囊预扩张

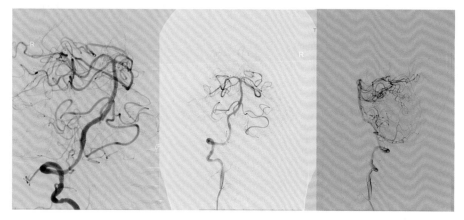

图 5.1.13　支架释放后造影提示支架贴壁良好

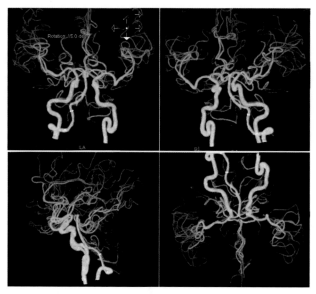

图 5.1.14　术后 CTA 示右椎动脉 V4 段支架内通畅

Neuroform EZ 自膨式支架（4.0 mm×20 mm），支架释放后造影提示支架贴壁良好，前向血流 mTICI 分级 3 级（图 5.1.13）。

术后立即复查头部 CT 未见出血，查体同前。

术后复查头颅 CTA：右椎动脉 V4 段支架内通畅（图 5.1.14）。

（五）讨论

对于较长的颅内动脉狭窄病变，经充分预扩张后，可放置尺寸较长的 off-label 自膨式支架。本例预扩张后，血管弹性回缩明显，放置完支架后狭窄程度明显改善，遂未行后扩张治疗。

（洪全龙　张义森　姜鹏　马宁）

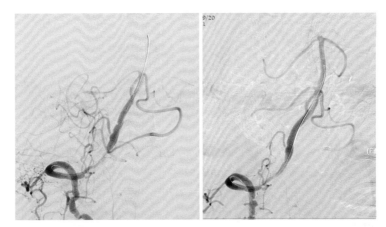

Fig. 5.1.12 The stenosis lesion in the V4 segment of right vertebral artery was dilated using a Gateway balloon

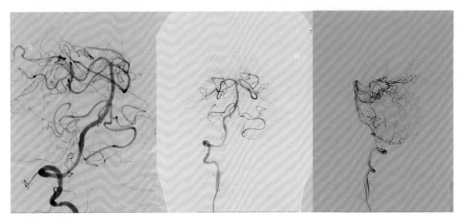

Fig. 5.1.13 The final angiogram exhibited outstanding stent wall apposition and grade 3 antegrade blood flow

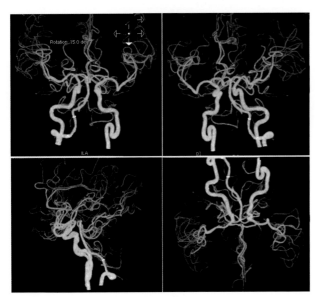

Fig. 5.1.14 Postprocedural CTA revealed the patency of the stent in the V4 segment of the right vertebral artery

self-expanding stent was utilized to address the lesion. Following the procedure, the final angiogram exhibited outstanding stent wall apposition and grade 3 antegrade blood flow (Fig. 5.1.13).

Postprocedural CT demonstrated absence of hemorrhage.

Postprocedural CTA revealed the patency of the stent in the V4 segment of the right vertebral artery (Fig. 5.1.14).

5. Comments

To treat severe, long-segment intracranial stenosis, the lesion was initially pre-dilated, after which an off-label, self-expanding stent of a prolonged size was employed. In the current case, there was an evident elastic recoil following balloon dilatation. However, the residual stenosis displayed a significant improvement following stent implantation.

(Translated by Rongrong Cui, Revised by Zhikai Hou)

第二节 成角病变

病例 11 右大脑中动脉成角病变

（一）临床病史及影像分析

患者，男性，40 岁，主因"发作性左侧肢体无力 5 个月"入院。

当地医院头颅 CT 未见颅内出血，予阿司匹林、他汀类药物治疗。入院前 10 天症状反复，再次就诊于当地医院。行头颅磁共振检查，DWI 未见急性梗死病灶（图 5.2.1 A）。头颅 CTA 示右大脑中动脉 M1 段重度狭窄，其远端分支稀疏（图 5.2.1 B）。予双联抗血小板治疗后仍有症状反复，为进一步行血管内治疗收入我院。

既往史：2 型糖尿病、脂蛋白代谢紊乱病史，通过药物控制良好 [低密度脂蛋白胆固醇（LDL-C）

1.6 mmol/L，糖化血红蛋白（HbA$_1$C）5.6%]。

查体：神经系统查体未见明显异常。

血栓弹力图：AA 抑制率 98.7%，ADP 抑制率 59.6%。

高分辨率磁共振管壁成像：右大脑中动脉 M1 段管腔偏心性变窄，血管前壁强化明显（图 5.2.1 C 和 D）。

头颅 CTP：右大脑中动脉供血区域低灌注，脑血流量（CBF）下降、脑血容量（CBV）正常，平均通过时间（MTT）以及达峰时间（TTP）延长（图 5.2.2）。

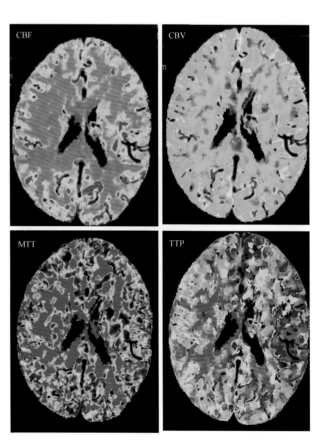

图 5.2.1 **A**. 头颅磁共振 DWI 未见急性梗死病灶；**B**. 头颅 CTA 提示右大脑中动脉 M1 段重度狭窄，其远端分支稀疏（箭头示）；**C** 和 **D**. 头颅高分辨率磁共振管壁成像提示右大脑中动脉 M1 段管腔偏心性变窄，血管前壁强化明显（箭头示）

图 5.2.2 头颅 CTP 提示右大脑中动脉供血区域低灌注，CBF 下降、CBV 正常，MTT 以及 TTP 延长

Section 2   Tortuous Stenoses

Case 11   Tortuous stenosis of the right middle cerebral artery

1. Clinical presentation and radiological studies

A 40-year-old man was hospitalized due to sudden episodes of paroxysmal left-limb hemiplegia for five months.

Non-contrast CT demonstrated no sign of hemorrhage. He was prescribed aspirin and statin after onset of the symptoms. He experienced recurrent symptoms in ten days prior to his current admission. MRI did not detect any acute cerebral infarction (Fig. 5.2.1 A). CTA showed severe stenosis in the M1 segment of the right middle cerebral artery with sparse distal branches (Fig. 5.2.1 B). His symptoms recurred despite receiving dual antiplatelet therapy.

The patient had a medical history of diabetes mellitus and dyslipidemia. The LDL-C level was maintained at 1.6 mmol/L and HbA1C was at 5.6%.

He was neurologically intact on admission.

Thromboelastography test indicated 59.6% inhibition of ADP and 98.7% inhibition of AA.

High-resolution MRI suggested an eccentrically thickened vessel wall with strong contrast enhancement on the anterior wall of the M1 segment of the right middle cerebral artery (Fig. 5.2.1 C, D).

CTP showed a prolongation of both MTT and TTP, with normal CBV and decreased CBF in the territory of the right middle cerebral artery (Fig. 5.2.2).

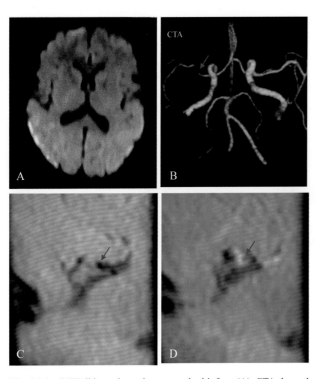

Fig. 5.2.1   DWI did not showed acute cerebral infarct (**A**). CTA showed severe stenosis in the M1 segment of the right middle cerebral artery (arrow) (**B**). High-resolution MRI suggested an eccentrically thickened vessel wall with strong contrast enhancement on the anterior wall of the M1 segment of the right middle cerebral artery (**C, D**)

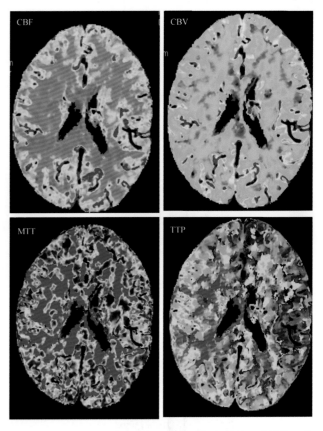

Fig. 5.2.2   CTP showed a prolongation of both MTT and TTP, with normal CBV and decreased CBF in the territory of the right middle cerebral artery

术前 DSA：右大脑中动脉 M1 段狭窄，狭窄率约为 90%，狭窄处成角，狭窄处有支豆纹动脉发出（图 5.2.3 A ～ C）。左前循环未见明显异常（图 5.2.3 D）。双椎动脉均衡型，右大脑后动脉通过软脑膜动脉向右大脑中动脉供血区域代偿（图 5.2.3 E 和 F）。

入院后给予双联抗血小板（阿司匹林 100 mg 1 次 / 日＋氯吡格雷 75 mg 1 次 / 日）、降脂（阿托伐他汀 20 mg 1 次 / 日）及降糖治疗。

（二）诊断

症状性右大脑中动脉 M1 段成角病变。

（三）术前讨论

患者右大脑中动脉 M1 段重度狭窄，同侧大脑后动脉经软脑膜动脉向其供血区域代偿，但 CT 灌注成像提示代偿不足。高分辨率磁共振管壁成像提示病变系动脉粥样硬化性狭窄。鉴于患者使用药物治疗仍有症状反复，考虑予以支架治疗。本例系成角病变，不适宜放置球囊扩张式支架，准备先行球囊扩张，再放置自膨式支架。考虑 Wingspan 推送系统头端在经过成角病变时有损伤血管的可能，拟放置经微导管释放的自膨式支架。治疗风险包括穿支闭塞和术后高灌注。

（四）治疗过程及随访

全麻下右股动脉穿刺置入 6F 动脉鞘，6F 导引导管放置于右颈内动脉 C1 段远端。送入 Transend 微导丝（0.014 in，300 cm）和 Echelon-10 微导管同轴通过右大脑中动脉 M1 段狭窄处至 M2 段下干（图 5.2.4 A 和 B）。导丝到位后造影显示成角血管被拉直，类似"拧毛巾样"改变（图 5.2.4 C）。使用 Gateway 球囊（2.0 mm×9 mm）于狭窄处扩张（图 5.2.4 D），后放置 XT-27 微导管至 M2 段下干（图 5.2.4 E），通过微导管在狭窄处释放 Neuroform EZ 支架（3.0 mm×15 mm）（图 5.2.4 F）。支架置入后三维血管造影见无明显残余狭窄（图 5.2.4 G 和 H）。观察 10 min 后无改变，遂结束治疗。

术后半年头部 CTP（图 5.2.5）：右大脑中动脉供血区域低灌注情况较前明显好转。

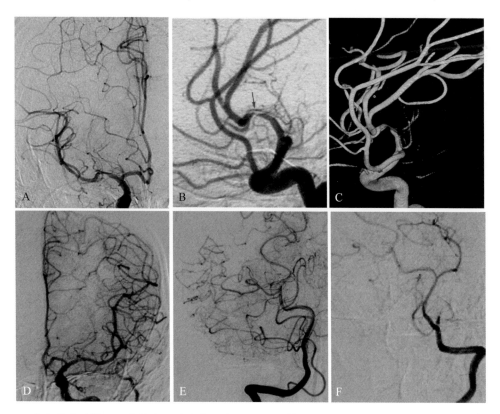

图 5.2.3　**A** ～ **C**. 右大脑中动脉 M1 段狭窄，狭窄率约为 90%，狭窄处成角，狭窄远端上壁有豆纹动脉发出（箭头示）；**D**. 左前循环未见明显异常；**E** 和 **F**. 双椎动脉均衡型，右大脑后动脉通过软脑膜动脉向右大脑中动脉供血区域代偿

The pre-procedure DSA depicted a tortuous 90% stenosis located in the M1 segment of the right middle cerebral artery, with a lenticulostriate artery arising from the stenotic lesion (Fig. 5.2.3 A – C). No significant abnormality was observed in the left anterior circulation (Fig.5.2.3D). Both vertebral arteries presented equivalent diameters. Moreover, it was observed that the existence of pial collaterals, which stemmed from the right posterior cerebral artery and compensated for the region of the right middle cerebral artery (Fig. 5.2.3 E, F).

Upon admission, he was prescribed a dual antiplatelet regimen, which included a daily dose of 100 mg aspirin and 75 mg clopidogrel, as well as a daily dose of 20 mg atorvastatin.

2. Diagnosis

Symptomatic stenosis of the M1 segment of the right middle cerebral artery.

3. Treatment schedule

The patient presented with a severe stenosis in the M1 segment of the right middle cerebral artery, along with inadequate collateral flow through the pial arteries from the right posterior cerebral artery. The high-resolution MRI indicated a severe stenosis in the M1 segment, attributed to the eccentric atherosclerotic plaque. The patient had an indication to undergo endovascular therapy considering he suffered from ischemic symptoms despite the aggressive medical treatment including dual antiplatelet therapy and excellent control of vascular risk factors.

Treatment approach: due to the tortuous nature of the stenotic lesion in the M1 segment of the right middle cerebral artery, implantation of a balloon-mounted stent was not deemed suitable. Instead, the lesion underwent pre-dilation with a balloon and subsequent treatment with a self-expanding stent. To reduce the risk of vessel injury during stent implantation, a self-expanding stent delivered through a micro-catheter was utilized. Possible complications of the procedure included perforator stroke and hyperperfusion syndrome.

4. Treatment and follow-up

Under general anesthesia, a 6F guide catheter was positioned at the C1 segment of the right internal carotid artery. A Transend microwire (0.014 in, 300 cm) and Echelon-10 microcatheter were coaxially navigated to the inferior division of the right middle cerebral artery (Fig. 5.2.4 A, B). After the microwire was advanced distal to the tortuous lesion, it was successfully straightened, resulting in the appearance of a "twisted-towel sign" (Fig. 5.2.4 C). The lesion was pre-dilated using a 2.0 mm×9 mm Gateway balloon (Fig. 5.2.4 D). An XT-27 microcatheter was positioned at the inferior division (Fig. 5.2.4 E), then a 3.0 mm×20 mm Neuroform EZ self-expanding stent was released to cover the entire lesion (Fig. 5.2.4 F). Following stent implantation, a three- dimensional angiogram showed absence of residual stenosis (Fig. 5.2.4 G, H). Ten minutes later, a final angiogram showed no alteration in the stented vessel.

Six months after the procedure, CTP results indicated a significant improvement in the hypoperfusion of the right middle cerebral artery territory (Fig. 5.2.5).

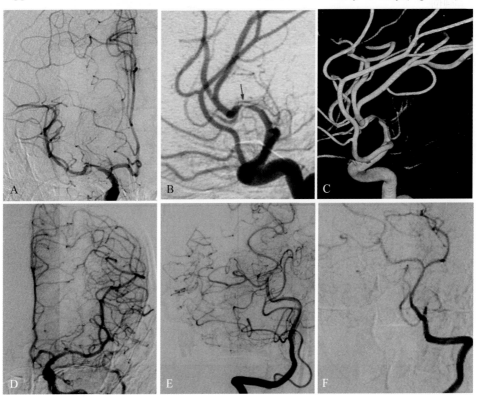

Fig. 5.2.3 The pre-procedure DSA depicted a tortuous 90% stenosis located in the M1 segment of the right middle cerebral artery (arrow), with a lenticulostriate artery arising from the stenotic lesion (**A** – **C**). No significant abnormalities were observed in the left anterior circulation (**D**). Both vertebral arteries presented equivalent diameters. Moreover, it was observed that the existence of pial collaterals, which stemmed from the right posterior cerebral artery and compensated for the region of the right middle cerebral artery (**E**, **F**)

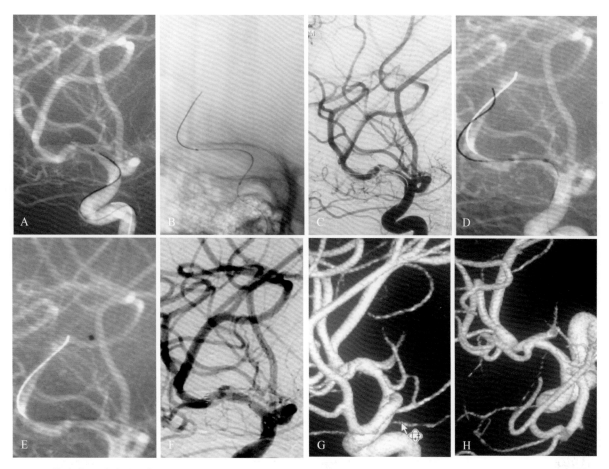

图 5.2.4　血管内介入治疗过程如下：**A** 和 **B**. Transend 微导丝和 Echelon-10 微导管同轴通过右大脑中动脉 M1 段狭窄处至下干 M2 段；**C**. 导丝到位后造影显示成角血管被拉直，类似"拧毛巾样"改变；**D**. Gateway 球囊扩张狭窄病变；**E**. 放置 XT-27 微导管至下干 M2 段；**F**. 释放 Neuroform EZ 支架；**G** 和 **H**. 支架置入后三维血管造影无明显残余狭窄

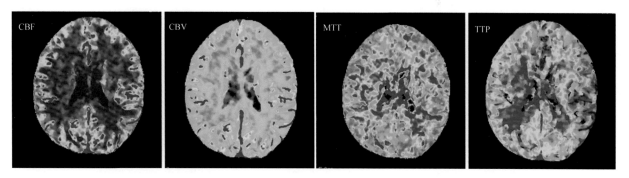

图 5.2.5　术后半年复查头部 CTP 提示右大脑中动脉供血区域低灌注情况较前明显好转

对比治疗前（图 5.2.6 A）与支架置入术后（图 5.2.6 B）右大脑中动脉图像，术后半年 DSA 显示支架内血流通畅，残余狭窄率约为 30%（图 5.2.6 C）。

（五）讨论

本例病变成角，如使用 Wingspan 系统，可能会对病变处血管造成损伤。经考虑我们选择 Neuroform EZ 支架，经导管释放和开环设计是其特点。与 Wingspan 支架相比，其支撑性稍差，且缺乏长度较短的型号（最短长度 15 mm）。本例术后半年造影复查提示残余狭窄率约为 30%，结合患者无任何临床症状，继续予以内科药物保守治疗。目前对诸如 Neuroform 及 Enterprise 等 off-label 动脉瘤辅助栓塞支架治疗狭窄性疾患的远期疗效尚不明了，我们还会继续加强相关病例的随访工作，特别是完善随访造影检查，以更好评价这类型支架的远期疗效。

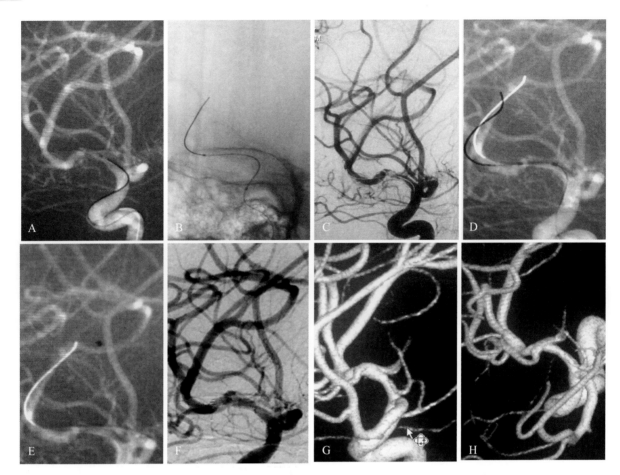

Fig. 5.2.4 A Transend microwire (0.014 in, 300 cm) and Echelon-10 microcatheter coaxially navigated to the inferior division of the right middle cerebral artery (**A, B**). The tortuous lesion was successfully straightened, resulting in the appearance of a "twisted-towel sign" (**C**). The lesion was pre-dilated using a 2.0 mm×9 mm Gateway balloon (**D**). An XT-27 microcatheter was positioned at the inferior division (**E**). The Neuroform EZ stent was employed to cover the lesion (**F**). A three- dimensional angiogram showed absence of residual stenosis (**G, H**)

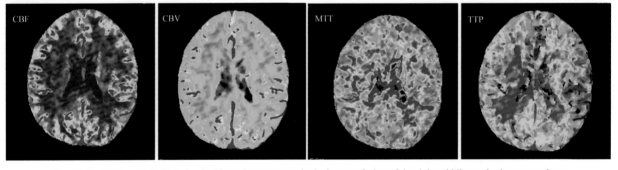

Fig. 5.2.5 CTP results indicated a significant improvement in the hypoperfusion of the right middle cerebral artery territory

The follow-up DSA conducted after six months from the procedure demonstrated a residual stenosis of 30% (Fig. 5.2.6).

5. Comments

In the case where the lesion assumes an angled shape, the employment of the Wingspan system may lead to vessel injury at the site of the lesion. The Neuroform EZ stent features an open-cell structure and is released via a microcatheter, thus reducing the potential risk of vessel injury. It is well-suited for treating an angled target vessel. In comparison to the Wingspan stent system, the Neuroform EZ stent has a lower radial strength and a longer segment, with a minimum length of 15 mm. It was discovered that there was still a 30% residual stenosis on the follow-up angiogram. As the patient was asymptomatic, medical treatment was suggested. The long-term effectiveness of endovascular treatment for intracranial stenosis utilizing off-label aneurysm-assisted embolization stents, such as the Neuroform and Enterprise stents, remain unclear. Further follow-up of alternative stent systems are warranted.

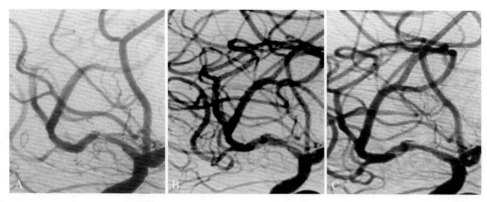

图 5.2.6 **A**.术前 DSA；**B**.支架置入术后 DSA；**C**.支架置入术后半年复查 DSA 提示支架内血流通畅，残余狭窄率约为 30%

（李红闪 吴岩峰 姚亮 左凤同 霍晓川 孙瑄）

5.2 手术操作视频（病例 11）

病例 12 左椎基底动脉交界区成角病变

（一）临床病史及影像分析

患者，男，50 岁，主因"头晕、视物成双 1 个月"入院。

当地医院头颅 MRI 未见新发及陈旧性梗死（图 5.2.7）。头颅 MRA 示左椎基底动脉交界区成角病变（图 5.2.8）。患者予以内科药物治疗后仍有症状反复，为进一步治疗就诊于我院。

既往史：冠心病、陈旧性心肌梗死，曾行冠状动脉支架置入术，糖尿病。吸烟 30 年，未戒烟。

查体：双眼右视可见水平眼震。

血栓弹力图：ADP 抑制率 33.1%，AA 抑制率 100%。

DSA：双侧后交通动脉开放（图 5.2.9 A 和 B），右椎动脉发出小脑后下动脉后未见显影（图 5.2.9 C），左椎基底动脉交界区成角病变（图 5.2.9 D）。

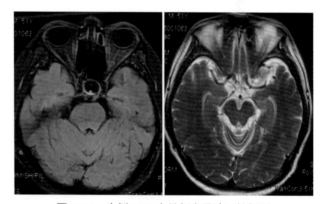

图 5.2.7 头颅 MRI 未见新发及陈旧性梗死

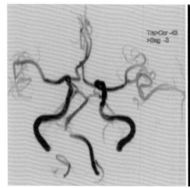
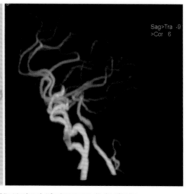

图 5.2.8 头颅 MRA 示左椎基底动脉交界区成角病变

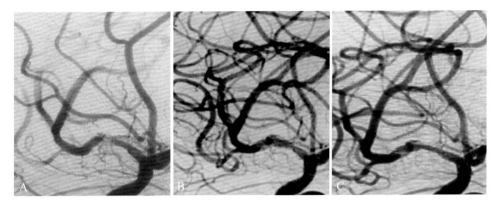

Fig. 5.2.6 (**A**) Baseline angiogram. (**B**) Angiogram after the stent implantation. (**C**) Follow-up angiogram six months after the procedure revealed a residual stenosis of 30%

(Translated by Rongrong Cui, Revised by Zhikai Hou)

5.2 Video of endovascular therapy (Case 11)

Case 12   Tortuous stenosis of the left vertebro-basilar junction

1. Clinical presentation and radiological studies

A 50-year-old man presented with dizziness and diplopia for a month.

The MRI indicated the absence of any acute infarction (Fig. 5.2.7). The MRA discovered the presence of tortuous stenosis at the left vertebro-basilar junction (Fig. 5.2.8). His symptoms persisted despite aggressive medical therapy.

The patient's medical history included coronary heart disease, a previous myocardial infarction, coronary artery stenting, and diabetes. Additionally, he had a 30-year history of cigarette smoking.

The physical examination revealed horizontal nystagmus when the patient gazes to the right.

The thromboelastography test showed 33.1% inhibition of ADP and 100% inhibition of AA.

DSA showed bilateral posterior communicating arteries being open (Fig. 5.2.9 A, B), termination of the right vertebral artery's V4 segment into PICA (Fig. 5.2.9 C), and tortuous stenosis at the junction of the left vertebro-basilar artery (Fig. 5.2.9 D).

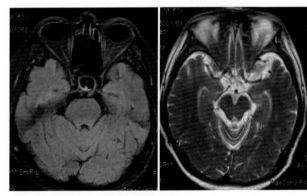

Fig. 5.2.7 MRI showed the absence of acute infarct

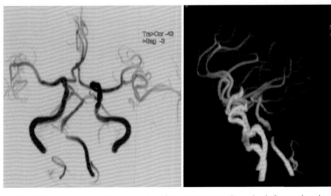

Fig. 5.2.8 MRA discovered the presence of tortuous stenosis at the left vertebro-basilar junction

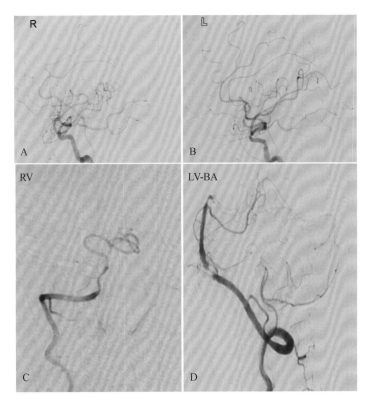

图 5.2.9　DSA 示双侧后交通动脉开放（**A** 和 **B**），右椎动脉发出小脑后下动脉后未见显影（**C**），左椎基底动脉交界区成角病变（**D**）

头部 CTP：后循环区域低灌注（图 5.2.10）。

患者因幽闭恐惧症未行高分辨率磁共振成像检查。

入院后给予双联抗血小板（阿司匹林 100 mg 1 次 / 日 ＋ 氯吡格雷 75 mg 1 次 / 日）、降脂（阿托伐他汀 10 mg 1 次 / 日）等治疗。

（二）诊断

症状性左椎基底动脉交界区成角病变。

（三）术前讨论

患者存在后循环缺血症状，药物治疗后仍有症状反复，责任血管明确，有血管内介入治疗指征。

治疗策略：拟球囊预扩张，再放置自膨式支架。

相关风险：穿支闭塞、动脉夹层、急性或亚急性血栓形成等。

（四）治疗过程

右股动脉入路置入 6F 动脉鞘，将 6F 导引导管置于左椎动脉 V2 段远端。Transend 微导丝（0.014 in，300 cm）越过狭窄段，放置于左大脑后动脉 P1 段。

沿微导丝送入 Gateway 球囊（2.5 mm×9 mm）至狭窄段预扩张一次（图 5.2.11 A）。扩张后撤出球囊，沿微导丝送入 Wingspan 自膨式支架（3.0 mm×15 mm）至狭窄段后释放支架。造影显示支架贴壁良好，残

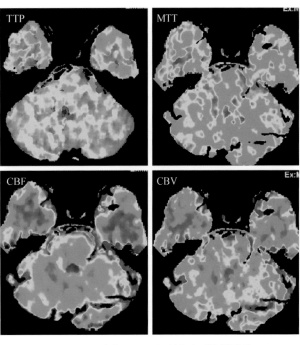

图 5.2.10　头部 CTP 示后循环区域低灌注

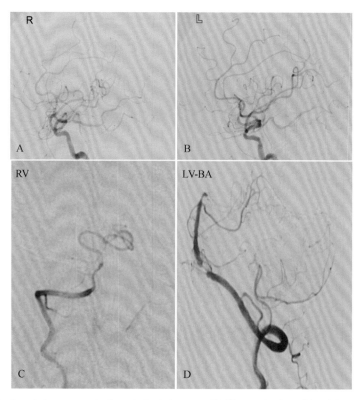

Fig. 5.2.9   DSA revealed bilateral posterior communicating arteries being open (**A, B**), termination of the right vertebral artery's V4 segment into PICA (**C**), and tortuous stenosis at the junction of the left vertebro-basilar artery (**D**)

The CT perfusion indicated hypoperfusion in the territory of the posterior circulation (Fig. 5.2.10).

The patient did not receive the high-resolution MRI due to being claustrophobic.

Following admission, he was prescribed a dual antiplatelet regimen consisting of daily aspirin (100 mg) and clopidogrel (75 mg) along with atorvastatin (10 mg) daily.

2. Diagnosis

Symptomatic tortuous stenosis of the left vertebro-basilar junction.

3. Treatment schedule

The patient presented with symptomatic stenosis at the left vertebro-basilar junction. Despite receiving aggressive medical treatment, he experienced recurrent symptoms. Consequently, the patient was indicated for endovascular treatment.

Treatment approach: the stenotic lesion was initially dilated using a balloon, then a self-expanding stent was implanted. Potential risks included perforating artery occlusion, arterial dissection, and acute/subacute in-stent thrombosis.

4. Treatment

Under general anesthesia, a 6 French guide catheter was positioned at the distal end of the V2 segment of the left vertebral artery. A Transend microwire (0.014 in, 300 cm)

was maneuvered into the P1 segment of the left posterior cerebral artery. The stenosis lesion was pre-dilated using a 2.5 mm×9 mm Gateway balloon (Fig. 5.2.11 A). Then, a 3.0 mm×15 mm Wingspan self-expanding stent was used to cover the lesion. After the stent was implanted, the

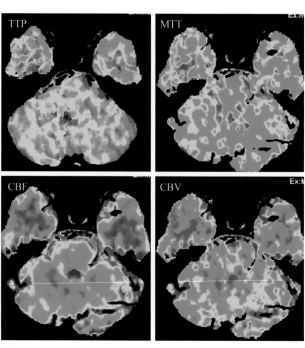

Fig. 5.2.10   CT perfusion indicated hypoperfusion in the territory of the posterior circulation

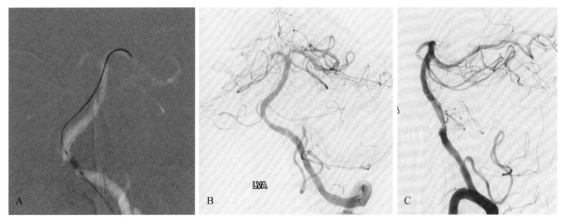

图 5.2.11　**A**.球囊在狭窄处预扩张；**B** 和 **C**.支架置入术后造影

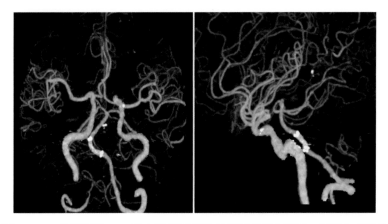

图 5.2.12　术后头部 CTA 示左椎基底动脉交界区支架内通畅，远端分支正常

余狭窄率约为 10%（图 5.2.11 B 和 C），观察 10 min 重复造影无变化后结束治疗。

术后即刻头部 CT 未见出血。

术后头部 CTA：左椎基底动脉交界区支架内通畅，远端分支正常（图 5.2.12）。

术后头部 CTP：后循环区域低灌注较术前改善（图 5.2.13）。

（五）讨论

本例左椎动脉 V4 段至基底动脉近段狭窄，病变长度较短（＜5 mm），但因病变成角，不太适合放置球囊扩张式支架。在使用小球囊充分预扩张的基础上，放置支撑性较好的自膨式支架，即刻疗效较为满意。

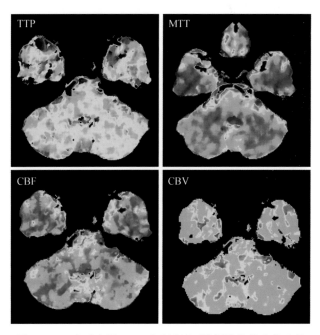

图 5.2.13　术后头部 CTP 示后循环区域低灌注较术前改善

（杨连琦　崔凯　张义森　姜鹏　马宁）

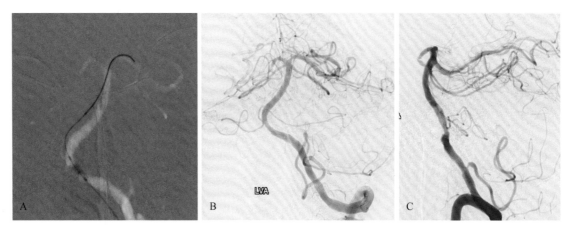

Fig. 5.2.11 (**A**) The lesion was pre-dilated using the Gateway balloon. (**B**, **C**) The angiogram performed post stent implantation

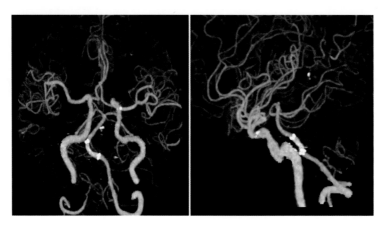

Fig. 5.2.12 Postprocedural CTA showed a patent stent located in the left vertebro-basilar artery junction

angiogram indicated excellent wall apposition of the stent with approximately 10% residual stenosis (Fig. 5.2.11 B, C).

The non-contrast CT scan after the procedure revealed no evidence of hemorrhage. The CTA revealed a patent stent located in the left vertebro-basilar artery junction (Fig. 5.2.12).

The post-procedure CTP demonstrated an improvement in the hypoperfusion within the posterior circulation territory (Fig. 5.2.13).

5. Comments

Due to the location of the stenosis at the junction of the left vertebro-basilar artery and its tortuous nature, a balloon-mounted stent was deemed inappropriate in the case of this patient's presentation. In such a case, we utilized a small-sized balloon to perform pre-dilation of the stenosed lesion, followed by implantation of a self-expanding stent.

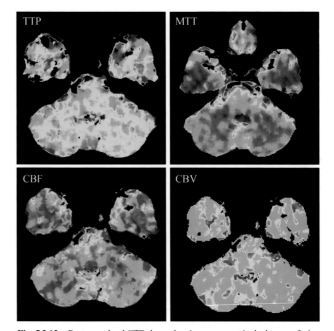

Fig. 5.2.13 Postprocedural CTP showed an improvement in the hypoperfusion within the posterior circulation territory

(Translated by Rongrong Cui, Revised by Zhikai Hou)

第三节　闭塞病变

病例 13　右颈内动脉 C6 段闭塞

（一）临床病史及影像分析

患者，女性，52 岁，主因"言语不利、反应迟钝 6 个月，加重 2 个月"入院。

6 个月前当地医院头部 MRI 示右侧丘脑梗死灶（图 5.3.1 A），MRA 示右颈内动脉颅内段狭窄（图 5.3.1 B）。2 个月前患者症状加重，复查头部 MRI 示右半卵圆中心多发梗死（图 5.3.1 C 和 D），MRA 示右颈内动脉颅内段显影欠佳，考虑闭塞（图 5.3.1 E）。CTA 示右颈内动脉颅外段显影欠佳，右大脑中动脉可见显影（图 5.3.1 F 和 G）。患者经内科药物治疗，症状仍有反复。为行介入治疗，就诊于我院。

既往史：高血压、卒中、支气管炎病史。

查体：神经系统查体未见明显异常。

入院后 DSA：右颈内动脉眼段（C6 段）闭塞（图 5.3.2 A 和 B）；前交通动脉开放，右大脑前动脉 A1 段未见显影，右大脑前动脉经软脑膜动脉及深穿支动脉向右大脑中动脉供血区域代偿（图 5.3.2 C ～ E）；后循环向前循环有少量软脑膜动脉代偿（图 5.3.2 F）。

CTP：右侧大脑半球低灌注（图 5.3.3 A）。

高分辨率 MRI：右颈内动脉末端闭塞，右大脑中动脉可见血管流空，考虑闭塞远端血管通畅（图 5.3.3 B 和 C）。

血栓弹力图：AA 抑制率 99%，ADP 抑制率 39.1%。

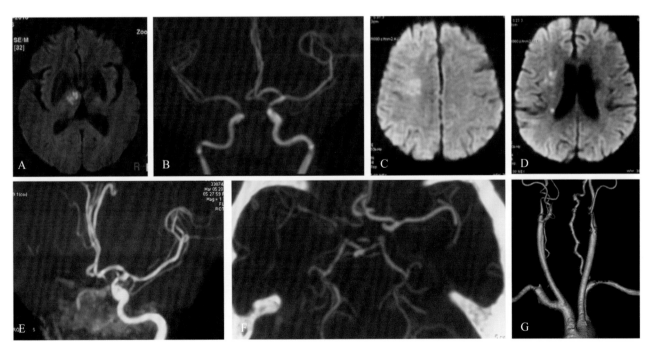

图 5.3.1　头部 MRI 示右侧丘脑梗死灶（**A**），MRA 示右颈内动脉颅内段狭窄（**B**）。复查头部 MRI 示右半卵圆中心多发梗死（**C 和 D**），MRA 示右颈内动脉颅内段闭塞（**E**）。头部 CTA 示右颈内动脉颅外段显影欠佳（**F 和 G**）

Section 3　Chronic Occlusions

Case 13　Right internal carotid artery ophthalmic segment occlusion

1. Clinical presentation and radiological studies

A 52-year-old female patient was admitted to the hospital due to speech impairment and delayed response for 6 months, worsening for 2 months.

Six months ago, the MRI indicated acute infarction in the right thalamus (Fig. 5.3.1 A). The MRA showed stenosis in the intracranial segment of the right internal carotid artery (Fig. 5.3.1 B). Within 2 months, her symptoms gradually worsened. Subsequent MRI scans showed multiple infarctions in the right centrum semiovale and periventricular area (Fig. 5.3.1 C, D). The MRA revealed occlusion in the intracranial segment of the right internal carotid artery (Fig. 5.3.1 E). Furthermore, CT angiography revealed severe stenosis in the extracranial segment of the right internal carotid artery (Fig. 5.3.1 F, G). Her symptoms gradually worsened despite receiving aggressive medical treatment.

Her medical history included hypertension, stroke, and bronchitis.

She exhibited no neurological deficits upon admission.

DSA revealed an occlusion in the ophthalmic segment of the right internal carotid artery (Fig. 5.3.2 A, B), while the anterior communicating artery remained open. The right anterior cerebral artery compensated for the occlusion in the right middle cerebral artery through the pia artery and deep perforating artery (Fig. 5.3.2 C–E). However, collateral circulation from the posterior circulation was not significant (Fig. 5.3.2 F).

The CT perfusion showed hypoperfusion in the territory supplied by the right internal carotid artery (Fig. 5.3.3 A).

The high-resolution MRI (HRMRI) revealed an occlusion at the end of the right internal carotid artery, as well as a flowing void in the right middle cerebral artery which suggests that the vessel lumen beyond the occluded segment remains unobstructed (Fig. 5.3.3 B, C).

Thromboelastography test indicated a 39.1% inhibition of ADP and 99% inhibition of AA.

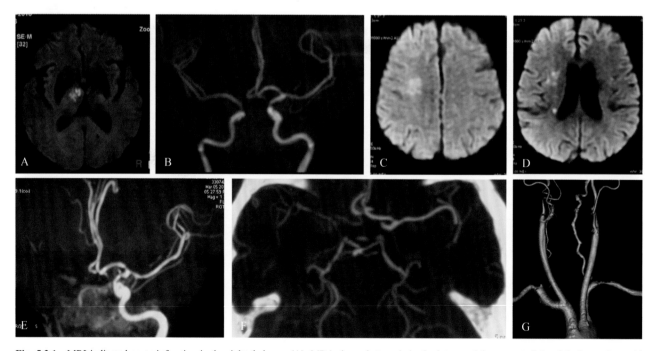

Fig. 5.3.1　MRI indicated acute infarction in the right thalamus (**A**), MRA showed stenosis in the intracranial segment of the right internal carotid artery (**B**). Follow-up MRI showed multiple infarctions in the right centrum semiovale and periventricular area (**C**, **D**). MRA revealed occlusion in the intracranial segment of the right internal carotid artery (**E**). CT angiography also revealed severe stenosis in the extracranial segment of the right internal carotid artery (**F**, **G**)

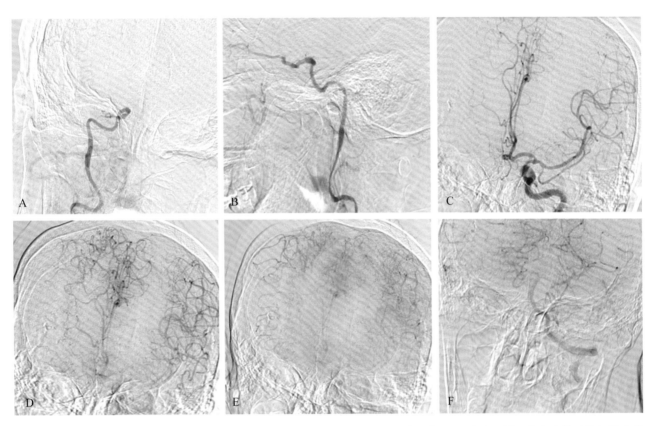

图 5.3.2　DSA 示右颈内动脉眼段闭塞（**A** 和 **B**），前交通动脉开放，右大脑前动脉 A1 段未见显影，右大脑前动脉经软脑膜动脉及深穿支动脉向右大脑中动脉供血区域代偿（**C ～ E**），后循环向前循环有少量软脑膜动脉代偿（**F**）

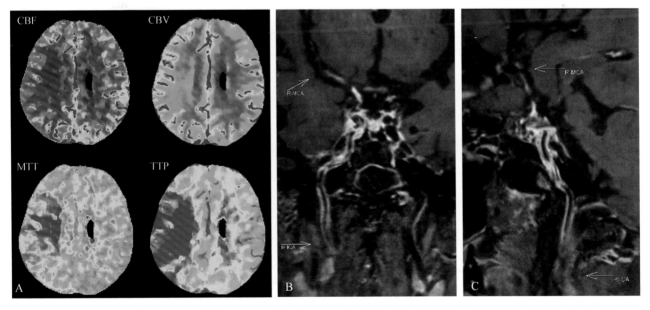

图 5.3.3　CTP 示右侧大脑半球低灌注（**A**）。高分辨率 MRI 示右颈内动脉末端闭塞，闭塞远端血管通畅（**B** 和 **C**）

入院后给予双联抗血小板（阿司匹林 100 mg 1 次 / 日＋氯吡格雷 75 mg 1 次 / 日）、降脂（阿托伐他汀 20 mg 1 次 / 日）及降压治疗。

（二）诊断

症状性右颈内动脉 C6 段闭塞。

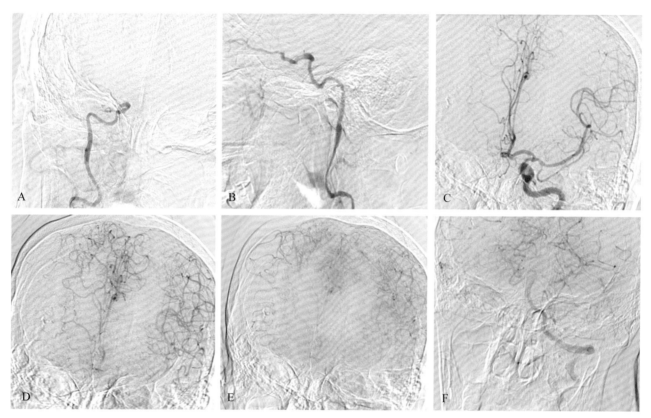

Fig. 5.3.2   DSA revealed an occlusion in the ophthalmic segment of the right internal carotid artery (**A**, **B**). The anterior communicating artery remained open. The right anterior cerebral artery compensated for the occlusion in the right middle cerebral artery through the pia artery and deep perforating artery (**C–E**). Collateral circulation from the posterior circulation was not significant (**F**)

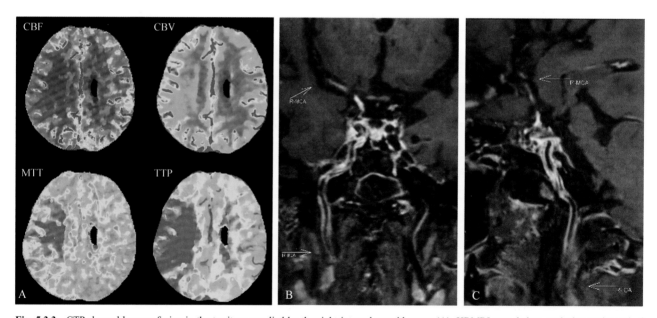

Fig. 5.3.3   CTP showed hypoperfusion in the territory supplied by the right internal carotid artery (**A**). HRMRI revealed an occlusion at the end of the right internal carotid artery, as well as a flowing void in the right middle cerebral artery which suggests that the vessel lumen beyond the occluded segment remains unobstructed (**B**, **C**)

Upon admission, she was prescribed a dual antiplatelet regimen comprising a daily dose of 100 mg Aspirin and 75 mg Clopidogrel, alongside a daily dose of 20 mg Atorvastatin.

2. Diagnosis

Symptomatic occlusion of the C6 segment of the right internal carotid artery.

（三）术前讨论

患者头部 MRI 提示右颈内动脉供血区域多发梗死，结合 CTP 所示的低灌注，考虑右颈内动脉眼段闭塞是本次发病的责任病变，有血管内介入治疗指征。

治疗策略：微导管结合微导丝通过病变，拟先单纯球囊扩张，择期再放置自膨式支架。

相关风险：开通失败、脑出血及夹层风险。

（四）治疗过程

全麻下右股动脉入路，将 6F 导引导管放置在右颈内动脉 C1 段。DSA 显示右颈内动脉 C6 段闭塞（图 5.3.4 A）。将 Synchro 微导丝（0.014 in，200 cm）与 SL-10 微导管同轴，通过闭塞病变困难（图 5.3.4 B）。更换为 Pilot 50 微导丝（0.014 in，190 cm）后经尝试通过闭塞段（图 5.3.4 C），跟进微导管困难，利用导管内球囊辅助技术撤出微导管（图 5.3.4 D），保留 Pilot 50 微导丝（图 5.3.4 E）。经微导丝输送 Mini TREK 球囊（1.5 mm×15 mm）和赛诺球囊（1.5 mm×15 mm），到位困难。采用 V-18 导丝增加支撑，也未获成功。遂改送 Maverick 球囊（2.0 mm×20 mm），最终越过闭塞段，并进行扩张（图 5.3.4 F）。扩张后造影显示残余狭窄率约为 60%（图 5.3.4 G 和 H）。

术后立即复查头部 CT 未见出血。

术后 CTA：右颈内动脉 C6 段残余狭窄率约为 60%（图 5.3.5 A）。

术后 CTP：右侧大脑半球低灌注较术前改善（图 5.3.5 B）。

（五）讨论

本例右颈内动脉眼段闭塞，结合病史和相关影像学检查，考虑近期闭塞，开通可能性较高。闭塞段较长，路径迂曲，使用两种快速交换球囊均未能到位，改用 V-18 导丝增加支撑后，更换通过性较

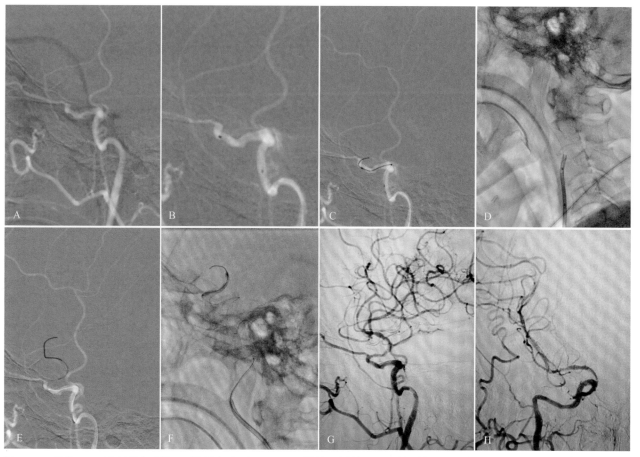

图 5.3.4 术前 DSA 示右颈内动脉 C6 段闭塞（**A**）。Synchro 微导丝同轴 SL-10 微导管通过闭塞病变困难（**B**），更换为 Pilot 50 微导丝后通过闭塞病变（**C**），撤出微导管（**D**），闭塞处保留 Pilot 50 微导丝（**E**），Maverick 球囊扩张闭塞病变（**F**），扩张后造影示残余狭窄率约为 60%（**G 和 H**）

3. Treatment schedule

The patient exhibited an occlusion in the C6 segment of the right internal carotid artery. The MRI results revealed multiple cerebral infarcts in the relevant territory. And CT perfusion further indicated hypoperfusion in the associated area. Despite receiving intensive medical treatment, the patient experienced recurrent ischemic events, with the stenotic lesion steadily deteriorating to an occlusion. As such, endovascular therapy was recommended to the patient.

Treatment approach: We plan to perform a primary balloon dilation to achieve recanalization of the occluded artery. Additionally, we conducted elective stent implantation to minimize the risk of hyperperfusion syndrome. Potential risks associated with the procedure include failed recanalization, cerebral hemorrhage, and iatrogenic dissection.

4. Treatment

Under general anesthesia, a 6F guide catheter was positioned at the C1 segment of the right internal carotid artery. Angiogram confirmed the occlusion in the C6 segment of the right internal carotid artery (Fig. 5.3.4 A). It is difficult to achieve coaxial advancement of the Synchro microwire (0.014 in, 200 cm) and the SL-10 microcatheter into the occluded segment (Fig. 5.3.4 B). We attempted to advance into the occluded segment by replacing the Pilot 50 microwire (0.014 in, 190 cm) (Fig. 5.3.4 C). However, It was difficult to deliver the microcatheter.

The intra-catheter balloon-assist technique was performed to withdraw the microcatheter (Fig. 5.3.4 D). Furthermore, the Pilot 50 microwire was left retained (Fig. 5.3.4 E). In addition, even with the V-18 guidewire providing increased support force, delivering the Mini TREK balloon (1.5mm×15mm) or Sino balloon (1.5mm×15mm) into the occluded segment proved to be challenging. Instead, The Maverick balloon (2.0 mm× 20 mm) was utilized to navigate through the occluded segment and dilate the lesion(Fig. 5.3.4 F). The angiogram after the balloon dilatation showed a 60% residual stenosis (Fig. 5.3.4 G, H).

Postprocedural CT showed absence of hemorrhage.

Postprocedural CTA showed a 60% residual stenosis in the C6 segment of the right internal carotid artery (Fig. 5.3.5 A).

Postprocedural CT perfusion demonstrated an improvement in hypoperfusion within the right cerebral hemisphere (Fig. 5.3.5 B).

5. Comments

This case presents a patient with occlusion in the ophthalmic segment of the right carotid artery. Based on the patient's medical history and radiographic findings, we presume that the occlusion in the ophthalmic segment of the right internal carotid artery is a recent development, thus increasing the probability of successful recanalization. The elongated occlusion and the tortuous arterial access pose challenges in the advancement of rapid exchange balloons into the occlusive lesion. Hence, we employed the V-18 guidewire to increase

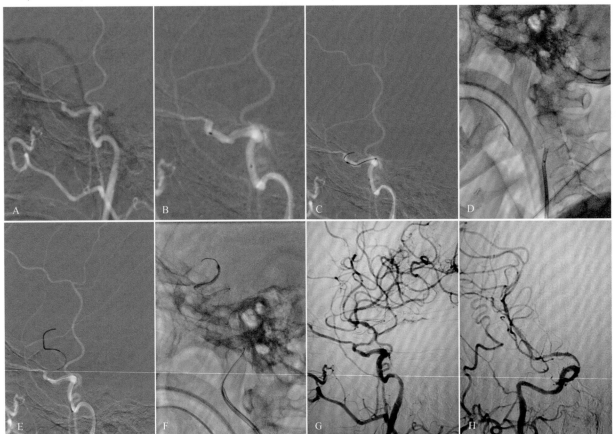

Fig. 5.3.4   Angiogram revealed an occlusion in the ophthalmic segment of the right internal carotid artery (**A**). It is difficult to achieve coaxial advancement of the Synchro microwire (0.014 in, 200 cm) and the SL-10 microcatheter into the occluded segment (**B**), a Pilot 50 microwire was advance into the occluded segment (**C**). The intra-catheter balloon-assist technique was performed to withdraw the microcatheter (**D**), the Pilot 50 microwire was left retained (**E**). A Maverick balloon was utilized to dilate the lesion (**F**). The angiogram after the balloon dilatation showed a 60% residual stenosis (**G, H**)

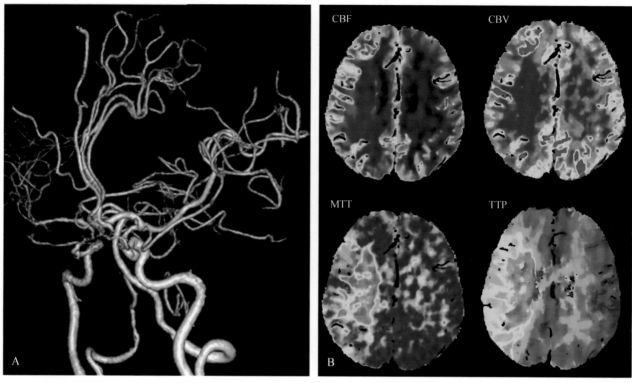

图 5.3.5 术后 CTA 示右颈内动脉 C6 段残余狭窄率约为 60%（**A**），CTP 示右侧大脑半球低灌注较术前改善（**B**）

好的 Maverick 球囊，才得以完成治疗过程。本例未选择更大直径的球囊扩张且未放置支架，主要考虑预防术后高灌注。后续将根据患者症状和血管情况再考虑是否择期置入支架。

本例治疗过程中，首过病变的微导丝系 190 cm 的短导丝，因微导管不能越过病变，这时如更换为 300 cm 的微导丝，也不能保证再次通过病变。这种情况下退管保留微导丝可以采用如下两种方法：①逐节剪短微导管，保留微导丝。②送入球囊至导引导管末端，回撤微导管至球囊近心端后充盈球囊，再回撤微导管，遂可留置微导丝。本例我们采用第二种方法顺利回撤微导管，保留了微导丝。

（苗春芝 王坤 姜鹏 马宁）

5.3 手术操作视频
（病例 13）

病例 14 左大脑中动脉 M1 段闭塞

（一）临床病史及影像分析

患者，男性，64 岁，主因"言语不利 2 个月"入院。

2 个月前当地医院头部 MRI 示左侧颞叶、基底节区、侧脑室旁、颞枕交界区多发急性梗死灶（图 5.3.6）。头部 CTA 及 CTP 提示左大脑中动脉 M1 段闭塞，闭塞远端分支稀疏；左大脑中动脉供血区域

低灌注（图 5.3.7）。患者经内科药物治疗仍有言语不利，为行血管内介入治疗而收入我院。

既往史：高血压病史。

查体：混合性失语，余体征阴性。

入院后头部 CT：左大脑中动脉供血区域多发梗死（图 5.3.8）。

DSA：左大脑中动脉 M1 段闭塞，动脉晚期见闭塞远端经穿支动脉吻合支代偿显影，此外大

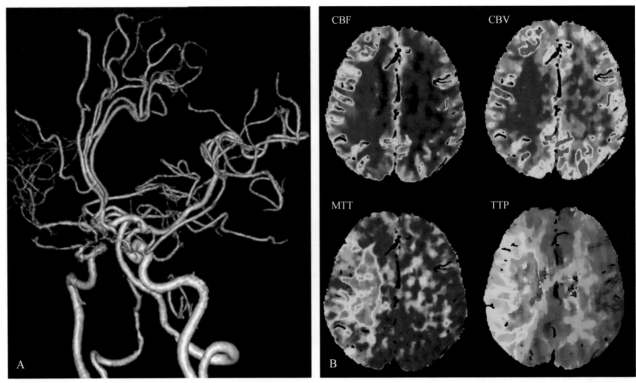

Fig. 5.3.5 Postprocedural brain CTA showed the residual stenosis rate of the C6 segment of the right internal carotid artery was 60% (**A**). CTP showed hypoperfusion in the right cerebral hemisphere was improved than before (**B**)

the support force and navigated through the occluded segment using a Maverick balloon, which has superior passage capacity compared to other balloons. Moreover, we avoided using a large-size balloon or performing stent implantation to prevent the occurrence of hyperperfusion syndrome. The decision to schedule stent implantation will depend on the patient's symptoms and vascular condition.

During the procedure, we utilized a 190 cm short microwire to traverse the occluded segment. If microcatheters fail to pass through the occlusion, replacing the short microwire with a longer 300 cm microwire would provide no guarantee of

successfully passing the lesion. The following two techniques may be employed to remove the microcatheter while retaining the microwire: 1) Gradually shorten the microcatheter section by section while retaining the microwire. 2) Advance the balloon to the end of the guide catheter, retract the microcatheter to the proximal end of the balloon, inflate the balloon, and withdraw the microcatheter. This will enable the microwire to be retained. We used the second method in this case.

(Translated by Rongrong Cui, Revised by Zhikai Hou)

5.3 Video of endovascular therapy (Case 13)

Case 14 Occlusion of the left middle cerebral artery M1 segment

1. Clinical presentation and radiological studies

A 64-year-old male patient was admitted to the hospital due to two months of dysarthria.

Two months ago, an MRI revealed the presence of multiple acute cerebral infarctions in the left temporal lobe, basal ganglia region, peri-ventricular area, and temporo-occipital junction (Fig. 5.3.6). CT angiography revealed occlusion in the M1 segment of the left middle cerebral artery, with only a few distal branches visible beyond the occluded segment. The CT

perfusion showed hypoperfusion within the territory of the left middle cerebral artery (Fig. 5.3.7). Despite receiving medical treatment, his symptoms continued to recur.

He had a medical history of hypertension.

On admission, the physical examination revealed mixed aphasia, with no other notable signs.

Subsequent CT scans after admission revealed multiple infarctions in the territory of the left middle cerebral artery. (Fig. 5.3.8).

DSA revealed an occlusion in the M1 segment of the left middle cerebral artery, with visualization of the distal end of

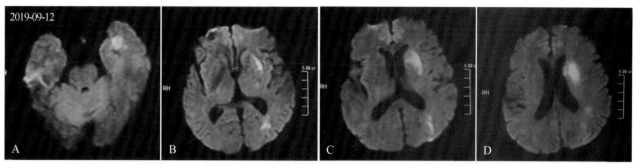

图 5.3.6　头部 MRI 示左侧颞叶、基底节区、侧脑室旁、颞枕交界区多发急性梗死灶（**A ～ D**）

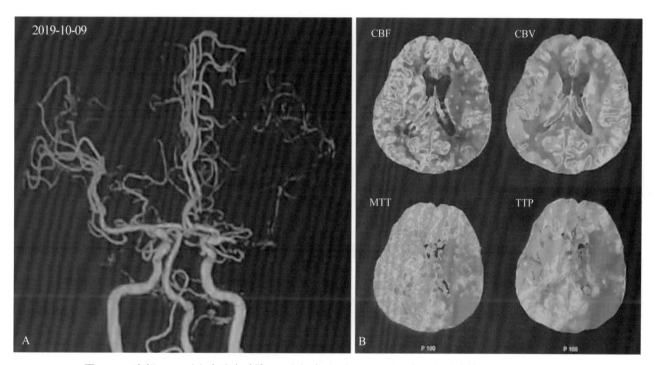

图 5.3.7　头部 CTA 示左大脑中动脉 M1 段闭塞（**A**），CTP 示左大脑中动脉供血区域低灌注（**B**）

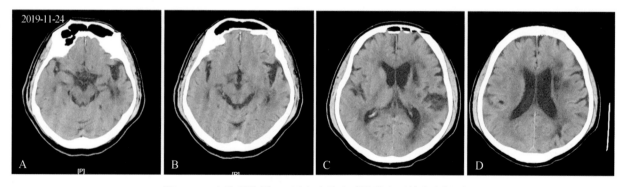

图 5.3.8　入院后头部 CT 示左大脑中动脉供血区域多发梗死

脑中动脉供血区域还可见同侧大脑前动脉经软脑膜动脉代偿逆行显影（图 5.3.9）。右颈内动脉 C6 段中度狭窄（图 5.3.10 A 和 B），未见明显后循环向左大脑中动脉供血区域代偿（图 5.3.10 C

和 D）。

目前予以双联抗血小板（阿司匹林 100 mg 1 次 / 日＋氯吡格雷 75 mg 1 次 / 日）、降脂（阿托伐他汀 20 mg 1 次 / 日）等治疗。

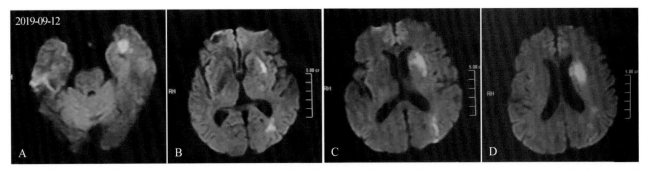

Fig. 5.3.6   MRI revealed the presence of multiple acute cerebral infarctions in the left temporal lobe, basal ganglia region, peri-ventricular area, and temporo-occipital junction (**A – D**)

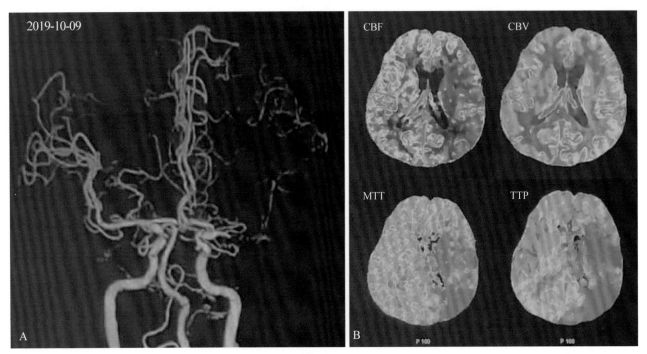

Fig. 5.3.7   CTA revealed occlusion in the M1 segment of the left middle cerebral artery (**A**). CTP demonstrated hypoperfusion in the left middle cerebral artery territory (**B**)

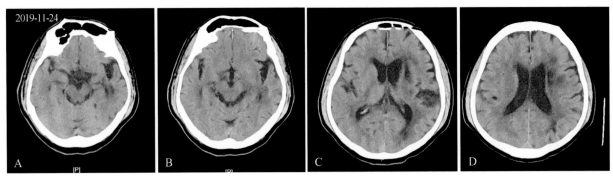

Fig. 5.3.8   Subsequent CT revealed multiple infarctions in the territory of the left middle cerebral artery

the occluded segment at the late-arterial phase. Furthermore, the ipsilateral anterior cerebral artery compensated for the middle cerebral artery territory through the pial anastomotic branch (Fig. 5.3.9). Moderate stenosis was also noted in the C6 segment of the right internal carotid artery. (Fig. 5.3.10 A, B). The compensation from the posterior circulation towards the occluded left middle cerebral artery was inadequate. (Fig. 5.3.10 C, D).

Upon admission, he was prescribed a dual antiplatelet comprising of a daily doses of 100 mg Aspirin and 75 mg Clopidogrel, as well as a daily dose of 20 mg Atorvastatin.

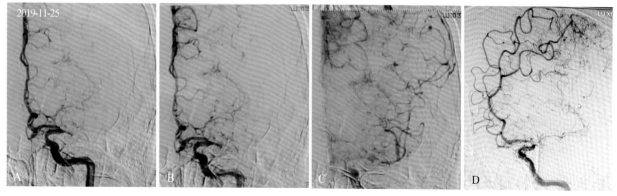

图 5.3.9 DSA 示左大脑中动脉 M1 段闭塞（**A**），闭塞远端经穿支动脉吻合支代偿显影（**B** 和 **C**），大脑中动脉供血区域还可见同侧大脑前动脉经软脑膜动脉代偿逆行显影（**D**）

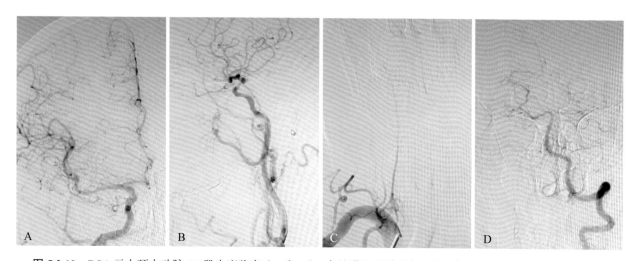

图 5.3.10 DSA 示右颈内动脉 C6 段中度狭窄（**A** 和 **B**），未见明显后循环向左大脑中动脉供血区域代偿（**C** 和 **D**）

（二）诊断

症状性左大脑中动脉 M1 段闭塞。

（三）术前讨论

患者症状为言语不利，结合 CTA 和 DSA，考虑责任病变为大脑中动脉 M1 段闭塞。因 CTP 提示相关供血区域低灌注，拟行血管内介入治疗。

治疗策略：微导丝结合微导管先通过闭塞病变，其后行球囊预扩张和置入自膨式支架。

相关风险：开通治疗失败、穿支动脉闭塞、急性或亚急性血栓形成、夹层等。

（四）治疗过程

全麻下右股动脉入路，将 6F 导引导管头端置于左颈内动脉 C1 段远端。DSA 示左大脑中动脉 M1 段中段闭塞，动脉晚期见烟雾状增生血管参与闭塞远端血管代偿（图 5.3.11 A 和 B）。在 SL-10 微导管辅助下，Synchro 微导丝（0.014 in，200 cm）无法通过闭塞段，遂更换 Pilot 50 微导丝（0.014 in，190 cm），多次尝试后微导丝通过闭塞段（图 5.3.11 C 和 D）。微导管送至大脑中动脉上干，造影证实微导管头端位于真腔内（图 5.3.12 A）。交换送入 Transend 微导丝（0.014 in，300 cm），撤出微导管，送入 Gateway 球囊（1.5 mm×15 mm），越过闭塞段，缓慢扩张（图 5.3.12 B）。其后造影示闭塞段管腔显影，远端仅有大脑中动脉上干显影（图 5.3.12 C），在动脉晚期可见大脑中动脉其他分支显影（图 5.3.12 D），此时考虑微导丝有可能经内膜下穿过闭塞段，稍前送球囊，再次缓慢扩张（图 5.3.13 A）。扩张后造影见大脑中动脉远端分支较前增多，外侧豆纹动脉显影，外侧豆纹动脉近心端见微导丝走行在内膜下（图 5.3.13 B），进一步证实有医源性夹层可能。经微导丝送入 Select Plus 微导管，释放

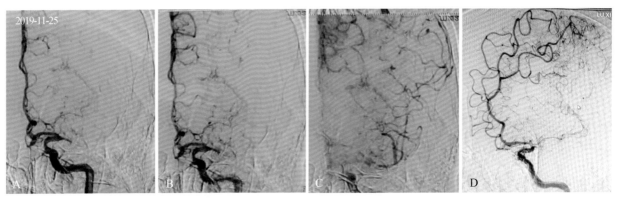

Fig. 5.3.9   DSA revealed an occlusion in the M1 segment of the left middle cerebral artery (**A**). The distal end of the occlusion can be visualized through the anastomosis branch of the perforating artery (**B**, **C**). The ipsilateral anterior cerebral artery compensated for the middle cerebral artery territory through the pial anastomotic branch (**D**)

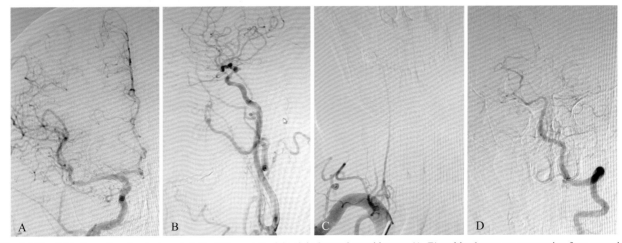

Fig. 5.3.10   DSA showed moderate stenosis in the C6 segment of the right internal carotid artery (**A**, **B**) and inadequent compensation from posterior circulation to the occluded left middle cerebral artery (**C**, **D**)

2. Diagnosis

Symptomatic occlusion of the M1 segment of the left middle cerebral artery.

3. Treatment schedule

This case involves a patient with occlusion in the M1 segment of the left middle cerebral artery who experienced recurrent symptoms despite intensive medical treatment. CT perfusion indicated hypoperfusion in the territory of the left middle cerebral artery. As such, the patient has an indication for endovascular treatment.

Treatment approach: The occluded lesion was traversed using a coaxially advanced microwire and microcatheter, and subsequently treated with balloon pre-dilation and implantation of a self-expanding stent. Potential risks of the procedure included failed recanalization, perforating artery occlusion, in-stent thrombosis, and iatrogenic dissection.

4. Treatment

Under general anesthesia, a 6F guide catheter was positioned at the C1 segment of the left internal carotid artery. The DSA examination confirmed that there was occlusion in the M1 segment of the left middle cerebral artery, and a smoky vascular collateral network was observed in the late arterial phase (Fig. 5.3.11 A, B). Advancing the Synchro microwire (0.014 in, 200 cm) and the SL-10 microcatheter coaxially into the occluded segment was proven to be difficult. As an alternative, we tried to advance the Pilot 50 microwire (0.014 in, 190 cm) into the occluded segment (Fig. 5.3.11 C, D). The microcatheter was placed at the upper branch of the middle cerebral artery. The angiogram verified that the microcatheter was positioned within the true lumen (Fig. 5.3.12 A). Then the Gateway balloon (1.5 mm×15 mm) was utilized to pre-dilate the occluded segment (Fig. 5.3.12 B). Following balloon dilatation, the angiogram revealed visualization of the upper branch of the middle cerebral artery (Fig. 5.3.12 C), while other branches of the middle cerebral artery may become visible in the late-arterial stage (Fig. 5.3.12 D). The balloon was further advanced and carefully re-inflated (Fig. 5.3.13 A). The following angiogram revealed the visualization of more distal branches of the middle cerebral artery, including the lateral lenticulostriate artery. At the proximal end of the latter, the microwire was observed beneath the intima. (Fig. 5.3.13 B), thus confirming the possibility of an iatrogenic dissection. A 4 mm×23 mm Enterprise self-expanding stent was utilized to fully cover the lesion (Fig. 5.3.13 C, D). The post-stent

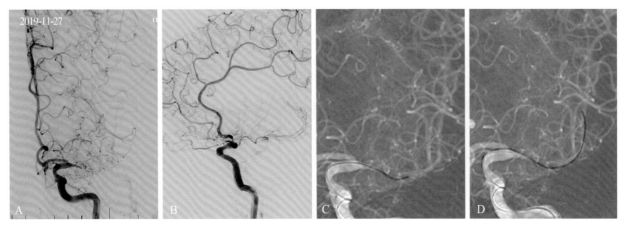

图 5.3.11　DSA 示左大脑中动脉 M1 段中段闭塞，动脉晚期见烟雾状增生血管参与闭塞远端血管代偿（**A** 和 **B**）；Synchro 微导丝无法通过闭塞段，更换为 Pilot 50 微导丝后经多次尝试通过闭塞段（**C** 和 **D**）

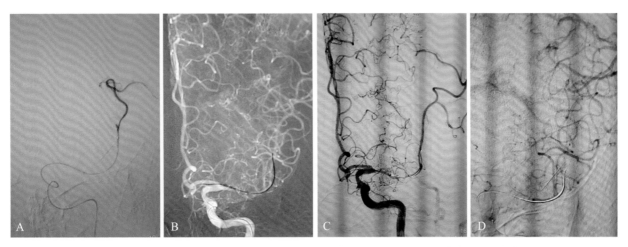

图 5.3.12　微导管送至大脑中动脉上干，造影证实微导管头端位于真腔（**A**），Gateway 球囊扩张闭塞病变（**B**），扩张后造影示闭塞段管腔显影，远端仅有大脑中动脉上干显影（**C**），动脉晚期可见大脑中动脉其他分支显影（**D**）

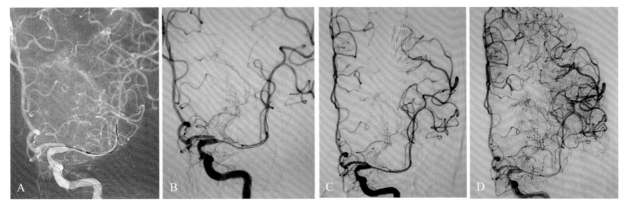

图 5.3.13　Gateway 球囊再次缓慢扩张病变（**A**）。扩张后造影见大脑中动脉远端分支较前增多，外侧豆纹动脉显影，外侧豆纹动脉近心端见微导丝走行于内膜下（**B**）。释放 Enterprise 自膨式支架（**C** 和 **D**）

Enterprise 自膨式支架（4 mm×23 mm）（图 5.3.13 C 和 D），其后造影显示原夹层贴合，大脑中动脉远端上、下干均有显影，未见颞极动脉显影，观察 10 min 未见变化后结束治疗。

术后第 2 日，患者言语功能较前改善。

术后 10 天 CTA 及 CTP 显示：左大脑中动脉支架术后管腔通畅，未见颞极动脉显影，左大脑中动脉供血区域低灌注较术前明显改善（图 5.3.14）。

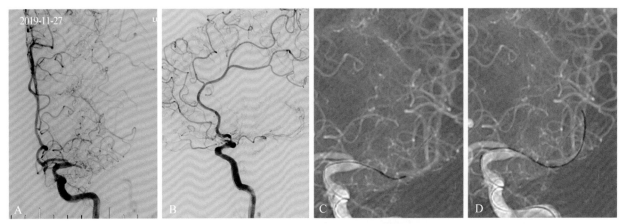

Fig. 5.3.11 DSA showed there was occlusion in the M1 segment of the left middle cerebral artery, and a smoky vascular collateral network was observed in the late arterial (**A**, **B**). Advancing the Synchro microwire into the occluded segment proved challenging, thus an alternative Pilot 50 microwire was employed to navigate through the occluded segment. (**C**, **D**)

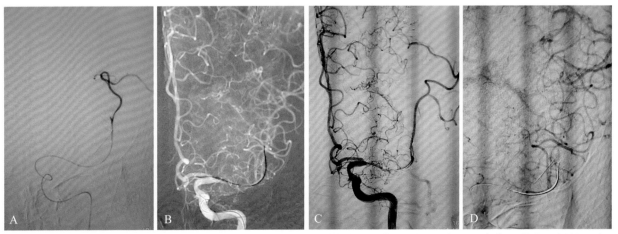

Fig. 5.3.12 The angiogram verified that the microcatheter was positioned within the true lumen (**A**). A Gateway balloon (1.5 mm×15 mm) was utilized to pre-dilate the occluded segment (**B**). The angiogram revealed visualization of the upper branch of the middle cerebral artery (**C**), while other branches of the middle cerebral artery may become visible in the late-arterial stage (**D**)

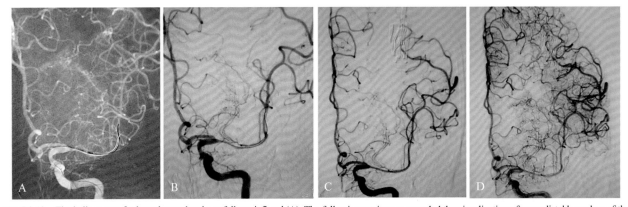

Fig. 5.3.13 The balloon was further advanced and carefully re-inflated (**A**). The following angiogram revealed the visualization of more distal branches of the middle cerebral artery, including the lateral lenticulostriate artery. At the proximal end of the latter, the microwire was observed beneath the intima (**B**). A 4 mm×23 mm Enterprise self-expanding stent was utilized to fully cover the lesion (**C**, **D**)

implantation angiogram indicates that the iatrogenic dissection vanished. Both the upper and lower branches of the left middle cerebral artery were discernible. However, the temporal polar artery remained imperceptible. After a lapse of ten minutes, a final angiogram manifested no alteration in the stented vessel.

The patient's alalia symptom improved on the second day following the procedure.

On the 10th day post-procedure, the CTA revealed patent stenting of the left middle cerebral artery, while the temporal polar artery was not visible. CT Perfusion indicated a substantial improvement in hypoperfusion within the territory of the left middle cerebral artery. (Fig. 5.3.14).

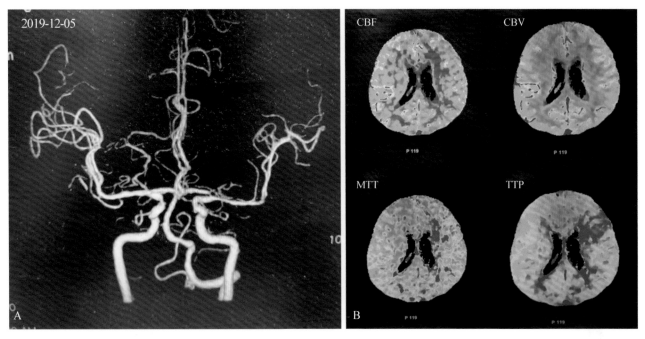

图 5.3.14　术后 10 天头部 CTA 示左大脑中动脉支架术后管腔通畅，颞极动脉未见显影（**A**）。CTP 示左大脑中动脉供血区域低灌注较术前明显改善（**B**）

（五）讨论

本例第一次球囊扩张后造影，仅见大脑中动脉上干显影，考虑存在夹层可能。因第一次球囊扩张位置稍靠近心端，远端夹层出口未完全扩开，我们结合术中操作，考虑夹层位于大脑中动脉下壁，遂将球囊前行后再次扩张。第二次球囊扩张后造影进一步佐证了术中医源性夹层。球囊扩张后夹层范围未进一步增大，故置入较长的自膨式支架以期完全覆盖病变。因夹层位于下壁，支架术后大脑中动脉上壁发出的分支未受影响。

（尤吉栋　何子骏　孙立倩　马宁）

病例 15　左椎动脉 V3 ～ V4 段闭塞

（一）临床病史及影像分析

患者，男性，35 岁，主因"眩晕、复视伴行走不稳 2 个月，加重伴言语不清 2 天"入院。

当地医院头部 MRI 示左侧小脑及双侧丘脑多发急性缺血病灶（图 5.3.15）。患者经内科药物治疗，症状仍有反复。为行血管内治疗，就诊于我院。

既往史：糖尿病、高血脂、高血压病史。

查体：左侧中枢性面瘫，四肢肌力 3 级。

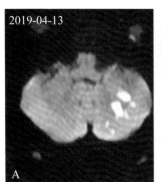
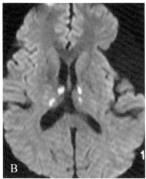

图 5.3.15　头部 MRI 示左侧小脑及双侧丘脑多发急性缺血病灶（**A** 和 **B**）

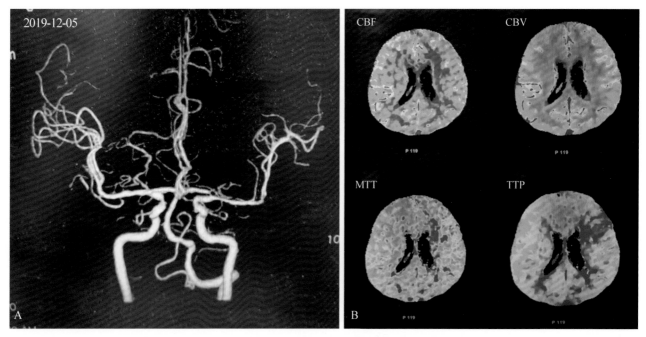

Fig. 5.3.14   CTA revealed patent stenting of the left middle cerebral artery, while the temporal polar artery was not visible (**A**). CT Perfusion indicated a substantial improvement in hypoperfusion within the territory of the left middle cerebral artery (**B**)

5. Comments

This case described a patient with occlusion in the left middle cerebral artery. Following the initial balloon angioplasty, the angiogram revealed that solely the upper branch of the middle cerebral artery was visible, thereby indicating the potential for iatrogenic dissection. The initial balloon angioplasty targeted the proximal occlusion segment of the middle cerebral artery, however, the distal segment of the dissection was not successfully dilated. Based on our suspicion of the arterial dissection being situated on the inferior wall of the middle cerebral artery, we decided to further advance the balloon and re-inflate it at the distal occlusion segment. Following the second balloon angioplasty, the angiogram verified the occurrence of an iatrogenic dissection. To address this, we employed a selfexpanding stent with a long segment to cover the lesion. As the dissection was situated on the inferior wall, the branches originating from the upper wall of the middle cerebral artery were unaffected after the stent placement.

(Translated by Rongrong Cui, Revised by Zhikai Hou)

Case 15   Occlusion of the left vertebral artery V3–V4 segments

1. Clinical presentation and radiological studies

A 35-year-old male was admitted to the hospital with complaints of dizziness, double vision, and unsteady walking persisting for two months, in addition to the onset of dysarthria in the last two days.

The MRI results revealed the presence of multiple infarcts located in the left cerebellar hemispheres as well as the bilateral thalamus (Fig. 5.3.15). Despite receiving medical treatment, his symptoms gradually deteriorated and recurred.

His medical history included diabetes, hyperlipidemia, and hypertension.

The physical examination revealed central facial paralysis on the left side and a muscle strength of grade 3 in all four limbs.

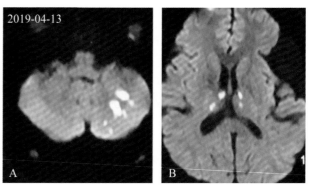

Fig. 5.3.15   MRI showed multiple infarcts in the left cerebellar hemispheres and bilateral thalamus (**A**, **B**)

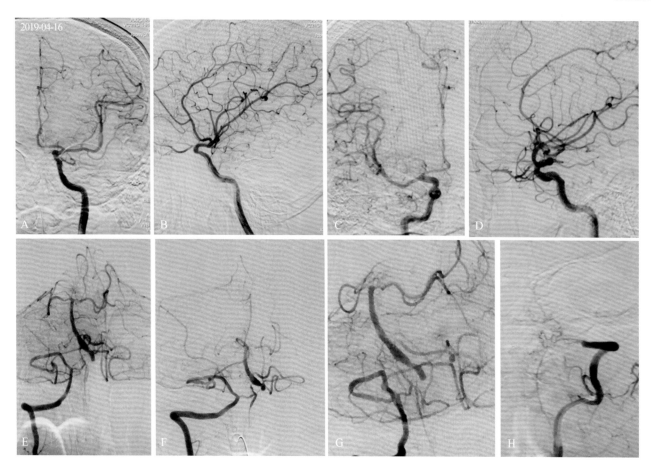

图 5.3.16 DSA 示双侧颈内动脉系统未见明显异常，双侧后交通动脉未开放（**A～D**）。右椎动脉终止于小脑后下动脉；左椎动脉为优势椎动脉，V3～V4 段闭塞；基底动脉及其分支通过右椎动脉的细小分支代偿显影，双侧大脑后动脉未见显影，左椎动脉末端可见残端（**E～H**）

血栓弹力图：ADP 抑制率 51.70%，AA 抑制率 66.90%。

DSA：双侧颈内动脉系统未见明显异常，双侧后交通动脉未开放（图 5.3.16 A～D）；右椎动脉终止于小脑后下动脉；左椎动脉为优势椎动脉，V3～V4 段闭塞；基底动脉及其分支通过右椎动脉的细小分支代偿显影，双侧大脑后动脉未见显影，左椎动脉末端可见残端（图 5.3.16 E～H）。

头部高分辨率磁共振成像：右椎动脉 V4 段先天发育不良，管径纤细；左椎动脉 V3～V4 段管腔内长条状短 T1 长 T2 信号，增强扫描未见强化，局部管腔闭塞，考虑血栓栓塞可能（图 5.3.17）。

目前予以双联抗血小板（阿司匹林 100 mg 1 次 / 日＋氯吡格雷 75 mg 1 次 / 日）、降脂（阿托伐他汀 40 mg 1 次 / 日）治疗。

（二）诊断

症状性左椎动脉 V3～V4 段闭塞。

（三）术前讨论

患者反复出现后循环缺血症状，DSA 提示左椎动脉 V3～V4 段闭塞，右椎动脉终止于小脑后下动脉。高分辨率磁共振血管成像提示右椎动脉 V4 段发育不良，左椎动脉 V3～V4 段亚急性血栓形成，故拟行左椎动脉开通治疗。若能通过病变，拟先球囊扩张，再放置自膨式支架。相关风险包括闭塞再通失败、穿支动脉闭塞、急性或亚急性血栓形成、高灌注综合征等。

（四）治疗过程

全麻下右股动脉入路，将 6F 导引导管头端置于左椎动脉 V2 段远端，造影显示左椎动脉 V3 段远端

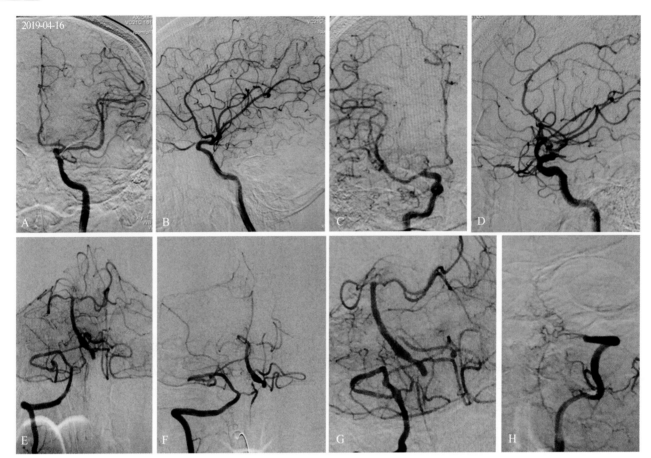

Fig. 5.3.16 DSA showed no significant abnormalities in the bilateral internal carotid artery system, unopen bilateral posterior communicating arteries (**A − D**), a right vertebral artery that terminated at the posterior inferior cerebellar artery, and occlusion of the V3 − V4 segments of the dominant left vertebral artery. The right vertebral artery provided collateral anastomosis to visualize the basilar artery. However, both the bilateral posterior cerebral arteries remained unobserved, and the left vertebral artery, which had been occluded, was left with a residual stump end (**E − H**)

The thromboelastography test revealed a 66.9% inhibition of AA and a 51.7% inhibition of ADP.

The DSA results demonstrated no significant abnormalities in the bilateral internal carotid artery system, unopen bilateral posterior communicating arteries (Fig. 5.13.16 A−D), a right vertebral artery that terminated at the posterior inferior cerebellar artery, and occlusion of the V3 − V4 segments of the dominant left vertebral artery. The right vertebral artery provided collateral anastomosis to visualize the basilar artery. However, both the bilateral posterior cerebral arteries remained unobserved, and the left vertebral artery, which had been occluded, was left with a residual stump end. (Fig. 5.3.16 E−H).

High-resolution MRI revealed a dysplastic V4 segment of the right vertebral artery, while the V3 − V4 segments of the left vertebral artery displayed occlusion, with a hyperintense substance observed in the occluded lumen. Contrast-enhanced T1 sequences provided no indication of lumen enhancement. (Fig. 5.3.17).

Upon admission, he was prescribed a dual antiplatelet consisting of a daily doses of 100mg Aspirin and 75 mg Clopidogrel, as well as a daily dose of 40mg of Atorvastatin.

2. Diagnosis

Symptomatic occlusion of the left vertebral artery V3−

V4 segments.

3. Treatment schedule

Despite receiving aggressive medical treatment, the patient's symptoms exhibited gradual deterioration and recurrence. The angiogram revealed an occlusion in the V3−V4 segments of the left vertebral artery. Furthermore, high-resolution MRI indicated dysplasia in the V4 segment of the right vertebral artery, as well as subacute thrombosis in the V3−V4 segments of the left vertebral artery. As a solution, it was recommended that the V3−V4 segments of the left vertebral artery be recanalized.Technical approach: The occluded lesion was traversed using a coaxially advanced microwire and microcatheter, and subsequently treated with balloon pre-dilation and implantation of a self-expanding stent. Pontential risks of the procedure included failed recanalization, perforating artery occlusion, in-stent thrombosis, and hyperperfusion syndrome.

4. Treatment

Under general anesthesia, a 6 F guide catheter was positioned at the V2 segment of the left vertebral artery. Angiogram confirmed occlusion in the V3 segment of the left

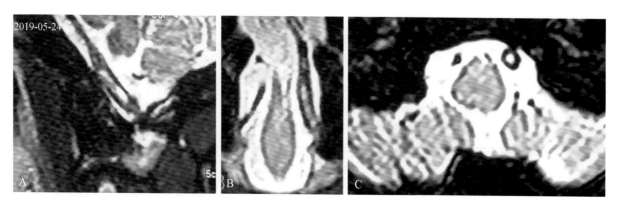

图 5.3.17　高分辨率磁共振成像示右椎动脉 V4 段先天发育不良，左椎动脉 V3 ～ V4 段管腔内长条状短 T1 长 T2 信号，增强扫描未见强化，局部管腔闭塞

闭塞（图 5.3.18 A）。Echelon-10 微导管与 Synchro 微导丝（0.014 in，200 cm）同轴，多次尝试后通过闭塞段。微导管造影证实处于真腔（图 5.3.18 B）。交换 Transend 微导丝（0.014 in，300 cm），将其头端置于右小脑上动脉中段，经微导丝送入 Maverick 球囊（2.0 mm×15 mm），由远及近分段扩张闭塞段（图 5.3.18 C）。造影见闭塞段再通（图 5.3.18 D）。

交换 Select Plus 微导管，经微导管送入 Enterprise 自膨式支架（4.5 mm×37 mm），释放后造影见支架近端未完全覆盖闭塞段（图 5.3.18 E），后在近端置入一枚 Apollo 球囊扩张式支架（2.5 mm×8 mm）。2 枚支架完全覆盖闭塞段，残余狭窄率为 15%。观察 15 min 无改变结束手术（图 5.3.18 F）。

术后立即复查头部 CT 未见出血。

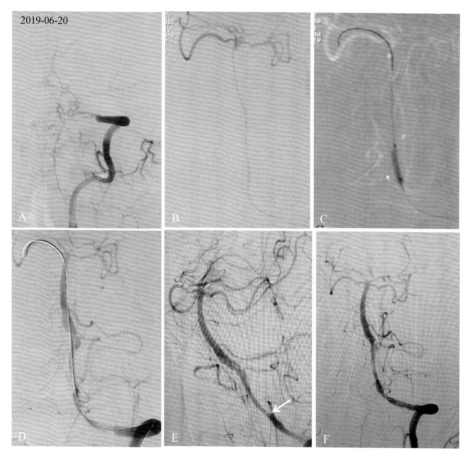

图 5.3.18　**A**. 术前造影；**B**. 微导管造影证实微导管进入真腔；**C**. Maverick 球囊扩张闭塞段；**D**. 球囊扩张后造影见闭塞段再通；**E**. 支架置入后，造影见支架近端未完全覆盖闭塞段（箭头示）；**F**. 植入第 2 枚支架后造影

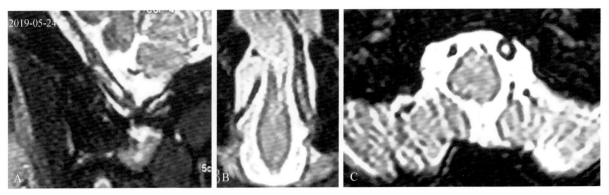

Fig. 5.3.17 HRMRI revealed a dysplastic V4 segment of the right vertebral artery, while the V3–V4 segments of the left vertebral artery displayed occlusion, with a hyperintense substance observed in the occluded lumen. Contrast-enhanced T1 sequences provided no indication of lumen enhancement

vertebral artery (Fig. 5.3.18 A). The Synchro microwire (0.014 in, 200 cm) and Echelon-10 microcatheter were advanced coaxially into the occluded segment. The transcatheter angiogram showed that the microcatheter was in the true lumen (Fig. 5.3.18 B). The Transend microwire (0.014 in, 300 cm) was exchanged and positioned in the middle segment of the right superior cerebellar artery. Next, a Maverick balloon (2.0 mm×15 mm) was used to dilate the occluded segment from distal to proximal (Fig. 5.3.18 C). The following angiogram revealed successful recanalization of the previously occluded artery. (Fig. 5.3.18 D). A 4.5 mm×37 mm Enterprise stent was utilized to cover the lesion. The post-stent implantation angiogram displayed an incomplete coverage of the occluded lesion at the proximal end of the stent (Fig. 5.3.18 E). The proximal occluded segment was covered using a 2.5 mm× 8 mm Apollo stent. The final angiogram exhibited a residual stenosis of 15% post-stent implantation (Fig. 5.3.18 F).

Post-procedural CT did not indicate any signs of hemorrhage.

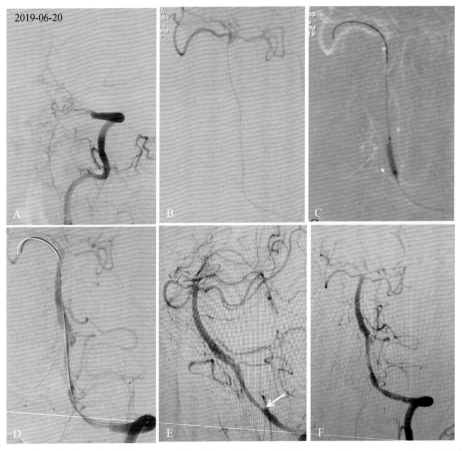

Fig. 5.3.18 Angiogram confirmed occlusion in the V3 segment of the left vertebral artery (**A**). The transcatheter angiogram showed that the microcatheter was in the true lumen (**B**). A Maverick balloon (2.0 mm×15 mm) was used to dilate the occluded segment from distal to proximal (**C**). The following angiogram revealed successful recanalization of the previously occluded artery (**D**). The post-stent implantation angiogram displayed an incomplete coverage of the occluded lesion at the proximal end of the stent (arrow) (**E**). The final angiogram exhibited a residual stenosis of 15% post-stent implantation (**F**)

（五）讨论

本例右椎动脉 V4 段发育不良，并经高分辨率磁共振成像证实，不宜开通治疗。左椎动脉 V3～V4 段闭塞，结合临床症状考虑近期闭塞，有开通可能。术中开通较为顺利，与闭塞时间较短相关。闭塞段用 2.0 mm 球囊预扩及置入支架后均未见明显弹性回缩，推测病变为亚急性血栓形成，较为松软且无钙化。本例在术后用替罗非班桥接双联抗血小板治疗，并且严格控制血压，积极预防后循环高灌注及急性支架内血栓形成。

（李郁芳　雒东江　马宁）

病例 16　基底动脉闭塞

（一）临床病史及影像分析

患者，男性，43 岁，主因"头晕伴言语不清 10 天"入院。予以内科药物治疗，仍有头晕发作。

既往史：高血压、糖尿病病史。

查体：左侧鼻唇沟略浅，左侧肌力 5- 级，左侧指鼻试验阳性，左侧跟-膝-胫试验阳性，左侧偏身针刺觉减退，左侧巴宾斯基征阳性。

头部 MRI：脑桥新发梗死（图 5.3.19 A）。

MRA：基底动脉未见显影，考虑闭塞可能（图 5.3.19 B）。

高分辨率 MRI：基底动脉中段未见血管流空影，增强呈等信号（图 5.3.20 A 和 B）；闭塞近端管壁未见明显增厚，强化不明显；闭塞远端管壁偏心性增厚（腹侧壁），强化明显（图 5.3.20 C～E）。

DSA：右大脑中动脉闭塞，右后交通动脉开放，右大脑前动脉和后动脉经软脑膜动脉向右大脑中动脉供血区域代偿，基底动脉中上段、左大脑后动脉及双侧小脑上动脉经后交通动脉代偿显影（图 5.3.21 A）。左大脑中动脉及前动脉未见明显异常（图 5.3.21 B）。右椎动脉非优势，发出右小脑后下动脉（PICA）以远未见显影（图 5.3.21 C 和 D）。左椎动脉优势，基底动脉发出双侧小脑前下动脉（AICA）后闭塞（图 5.3.21 E 和 F）。

予以双联抗血小板（阿司匹林 100 mg 1 次 / 日＋氯吡格雷 75 mg 1 次 / 日）及降脂（阿托伐他汀

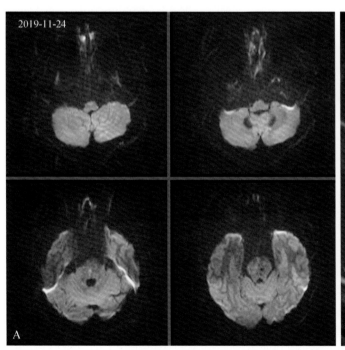
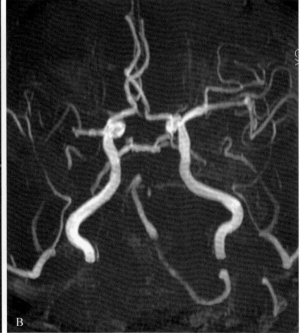

图 5.3.19　**A**. MRI 示脑桥新发梗死；**B**. MRA 示基底动脉未见显影，考虑闭塞

5. Comments

This case involves a patient presenting with symptomatic occlusion in the V3–V4 segment of the left vertebral artery, as well as dysplasia in the V4 segment of the right vertebral artery, which was confirmed by high-resolution vessel wall imaging. Consequently, a decision was made to recanalize the left vertebral V3–V4 segment. Successful recanalization of the occlusion was associated with a short time interval from occlusion to recanalization. During the procedure, there was no significant elastic recoil observed in the occlusion segment after balloon angioplasty and stent implantation. The occlusion of the lesion was suspected to result from thrombus formation, with no evidence of focal vessel wall calcification. To prevent acute in-stent thrombosis, a bridging protocol was implemented involving the intravenous administration of tirofiban followed by oral dual antiplatelet therapy. Additionally, strict blood pressure control was implemented to prevent hyperperfusion syndrome.

(Translated by Rongrong Cui, Revised by Zhikai Hou)

Case 16   Occlusion of the basilar artery

1. Clinical presentation and radiological studies

A 43-year-old man was admitted to the hospital due to vertigo and dysarthria for 10 days. Despite receiving medical treatment, his symptoms continued to persist.

He had a medical history of diabetes and hypertension.

Physical examination showed a central facial paralysis on the left side, muscle strength in the left limbs at grade 5 minus, inaccurate coordination on left finger-to-nose and heel-to-shin testing, decreased pinprick sensation in left limbs, and a positive Babinski sign on the left side.

MRI revealed acute infarction in the pontine (Fig. 5.3.19 A).

MRA showed an occlusion of the basilar artery (Fig. 5.3.19 B).

High-resolution MRI showed an occlusion at the middle segment of the basilar artery. There was no contrast enhancement in the occluded segment (Fig. 5.3.20 A, B). The vessel wall proximal to the occlusion did not display any evident thickening or enhancement. The vessel wall distal to the occlusion was eccentric thickening (ventral wall), with strong enhancement (Fig. 5.3.20 C–E).

DSA indicated occlusion of the right middle cerebral artery, while the right posterior communicating artery remained patency. The area supplied by the right middle cerebral artery was compensated by collateral circulation through the pial arteries by the right anterior and posterior cerebral arteries. The posterior communicating artery provided collateral blood flow, enabling visualization of the middle-upper segment of the basilar artery, as well as the left posterior cerebral artery and both superior cerebellar arteries. (Fig. 5.3.21 A). The left middle and anterior cerebral arteries did not exhibit obvious abnormalities (Fig. 5.3.21 B). The right vertebral artery terminated at the right PICA (Fig. 5.3.21 C, D), while the basilar artery was occluded after originating from the bilateral AICA (Fig. 5.3.21 E, F).

After admission, he was prescribed a dual-antiplatelet regime consisting of Aspirin 100 mg daily and Clopidogrel

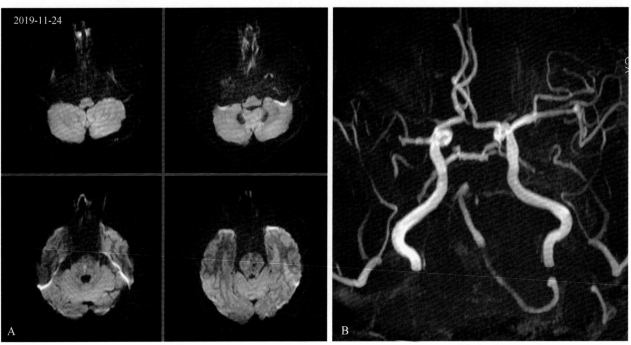

Fig. 5.3.19   MRI revealed acute infarction in the pontine (**A**). MRA showed an occlusion of the basilar artery (**B**)

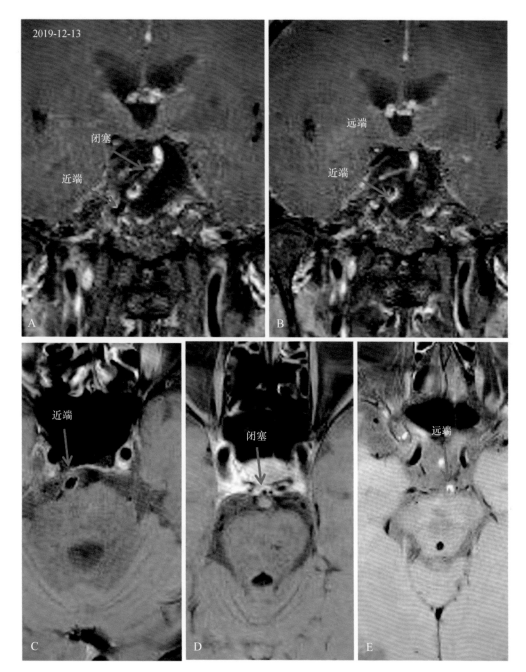

图 5.3.20　高分辨率磁共振成像示：**A** 和 **B** 基底动脉中段未见血管流空影，增强呈等信号（箭头示）；**C** 至 **E**.闭塞近端管壁未见明显增厚，强化不明显；闭塞远端管壁偏心性增厚（腹侧壁），强化明显（箭头示）

20 mg 1 次 / 日）等治疗。

（二）诊断

症状性基底动脉闭塞。

（三）术前讨论

患者后循环新发脑梗死，多项影像学检查提示基底动脉闭塞。经内科药物治疗后依然有症状反复，考虑致病机制系基底动脉闭塞所致的相关

供血区域低灌注，拟行血管内介入治疗。闭塞段相对较长，高分辨率磁共振成像提示闭塞段斑块成分较多，有开通不成功可能。此外，通过闭塞段病变有引发医源性夹层、穿支卒中以及急性或亚急性血栓形成等风险。

（四）治疗过程

全麻下右股动脉入路，将 6F 导引导管头端置于左椎动脉 V2 段，造影显示基底动脉中段闭塞，动

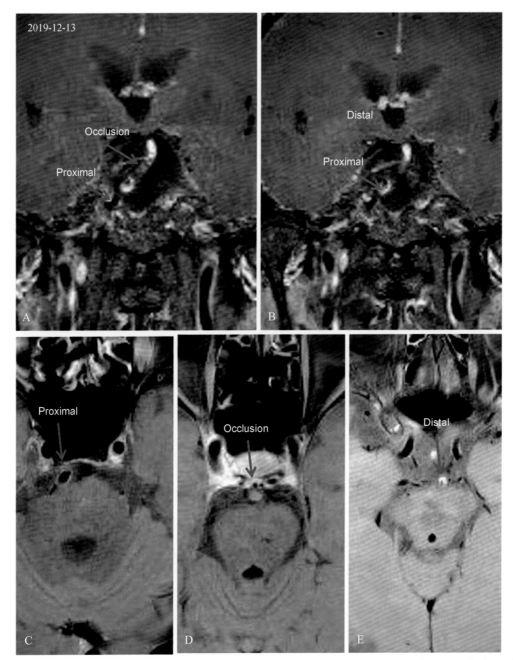

Fig. 5.3.20 HRMRI showed an occlusion at the middle segment of the basilar artery. There was no contrast enhancement in the occluded segment (arrow) (**A, B**). The vessel wall proximal to the occlusion did not display any evident thickening or enhancement. The vessel wall distal to the occlusion was eccentric thickening (ventral wall), with strong enhancement(arrow) (**C–E**)

75 mg daily, as well as Atorvastatin 20 mg daily.

2. Diagnosis

Symptomatic occlusion of the basilar artery.

3. Treatment schedule

This case involves a patient with acute cerebral infarction in the posterior circulation. Multi-modal imaging revealed the occlusion of the basilar artery. The aggressive medical treatment was unsuccessful, and the patient continued to experience recurrent symptoms. Endovascular treatment was recommended to recanalize the occluded

basilar artery. HRMRI showed that the occluded segment of the basilar artery was lengthy, thus increasing the risk of unsuccessful recanalization. Potential risks of the procedure included iatrogenic dissection, perforating artery occlusion, and acute/subacute in-stent thrombosis.

4. Treatment

Under general anesthesia, a 6F guide catheter was positioned at the V2 segment of the left vertebral artery. Angiogram revealed the middle-upper segment of the basilar artery was occluded. The upper segment of the basilar artery was visualized in the late-arterial phase, which was compensated

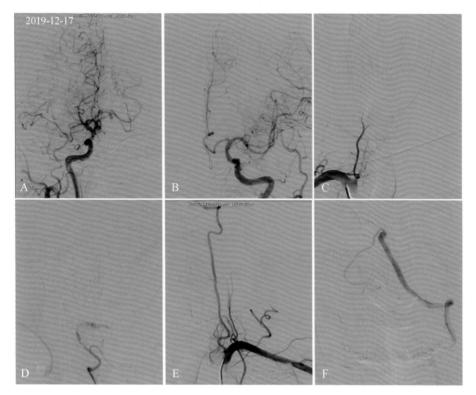

图 5.3.21 DSA 示：**A**. 右大脑中动脉闭塞，右后交通动脉开放，右大脑前动脉和后动脉经软脑膜动脉向右大脑中动脉供血区域代偿，基底动脉中上段、左大脑后动脉及双侧小脑上动脉经后交通动脉代偿显影；**B**. 左大脑中动脉及前动脉未见明显异常；**C** 和 **D**. 右椎动脉非优势，发出右 PICA 以远未见显影；**E** 和 **F**. 左椎动脉优势，基底动脉发出双侧 AICA 后闭塞

脉晚期基底动脉远段经右 AICA 与右小脑上动脉见代偿显影（图 5.3.22 A 和 B）。将 Synchro 微导丝（0.014 in，300 cm）与 SL-10 微导管同轴，微导丝首次通过闭塞段后，微导丝头端摆动欠佳，跟进微导管，注射器未回吸出血液，考虑进入夹层（图 5.3.22 C）。撤出微导管至闭塞近端，路径图显示闭塞段部分再通，闭塞远段经夹层显影（图 5.3.22 D）。再次送入微导丝及微导管越过病变至右小脑上动脉（图 5.3.23 A 和 B）。撤出微导管，经微导丝送入 Gateway 球囊（1.5 mm×15 mm）扩张闭塞段（图 5.3.23 C），见基底动脉闭塞段远端部分显影（图 5.3.23 D）。再次予以 Gateway 球囊（2.0 mm×15 mm）扩张（图 5.3.24 A）。扩张后造影可见弹性回缩明显，残余狭窄率约为 60%（图 5.3.24 B）。将微导丝调整至右大脑后动脉，其后放置 Wingspan 支架（3.5 mm× 15 mm）。释放后造影提示残余狭窄率约为 40%，前向血流 mTICI 分级 3 级（图 5.3.24 C 和 D）。观察 10 min 无改变，结束手术。

患者术后头晕症状明显缓解。

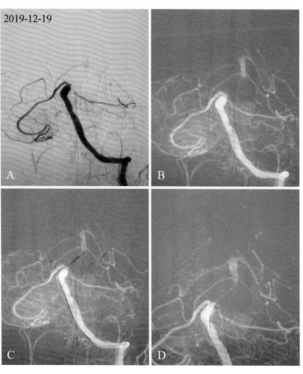

图 5.3.22 血管内介入治疗过程如下：**A**. 术前造影显示基底动脉中段闭塞；**B**. 动脉晚期基底动脉远段经右 AICA 与右小脑上动脉见代偿显影；**C**. 微导丝与微导管进入夹层；**D**. 撤出微导管，闭塞段部分再通，闭塞远段经夹层显影

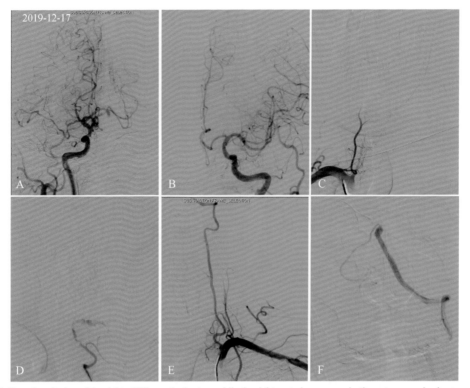

Fig. 5.3.21 DSA indicated occlusion of the right middle cerebral artery, while the right posterior communicating artery remained patency. The area supplied by the right middle cerebral artery was compensated by collateral circulation through the pial arteries by the right anterior and posterior cerebral arteries. The posterior communicating artery provided collateral blood flow, enabling visualization of the middle-upper segment of the basilar artery, as well as the left posterior cerebral artery and both superior cerebellar arteries (**A**). The left middle and anterior cerebral arteries did not exhibit obvious abnormalities (**B**). The right vertebral artery terminated at the right PICA (**C**, **D**). The basilar artery was occluded after originating from the bilateral AICA (**E**, **F**)

through collateral blood from the right superior cerebellar artery and the right AICA (Fig. 5.3.22 A, B). The Synchro microwire (0.014 in, 300 cm) and SL-10 microcatheter coaxially advanced through the occluded segment. Following the microwire's passage through the occlusion segment, the tip did not move effectively. Attempts to advance the microcatheter and draw blood back with a syringe were unsuccessful. It was speculated that the microwire had advanced into the false lumen of an iatrogenic dissection (Fig. 5.3.22 C). Retracting the microcatheter to the proximal segment of the occlusion revealed partial recanalization of the distal portion of the occlusion on the roadmap (Fig. 5.3.22 D). The microwire and microcatheter were navigated to the right superior cerebellar artery (Fig. 5.3.23 A, B). The occlusion was dilated using a 1.5 mm×15 mm Gateway balloon (Fig. 5.3.23 C), allowing visualization of the distal segment (Fig. 5.3.23 D). A 2.0 mm×15 mm Gateway balloon was then employed to further dilate the lesion (Fig. 5.3.24 A). Though post-dilation angiography revealed significant elastic recoil and residual stenosis of 60% (Fig. 5.3.24 B). To fully cover the lesion, a 3.5 mm×15 mm Wingspan stent was implanted. Subsequent angiography indicated a reduction to 40% residual stenosis following stent implantation (Fig. 5.3.24 C, D). Ten minutes later, A final follow-up angiogram showed a patent basilar artery with successful stent placement.

The patient experienced notable alleviation of his dizziness following the procedure.

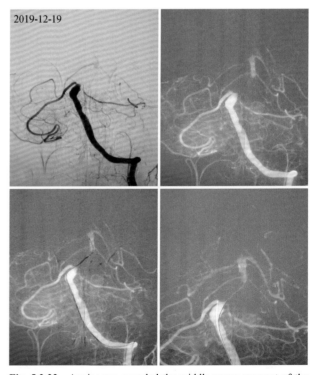

Fig. 5.3.22 Angiogram revealed the middle-upper segment of the basilar artery was occluded (**A**). The upper segment of the basilar artery was visualized in the late-arterial phase, which was compensated through collateral blood from the right superior cerebellar artery and the right AICA (**B**). The Synchro microwire (0.014 in, 300 cm) and SL-10 microcatheter coaxially advanced through the occluded segment (**C**). Retracting the microcatheter to the proximal segment of the occlusion revealed partial recanalization of the distal portion of the occlusion on the roadmap (**D**)

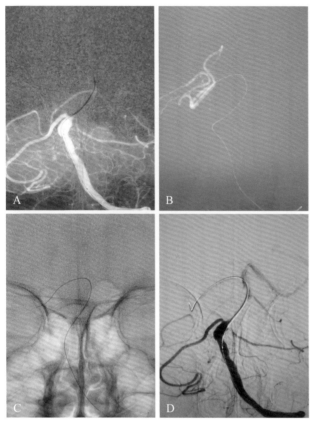

图 5.3.23　**A** 和 **B**. 再次将微导丝及微导管送至右小脑上动脉；**C**. Gateway 球囊扩张闭塞段；**D**. 球囊扩张后造影示闭塞段远端部分显影

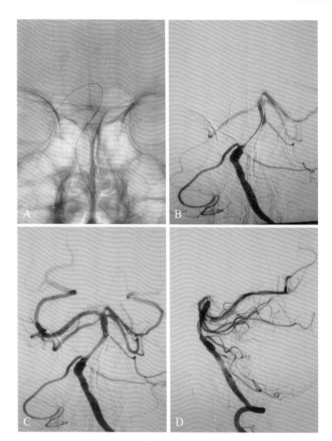

图 5.3.24　**A**. Gateway 球囊再次扩张病变；**B**. 球囊扩张后造影示弹性回缩明显，残余狭窄率约为 60%；**C** 和 **D**. 释放支架后造影示残余狭窄率约为 40%，前向血流 mTICI 分级 3 级

术后第 2 日复查 CTA：基底动脉支架置入术后，管腔通畅（图 5.3.25）。

（五）讨论

本例基底动脉闭塞，治疗过程中首过病变后微导丝头端摆动欠佳，跟进微导管，注射器未回吸出血液，考虑进入夹层，此时应避免微导管造影导致夹层进一步撕裂。第二次尝试进入真腔后，弹性回缩明显，遂选择支撑性较强的 Wingspan 支架，虽残余狭窄率较高，但考虑斑块负荷加重，为避免重要边支血管（AICA 和小脑上动脉）损伤，未予后扩张。

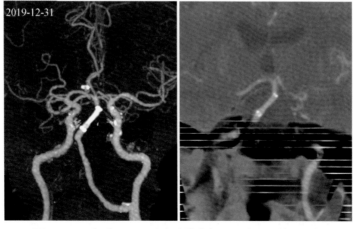

图 5.3.25　术后 CTA。基底动脉支架置入术后，管腔通畅

（王贤军　孙洪扬　陈旺　朱其义　马宁）

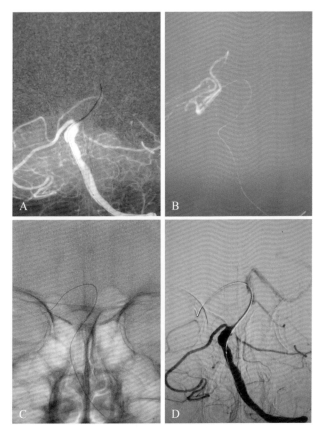

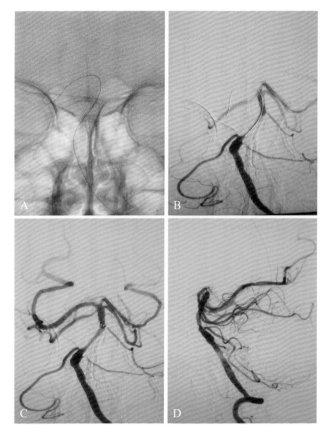

Fig. 5.3.23 The microwire and microcatheter were navigated to the right superior cerebellar artery (**A**, **B**). The occlusion was dilated using a 1.5 mm×15 mm Gateway balloon (**C**) the distal segment of the occlusion was visualized (**D**)

Fig. 5.3.24 A 2.0 mm×15 mm Gateway balloon was then employed to further dilate the lesion (**A**). Though post-dilation angiography revealed significant elastic recoil and residual stenosis of 60% (**B**). To fully cover the lesion, a 3.5 mm×15 mm Wingspan stent was implanted. Subsequent angiography indicated a reduction to 40% residual stenosis following stent implantation (**C**, **D**)

Post-procedural CTA indicated that the stent in the basilar artery was unobstructed (Fig. 5.3.25).

5. Comments

This case presented a patient with symptomatic basilar artery occlusion. During the procedure, the microwire encountered ineffective movement of the microwire tip while passing through the occluded segment. The microcatheter was advanced to a position close to the lesion, but attempts to draw blood back with a syringe proved unsuccessful. It was hypothesized that the microwire had caused damage to the arterial intima, resulting in an iatrogenic dissection. In order to prevent exacerbation of the dissection, we did not perform an angiogram via the transcatheter. After the balloon angioplasty, obvious elastic recoil was observed, prompting the selection of a Wingspan stent to cover the lesion. Despite the residual stenosis being significant, we refrained from performing balloon postdilatation in order to protect the basilar branch (including the AICA and superior cerebellar artery) from any potential damage.

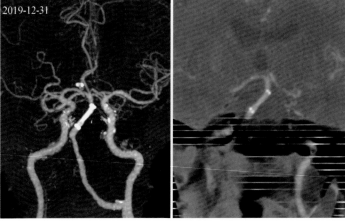

Fig. 5.3.25 Post-procedural CTA indicated that the stent in the basilar artery was unobstructed

(Translated by Rongrong Cui, Revised by Zhikai Hou)

第四节　路径迂曲病变

病例 17　路径迂曲的左椎动脉 V4 段重度狭窄

（一）临床病史及影像分析

患者，女性，61 岁，主因"发作性眩晕 3 个月"入院。

当地医院头部 MRI 示无新发梗死灶。头颅 CTA 示左椎动脉 V4 段重度狭窄（图 5.4.1）。予氯吡格雷、阿司匹林抗血小板聚集以及阿托伐他汀降脂治疗后症状仍有发作。现为进一步行血管内治疗来我院。

既往史：高血压、糖耐量异常以及脂蛋白代谢紊乱病史。

查体：入院神经系统查体无阳性体征。

血栓弹力图：AA 抑制率 88%，ADP 抑制率 32%。

高分辨率 MRI：左椎动脉 V4 段后外侧管壁不规则增厚，增强可见局部不规则强化，局部管腔不规则狭窄（图 5.4.2）。

CTA：双椎动脉、基底动脉、左大脑后动脉多发局部狭窄，以左椎动脉 V4 段为著（图 5.4.3）。

CTP：左侧颞枕叶和脑干低灌注（图 5.4.4）。

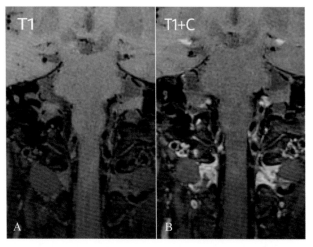

图 5.4.2　高分辨率 MRI 示左椎动脉 V4 段后外侧管壁不规则增厚，增强可见局部不规则强化，局部管腔不规则狭窄（A 和 B）

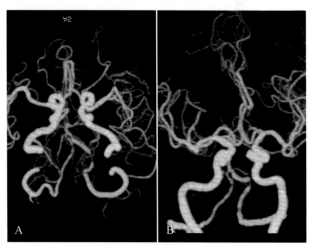

图 5.4.3　CTA 示双椎动脉、基底动脉、左大脑后动脉多发局部狭窄，以左椎动脉 V4 段为著（A 和 B）

DSA：左椎动脉优势，V1 和 V2 段迂曲，V4 段狭窄（图 5.4.5），右椎动脉 V2 段迂曲（图 5.4.6）。右前循环通过后交通动脉向后循环部分区域代偿（图 5.4.7）。

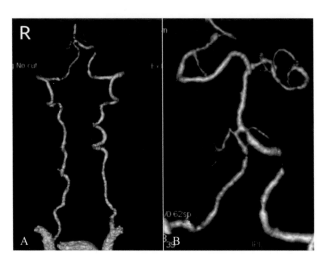

图 5.4.1　头颅 CTA 示左椎动脉 V4 段重度狭窄（A 和 B）

Section 4 Tortuous Proximal Anatomy

Case 17 Severe stenosis of the V4 segment of the left vertebral artery with tortuous proximal anatomy

1. Clinical presentation and radiological studies

A 61-year-old woman presented with paroxysmal dizziness for 3 months.

MRI indicated the lack of any recent infarction. CT angiography showed severe stenosis at the V4 segment of the left vertebral artery (Fig. 5.4.1). Despite undergoing intensive medical treatment, the patient's symptoms persisted. Her medical history included hypertension, impaired glucose tolerance, and lipoprotein metabolism disorder.

She was neurologically intact on admission.

Thromboelastography test revealed an 8.8% inhibition of AA and 32% inhibition of ADP.

High-resolution MRI showed severe stenosis at the V4 segment of the left vertebral artery, with the focal wall thickening. Contrasted-enhancement sequence indicated irregular enhancement of the lesion wall (Fig. 5.4.2).

CTA revealed multiple stenosis of the bilateral vertebral arteries, basilar artery, and left posterior cerebral artery, with the most severe stenosis at the V4 segment of the left vertebral artery (Fig. 5.4.3).

CT perfusion showed hypoperfusion in the left temporal occipital lobe and brain stem (Fig. 5.4.4).

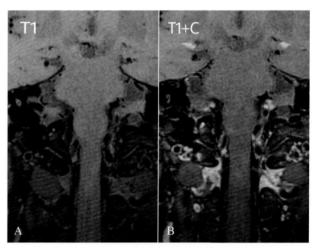

Fig. 5.4.2 HRMRI indicated severe stenosis at the V4 segment of the left vertebral artery, with the focal wall thickening. Contrastedenhancement sequence indicated irregular enhancement of the lesion wall (**A, B**)

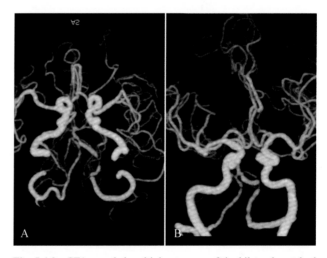

Fig. 5.4.3 CTA revealed multiple stenoses of the bilateral vertebral arteries, basilar artery, and left posterior cerebral artery, with the most severe stenosis at the V4 segment of the left vertebral artery (**A, B**)

DSA demonstrated a dominant left vertebral artery with tortuous V1–V2 segments, and a severe stenosis at the V4 segment of the left vertebral artery (Fig. 5.4.5). The V2 segment of the right vertebral artery was tortuous (Fig. 5.4.6). The right carotid artery provided compensatory blood flow to the posterior circulation territory through the patent posterior communicating artery (Fig. 5.4.7).

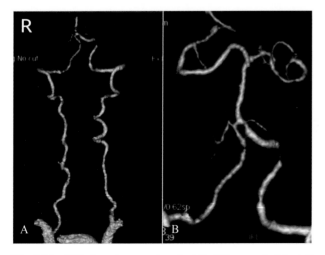

Fig. 5.4.1 CTA showed severe stenosis at the V4 segment of the left vertebral artery (**A, B**)

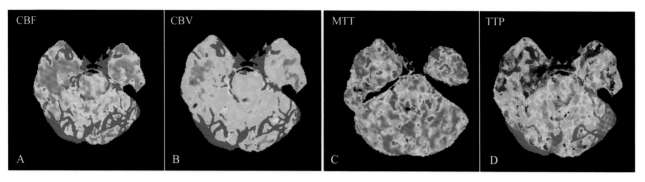

图 5.4.4 CTP 示左侧颞枕叶和脑干低灌注（**A ~ D**）

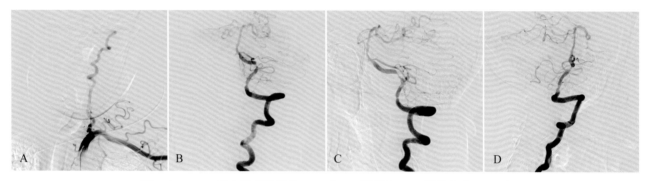

图 5.4.5 DSA 示左椎动脉优势，V1 和 V2 段迂曲，V4 段狭窄（**A ~ D**）

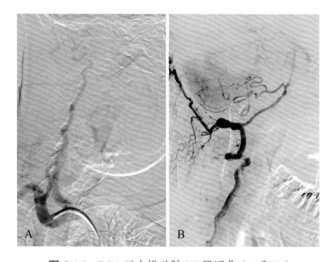

图 5.4.6 DSA 示右椎动脉 V2 段迂曲（**A 和 B**）

入院后给予双联抗血小板（阿司匹林 100 mg 1 次 / 日＋氯吡格雷 75 mg 1 次 / 日）以及降脂（阿托伐他汀 20 mg 1 次 / 日）等治疗。

（二）诊断

路径迂曲的症状性左椎动脉 V4 段狭窄。

（三）术前讨论

患者左椎动脉优势，V4 段重度狭窄，高分辨率 MRI 提示管腔内系动脉粥样硬化斑块，在口服双联抗血小板药物治疗下仍有反复短暂性脑缺血发作（TIA），考虑药物治疗效果欠佳，有介入治疗指征。

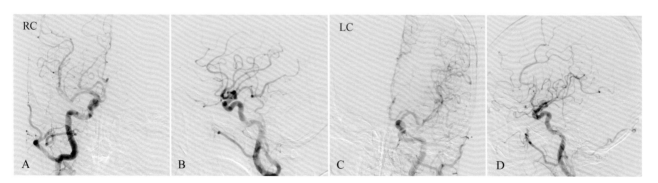

图 5.4.7 DSA 示右前循环通过后交通动脉向后循环部分区域代偿（**A ~ D**）

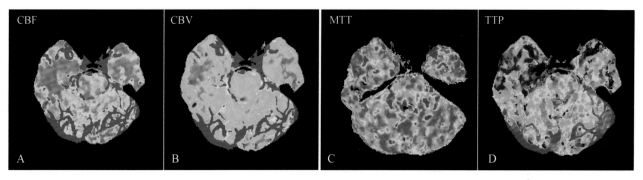

Fig. 5.4.4 CT perfusion showed hypoperfusion in the left temporal occipital lobe and brain stem (**A–D**)

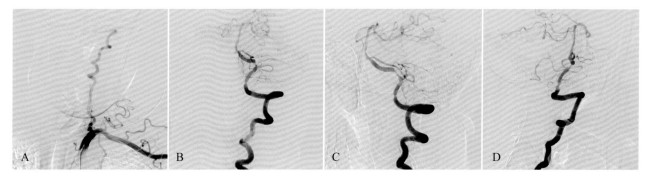

Fig. 5.4.5 DSA demonstrated a dominant left vertebral artery with tortuous V1–V2 segments, and a severe stenosis at the V4 segment of the left vertebral artery (**A–D**)

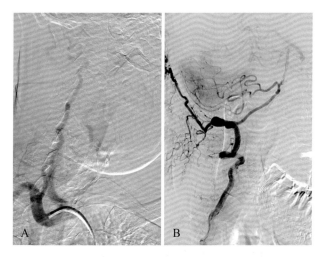

Fig. 5.4.6 The V2 segment of the right vertebral artery was tortuous (**A, B**)

Upon admission, she was prescribed a dual antiplatelet regimen comprising of daily doses of Aspirin 100 mg and Clopidogrel 75 mg, as well as Atorvastatin 20 mg.

2. Diagnosis

Symptomatic stenosis of the V4 segment of the left vertebral artery with tortuous proximal anatomy.

3. Treatment schedule

In this particular case, the patient presented a severe stenosis at the V4 segment of the dominant left vertebral artery, resulting from atherosclerotic plaques as evidenced by HRMRI. Despite receiving intensive medical treatment, the patient's symptoms persisted. As a result, undergoing interventional treatment was recommended. Treatment approach: In light of the tortuous access, a 7F long sheath

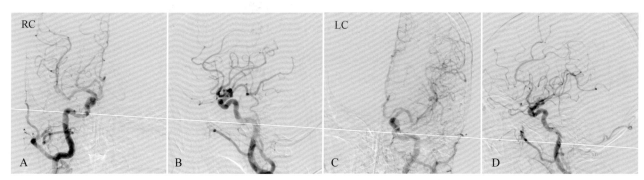

Fig. 5.4.7 The right carotid artery provided compensatory blood flow to the posterior circulation territory through the patent posterior communicating artery (**A–D**)

术前造影提示入路迂曲，拟使用 7F 长鞘（70 cm）结合 6F Navien 导引导管（115 cm）降低迂曲路径所致的技术难度。治疗风险包括穿支闭塞、高灌注、支架内急性或亚急性血栓形成等。

（四）治疗过程

全麻下右股动脉穿刺置入 8F 动脉鞘，交换技术送入 7F Cook 长鞘（70 cm）+ 6F Navien 导引导管（115 cm），Cook 长鞘置于左锁骨下动脉近端，Navien 导管置于左椎动脉开口处。沿 Navien 导管送入 Traxcess 微导丝（0.014 in，200 cm）+ Echelon-10 微导管至左椎动脉 V3 段，此时拟跟进 Navien 导管进入左椎动脉 V2 段，但反复尝试均未获成功（图 5.4.8）。

遂撤出 Navien 导管，将 Cook 长鞘置于左椎动脉开口部，Traxcess 微导丝（0.014 in，200 cm）+ Echelon-10 微导管结合将微导管置于左大脑后动脉 P2 段，交换 Transend 微导丝（0.014 in，300 cm）至左大脑后动脉 P2 段，Gateway 球囊（2.25 mm×

15 mm）于狭窄段预扩张（图 5.4.9）。其后放置 Wingspan 自膨式支架（3.5 mm×15 mm），释放后造影见支架贴壁良好，前向血流 mTICI 分级 3 级（图 5.4.10）。

（五）讨论

本例拟使用柔顺的导引导管克服路径迂曲的困难，但在具体操作时由于入路迂曲太严重而无法顺利到位，不得以将长鞘放置在左椎动脉开口处完成本次治疗过程，幸运的是导丝到位后球囊和支架系

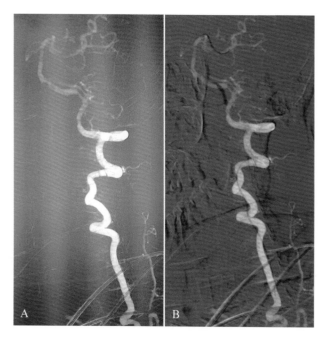

图 5.4.9　Gateway 球囊扩张狭窄病变（**A** 和 **B**）

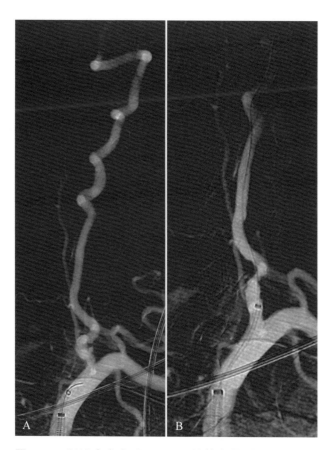

图 5.4.8　经过多次尝试，Navien 导管未能到达左椎动脉 V2 段（**A** 和 **B**）

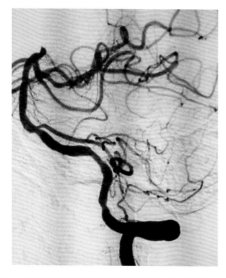

图 5.4.10　支架释放后造影示支架贴壁良好，前向血流 mTICI 分级 3 级

(70 cm) was employed in combination with a 6F Navien guide catheter (115 cm) to enhance the support force to the balloon and stent system. Potential risks associated with this procedure included perforating artery occlusion, hyperperfusion syndrome, and in-stent thrombosis.

4. Treatment

Under general anesthesia, an 8F arterial sheath was inserted through the right femoral artery. A 7F Cook long sheath (70 cm) and a 6F Navien guide catheter (115 cm) were positioned at the proximal left subclavian artery and the left vertebral artery origin, respectively. The Traxcess microwire (0.014 in, 200 cm) was advanced along with the Echelon-10 microcatheter to the V3 segment of the left vertebral artery. After multiple attempts, the Navien catheter was unable to reach the V2 segment of the left vertebral artery (Fig. 5.4.8). Consequently, the Navien catheter was withdrawn.

A Cook long sheath was inserted at the origin of the left vertebral artery. The Traxcess microwire (0.014 in, 200 cm) and the Echelon-10 microcatheter were coaxially advanced through the stenotic lesion to the P2 segment of the left posterior cerebral artery. Subsequently, a Gateway balloon (2.25 mm × 15 mm) was utilized to pre-dilate the lesion (Fig. 5.4.9). After balloon angioplasty, a 3.5 mm × 15 mm Wingspan stent was used to cover the lesion. The post-stent

implantation angiogram exhibited exceptional stent wall apposition and the antegrade blood flow was grade 3 (Fig. 5.4.10).

5. Comments

Initially, a flexible guide catheter was utilized to address the tortuous access, but unfortunately, it was not successfully placed. To insert the stent into the stenotic lesion, the long sheath was positioned at the origin of the left vertebral artery. Upon successful placement of the microwire in the P2 segment, the Gateway balloon was smoothly positioned, pre-dilated, retracted, and the Wingspan stent system was successfully released and retracted.

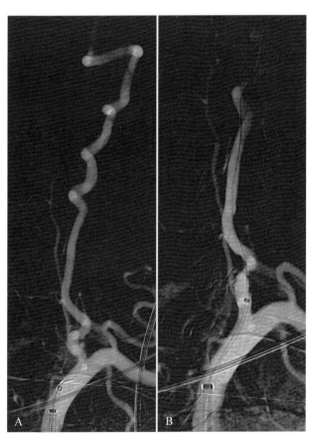

Fig. 5.4.8 The Navien catheter was unable to reach the V2 segment of the left vertebral artery (**A, B**)

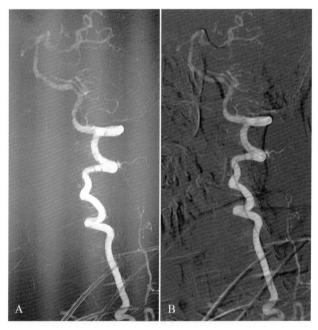

Fig. 5.4.9 A Gateway balloon (2.25 mm × 15 mm) was utilized to pre-dilate the lesion (**A, B**)

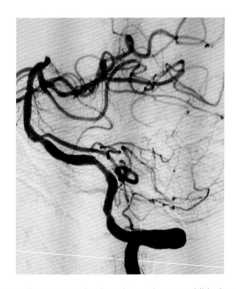

Fig. 5.4.10 The post-stent implantation angiogram exhibited exceptional stent wall apposition and the antegrade blood flow was grade 3

统到位、释放及回收过程均比较顺利。

　　对于类似病例，治疗过程中有以下细节需要注意：①选择大尺寸路途，最好囊括导引导管、长鞘开口到微导丝着陆区全程，了解输送过程中的近端导引导管、长鞘开口的位置变化，及时调整输送球囊或者支架系统的力道大小。②绝对避免重复路途，因为微导丝一旦到达着陆区后，迂曲血管被拉直，导致前向血流进一步减慢甚至停

滞，这会给后续球囊或者支架的定位造成巨大困难。③要充分考虑到自膨式支架系统释放或者回收困难的可能。④如果球囊都到位困难，适时终止治疗也是一种选择。

5.4　手术操作视频
（病例 17）

（姚亮　吴岩峰　霍晓川
宋立刚　马宁）

病例 18　路径迂曲的左椎动脉 V4 段重度狭窄

（一）临床病史及影像分析

　　患者，男性，因"头晕1月余"入院。

　　既往史：高血压和糖尿病病史1年，饮酒史30年。

　　查体：神经系统查体未见明显异常。

　　头部 MRI：右侧小脑半球及小脑蚓部多发梗死（图 5.4.11 A 和 B）。

　　头颈部 CTA：左椎动脉优势，双椎动脉 V4 段狭窄（图 5.4.11 C 和 D）。

　　DSA：右颈动脉造影显示海绵窦段迂曲（图 5.4.12 A 和 B）。左颈动脉造影显示后交通动脉

开放，向基底动脉尖及双侧大脑后动脉供血（图 5.4.12 C 和 D）。右椎动脉起始处闭塞，甲状颈干颈升支向右椎动脉 V2 段远端代偿供血（图 5.4.13 A 和 B）。左椎动脉 V1、V2 及 V3 段迂曲，V4 段重度狭窄，见小脑后下动脉向小脑前下动脉代偿供血（图 5.4.13 C ～ E）。

　　高分辨率 MRI：左椎动脉 V4 段走行变异，位于右椎动脉 V4 段腹侧。左椎动脉 V4 段管壁环形增厚，管腔重度狭窄（图 5.4.14）。

　　入院后口服阿司匹林 100 mg 1 次 / 日、氯吡格雷 75 mg 1 次 / 日、阿托伐他汀 40 mg 1 次 / 日，并给予降压、降糖治疗。

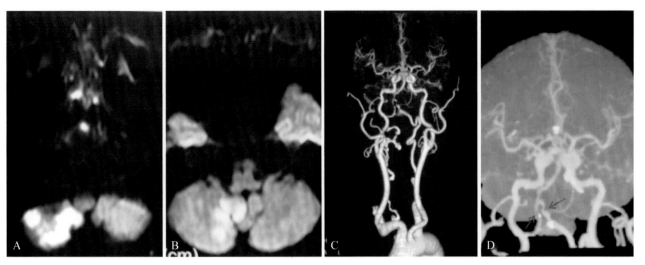

图 5.4.11　**A** 和 **B**. 头颅磁共振 DWI 示右小脑半球及小脑蚓部多发梗死；**C** 和 **D**. CTA 示左椎动脉优势，双椎动脉 V4 段狭窄（箭头示）

During similar procedures, attention should be paid to the following details: 1). It would be better to select a roadmap with a larger size containing the guide catheter, long sheath, and microwire in the landing area. This will help the neurointerventionist to monitor any changes in the positioning of the guide catheter and long sheath, allowing for adjustments in the balloon or stent system's delivery process. 2). It is advisable to avoid repeating the same roadmap. This is because the tortuous vessel tends to straighten out when the microwire reaches the landing zone, which may result in a slowdown in the antegrade blood flow. These factors can make the subsequent positioning of the balloon and stent more difficult. 3). The challenges related to releasing and retracting the self-expanding stent system should also be considered. 4). If the balloon is difficult to position correctly, it may be advisable to consider terminating the treatment.

(Translated by Rongrong Cui, Revised by Zhikai Hou)

5.4　Video of endovascular therapy (Case 17)

Case 18　Severe stenosis of the V4 segment of the left vertebral artery with tortuous proximal anatomy

1. Clinical presentation and radiological studies

A male patient was admitted to our hospital with a complaint of dizziness lasting over a month.

He had a medical history of diabetes and hypertension for a year, and had been consuming alcohol for more than 30 years.

Upon admission, his neurological status was deemed intact.

The MRI revealed the presence of multiple infarctions in both the cerebellar vermis and right hemisphere. (Fig. 5.4.11 A, B).

The CT angiography revealed that the left vertebral artery was dominant and bilateral vertebral arteries exhibited severe stenosis at the V4 segment (Fig. 5.4.11 C, D).

On DSA imaging, the cavernous segment of the right carotid artery exhibited tortuous access (Fig. 5.4.12 A, B). The left posterior communicating artery was patent and provided compensation for blood flow to the territory of the basilar artery (Fig. 5.4.12 C, D). The right vertebral artery was occluded at its origin, and compensation to the distal part of the V2 segment was provided by the ascending branch of the thyrocervical trunk (Fig. 5.4.13 A, B). The extracranial segments of the left vertebral artery were tortuous and the V4 segment exhibited severe stenosis. The left posterior inferior cerebellar artery provided compensation for the anterior inferior cerebellar artery (Fig. 5.4.13 C–E).

On high-resolution MRI, the V4 segment of the left vertebral artery displayed directional variation and was situated ventrally to the V4 segment of the right vertebral artery. The V4 segment of the left vertebral artery was severely stenosed, with circumferential thickening of the vessel wall (Fig. 5.4.14).

After admission, a dual-antiplatelet regimen was prescribed for him, which included a daily intake of 100 mg Aspirin, 75 mg Clopidogrel, together with a daily dose of 40 mg Atorvastatin.

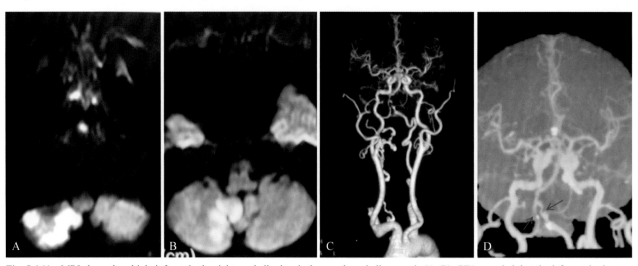

Fig. 5.4.11 MRI showed multiple infarcts in the right cerebellar hemisphere and cerebellar vermis (**A**, **B**). CTA revealed that the left vertebral artery was dominant and bilateral vertebral arteries exhibited severe stenosis at the V4 segment (arrow) (**C**, **D**)

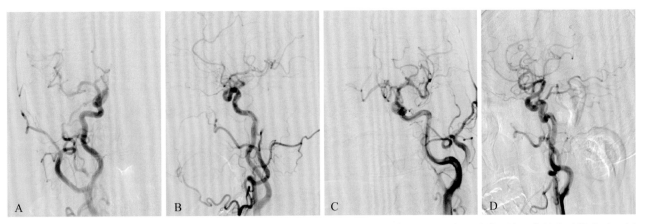

图 5.4.12　DSA 示：**A** 和 **B**. 右颈动脉造影见海绵窦段迂曲；**C** 和 **D**. 左颈动脉造影见后交通动脉开放，向基底动脉尖及双侧大脑后动脉供血

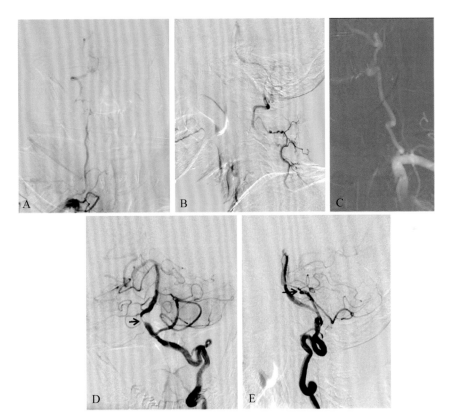

图 5.4.13　DSA 示：**A** 和 **B**. 右椎动脉起始处闭塞，甲状颈干颈升支向右椎动脉 V2 段远端代偿供血；**C ～ E**. 左椎动脉 V1、V2 及 V3 段迂曲，V4 段重度狭窄（箭头示），见小脑后下动脉向小脑前下动脉代偿供血（箭头示）

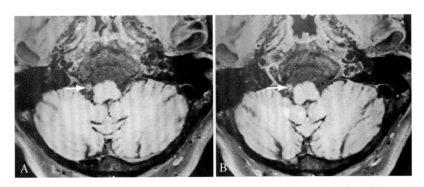

图 5.4.14　高分辨率 MRI 提示左椎动脉 V4 段管壁环形增厚，管腔重度狭窄（箭头示）（**A** 和 **B**）

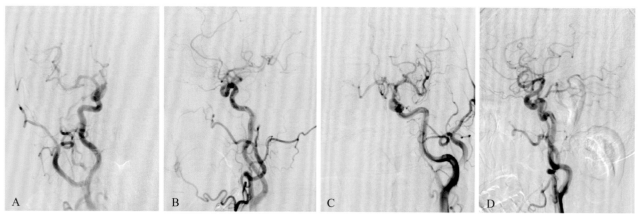

Fig. 5.4.12 The DSA showed the tortuous access in the cavernous segment of the right carotid artery (**A, B**), the left posterior communicating artery was patent and provided compensation for blood flow to the territory of the basilar artery (**C, D**)

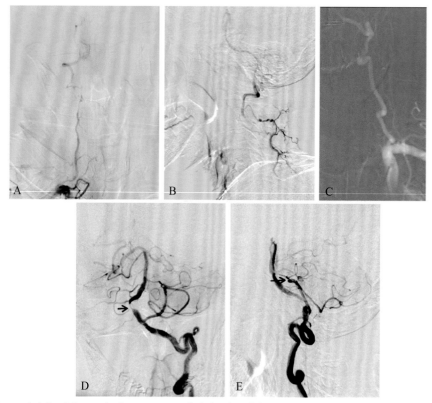

Fig. 5.4.13 The DSA revealed the right vertebral artery was occluded at its origin, and compensation to the distal part of the V2 segment was provided by the ascending branch of the thyrocervical trunk (**A, B**). The extracranial segments of the left vertebral artery were tortuous and the V4 segment exhibited severe stenosis. The left posterior inferior cerebellar artery provided compensation for the anterior inferior cerebellar artery (arrow) (**C–E**)

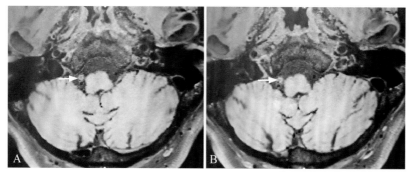

Fig. 5.4.14 The HRMRI showed the V4 segment of the left vertebral artery was severely stenosed, with circumferential thickening of the vessel wall (arrow) (**A, B**)

（二）诊断

路径迂曲的症状性左椎动脉 V4 段狭窄。

（三）术前讨论

结合患者病史及相关影像学检查，考虑右椎动脉 V1 和 V2 段闭塞系本次发病责任病变，血管内介入治疗开通困难。结合患者存在左椎动脉 V4 段重度狭窄，解除狭窄有利于改善后循环低灌注，故选择治疗左椎动脉 V4 段狭窄。但因左椎动脉 V2 和 V3 段路径迂曲，增加血管内介入治疗难度，拟采用长鞘结合中间导管。相关风险包括医源性夹层、急性血栓形成、动脉破裂等。

（四）治疗过程

全麻下右股动脉穿刺入路，置入 7F Cook 长鞘（90 cm），送至左锁骨下动脉，经长鞘送入 6F Navien 导管（115 cm）至左椎动脉 V2 段远端迂曲的近端（图 5.4.15 A 和 B）。造影显示左椎动脉 V4 段重度狭窄（图 5.4.15 C 和 D）。Synchro 微导丝（0.014 in，300 cm）结合 Echelon-10 微导管至基底动脉近端，撤出 Synchro 微导丝，送入 Transend 微导丝（0.014 in，300 cm）至右小脑上动脉（图 5.4.16 A）。撤出微导管，沿微导丝送入赛诺球囊（2.25 mm×10 mm）扩张病变，期间利用球囊锚定，跟进 Navien 导管越过左椎动脉 V2 段远端迂曲（图 5.4.16 B），撤出球囊，路径图显示残余狭窄率约为 40%（图 5.4.16 C），沿微导丝送入 Apollo 球囊扩张式支架（2.5 mm×13 mm）（图 5.4.17 A），对位准确后球囊加压释放支架（图 5.4.17 B），可见支架顺利张开，快速抽瘪球囊，造影示狭窄明显改善，残余狭窄率约为 20%，支架贴壁良好（图 5.4.17 C），

前向血流良好（mTICI 分级 3 级）。观察 10 min 后造影，显示无异常后结束治疗。

（五）讨论

对于路径严重迂曲的颅内动脉狭窄，如果导引导管位置不佳，微导丝及微导管会存在操纵困难，即便微导丝到位，由于导引导管不能提供有效支撑，后续的球囊或支架系统也很难到位。本例选择 Cook 长鞘结合中间导管，将系统远端置于左椎动脉 V2 段，期间使用球囊锚定继续跟进中间导管越过远端迂曲。对于类似病变，只有导引导管解剖位置足够高，才能克服操作困难，顺利完成治疗。

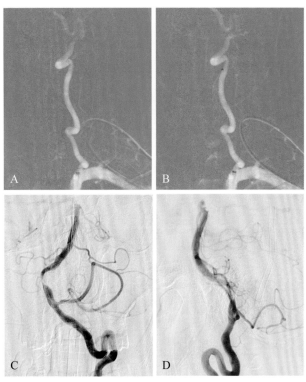

图 5.4.15　**A** 和 **B**. 置入长鞘，经长鞘送入导管至左椎动脉 V2 段；**C** 和 **D**. 术前造影显示左椎动脉 V4 段重度狭窄

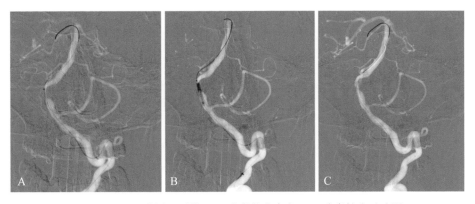

图 5.4.16　**A**. 微导丝到位；**B**. 球囊扩张病变；**C**. 球囊扩张后造影

2. Diagnosis

Symptomatic stenosis in the V4 segment of the left vertebral artery with tortuous proximal anatomy.

3. Treatment schedule

The case involved a patient with multiple infarcts located in the right cerebellar hemisphere and cerebellar vermis. The qualifying artery of the ischemic event was the V1–V2 segments of the right vertebral artery. However, the endovascular recanalization of the right vertebral artery proven to be challenging. The radiological studies revealed severe stenosis in the V4 segment of the dominant left vertebral artery. Stent implantation of the left V4 segment will improve the cerebral perfusion of posterior circulation. The endovascular treatment of the V4 segment of the left vertebral artery was indicated. Treatment approach: In light of the tortuous access at the V2–V3 of the left vertebral artery, a long sheath was employed in combination with an intermediate catheter to enhance the support force to the balloon and stent system. Potential risks associated with this procedure included iatrogenic dissection, acute in-stent thrombosis, arterial rupture, etc.

4. Treatment

Under general anesthesia, a 6F Navien catheter (115 cm) was navigated through the 7F Cook long sheath (90 cm) to access the V2 segment of the left vertebral artery (Fig. 5.4.15 A, B). The angiogram revealed significant stenosis in the V4 segment of the left vertebral artery (Fig. 5.4.15 C, D). With the assistance of Synchro microwire (0.014 in, 300 cm), the Echelon-10 microcatheter was navigated the proximal segment of the basilar artery. Following this, a Transend microwire (0.014 in, 300 cm) was advanced to the right superior cerebellar artery (Fig. 5.4.16 A). A Sino balloon (2.25 mm × 10 mm) was utilized to dilate the stenosis lesion (Fig. 5.4.16 B). By using the balloon anchoring technique, the Navien catheter was subsquently pass through the tortuous segment to access the proximal of the lesion. The roadmap angiogram showed a 40% residual stenosis (Fig. 5.4.16 C). A 2.5 mm × 13 mm Apollo stent was employed to cover the lesion (Fig. 5.4.17 A, B). Post-stent implantation angiogram showed excellent stent wall apposition and residual stenosis of 20%, with grade 3 antegrade blood flow (Fig. 5.4.17 C). Ten minutes later, a final angiogram demonstrated the patency of the stented vessel.

5. Comments

When dealing with the intracranial stenosis and severely tortuous proximal access, navigating the microwire and microcatheter can be challenging without proper guide catheter positioning. Even with the microwire in place, it remains difficult to deploy the balloon or stent system due to the insufficient support force provided by the guide catheter. In this case, the intermediate catheter was positioned at the V2 segment of the left vertebral artery through the 7F long sheath. By using the balloon anchoring technique, the intermediate catheter was subsequently pass through the tortuous segment to access the proximal of the lesion during the procedure. For similar lesions, it is recommended to place the guide catheter as proximal to the lesion as possible to provide sufficient support force to the balloon and stent system.

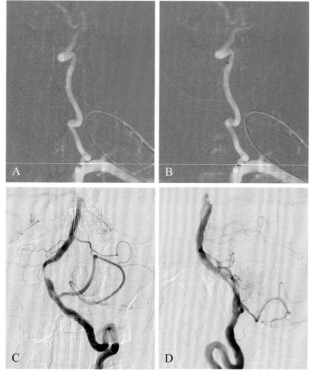

Fig. 5.4.15 A Navien catheter was navigated through the long sheath to access the V2 segment of the left vertebral artery (**A, B**). The angiogram revealed severe stenosis in the V4 segment of the left vertebral artery (**C, D**)

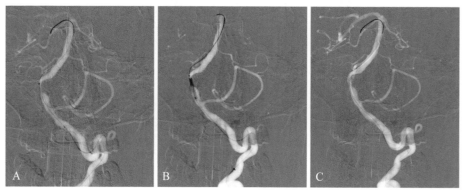

Fig. 5.4.16 (**A**) The Transend microwire was navigated into the right superior cerebellar artery. (**B**) The lesion was dilated with a Sino balloon. (**C**) The angiogram after balloon dilatation

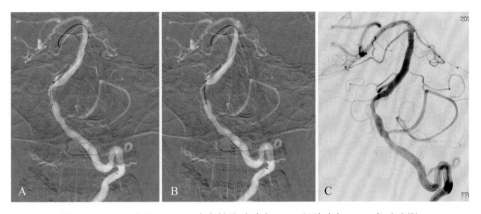

图 5.4.17　**A**.送入 Apollo 球囊扩张式支架；**B**.释放支架；**C**.术后造影

（宋佳　杨明　贾白雪　江裕华　马宁）

病例 19　路径迂曲的右大脑中动脉 M1 段重度狭窄

（一）临床病史及影像分析

患者，男性，58 岁，因"发作性左上肢无力 2 个月"入院。

当地医院头部 CTA 显示右大脑中动脉 M1 段重度狭窄（图 5.4.18）。给予口服阿司匹林、氯吡格雷及阿托伐他汀治疗后症状仍有反复。为进一步治疗来我院就诊。

既往史：高血压病史 20 余年，糖尿病、高脂血症病史 1 年。吸烟 40 年。

查体：左侧肢体轻瘫试验阳性，余无阳性体征。

糖化血红蛋白 7.5%，甘油三酯 2.3 mmol/L。

血栓弹力图：AA 抑制率 54.9%，ADP 抑制率 25.4%。

高分辨率 MRI：右大脑中动脉 M1 段管腔内前下壁偏心性斑块（图 5.4.19），伴明显强化（图 5.4.20）。

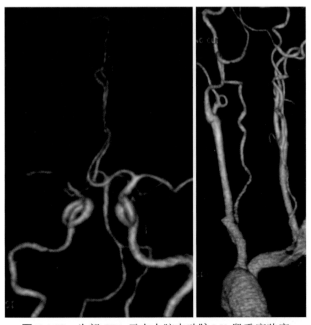

图 5.4.18　头部 CTA 示右大脑中动脉 M1 段重度狭窄

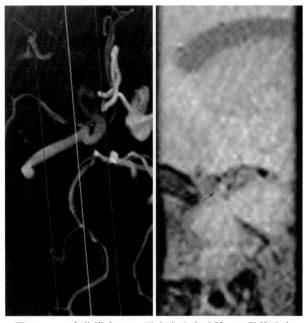

图 5.4.19　高分辨率 MRI 示右大脑中动脉 M1 段管腔内前下壁偏心性斑块

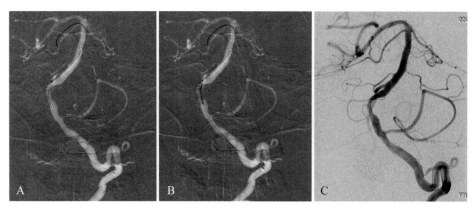

Fig. 5.4.17 (**A, B**) The Apollo balloon-expandable stent was used to cover the lesion. (**C**) The angiogram after stent implantation

(Translated by Rongrong Cui, Revised by Zhikai Hou)

Case 19   Severe stenosis of the M1 segment of the right middle cerebral artery with tortuous proximal anatomy

1. Clinical presentation and radiological studies

A 58-year-old man presented with paroxysmal weakness in the left upper limb for two months.

The CT angiography showed severe stenosis in the M1 segment of the right middle cerebral artery (MCA) (Fig. 5.4.18). Despite receiving aggressive medical treatment, the symptom of weakness in his left upper limb continued to recur.

He had suffered from hypertension for more than 20 years, and had been diagnosed with diabetes and hyperlipidemia for one year. Additionally, he had been a smoker for 40 years.

Physical examination showed left extremity paralysis test was positive.

The Glycated hemoglobin level was record as 7.5%. The concentration of the triglycerides was measured at 2.3 mmol/L.

Thromboelastography showed a 54.9% inhibition of AA and a 25.4% inhibition of ADP.

The high-resolution MRI (HRMRI) scan detected an eccentric plaque located in the anteroinferior wall of the M1 segment of the right MCA (Fig. 5.4.19), exhibiting strong enhancement within the plaque on the contrast-enhanced sequence (Fig. 5.4.20).

Fig. 5.4.18   CTA showed severe stenosis in the M1 segment of the right middle cerebral artery

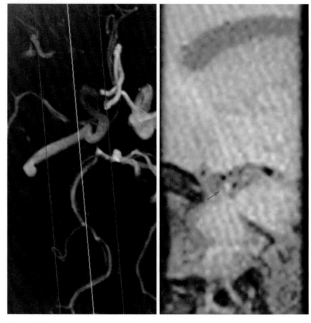

Fig. 5.4.19   HRMRI revealed an eccentric plaque in the anteroinferior wall of the M1 segment of the right MCA

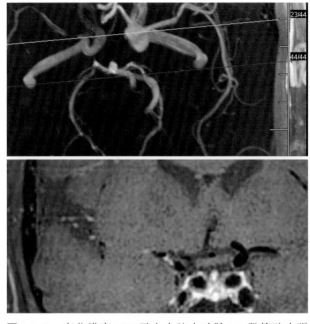

图5.4.20　高分辨率MRI示右大脑中动脉M1段管腔内强化斑块

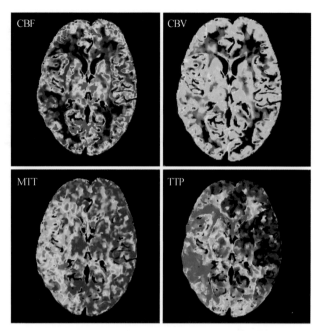

图5.4.22　CTP示右大脑中动脉分布区低灌注

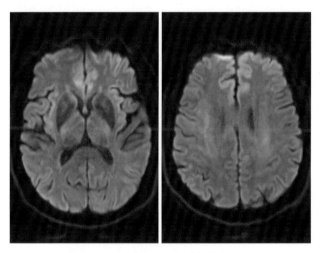

图5.4.21　头部MRI未见急性梗死灶

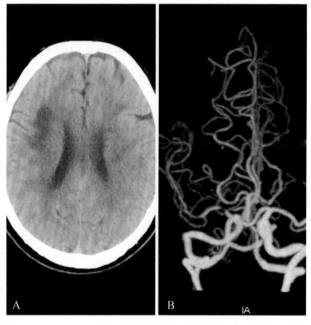

图5.4.23　**A.** CT平扫示右侧额叶、基底节区斑片状梗死灶；**B.** CTA示右大脑中动脉M1段重度狭窄

　　头部MRI：未见急性梗死灶（图5.4.21）。

　　CTP：右大脑中动脉分布区低灌注（图5.4.22）。

　　CT平扫：右侧额叶、基底节区斑片状梗死灶（图5.4.23 A）。

　　CTA：右大脑中动脉M1段重度狭窄（图5.4.23 B）。

　　DSA示右大脑中动脉M1段及右大脑前动脉A1段起始处重度狭窄，右大脑前动脉及右大脑后动脉通过软脑膜支向同侧大脑中动脉代偿供血（图5.4.24），前交通动脉开放（图5.4.25），左椎动脉开口处重度狭窄（图5.4.26）。

（二）诊断

　　路径迂曲的症状性右大脑中动脉重度狭窄。

（三）术前讨论

　　患者右大脑中动脉M1段及右大脑前动脉A1段起始处重度狭窄，同侧大脑前动脉及大脑后动脉经软脑膜动脉向右大脑中动脉供血区域代偿，但代

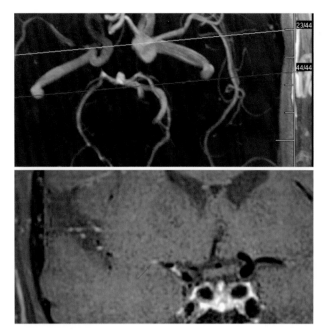

Fig. 5.4.20   The contrast-enhanced scan showed strong enhancement within the plaque

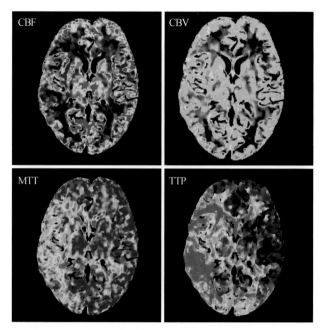

Fig. 5.4.22   CT perfusion demonstrated hypoperfusion in the right middle cerebral artery territory

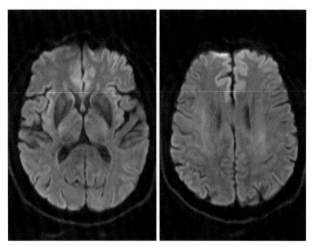

Fig. 5.4.21   The MRI results indicated no presence of acute cerebral infarction

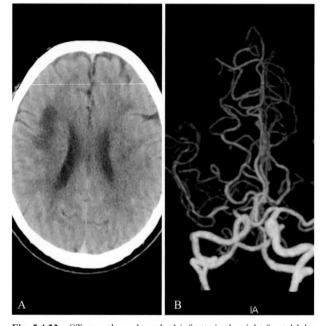

Fig. 5.4.23   CT scan showed cerebral infarcts in the right frontal lobe and basal ganglia (**A**), and CTA showed severe stenosis in the M1 segment of the right MCA (**B**)

The MRI result showed no evidence of an acute cerebral infarction (Fig. 5.4.21).

CT perfusion revealed hypoperfusion in the right middle cerebral artery territory (Fig. 5.4.22).

CT scan showed multiple cerebral infarcts in the right frontal lobe and basal ganglia (Fig. 5.4.23 A).

CTA showed severe stenosis of the M1 segment of the right MCA (Fig. 5.4.23 B).

DSA results showed severe stenosis in the M1 segment of the right MCA and the A1 segment of the right anterior cerebral artery (ACA). The territory of right MCA was compensated by the right ACA and posterior cerebral artery (PCA), through the pial collaterals (Fig. 5.4.24). The anterior communicating artery was patent (Fig. 5.4.25). Additionally, there was a severe stenosis at the origin of the left vertebral artery (Fig. 5.4.26)

2. Diagnosis

Symptomatic severe stenosis of the right middle cerebral artery with tortuous proximal anatomy.

3. Treatment schedule

The patient suffered from severe stenosis in the M1 segment of the right MCA and the A1 segment of the right ACA, and there was inadequate collateral compensation from the right ACA and PCA. According to high-resolution MRI, the stenosis in the

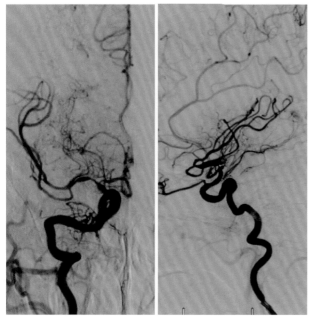

图 5.4.24 DSA 示右大脑中动脉 M1 段及右大脑前动脉 A1 段起始处重度狭窄，右大脑前动脉及右大脑后动脉通过软脑膜支向同侧大脑中动脉代偿供血

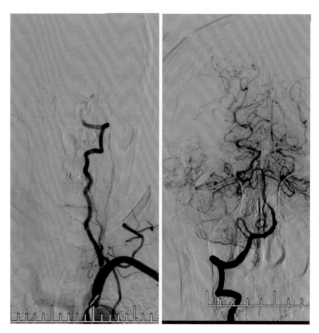

图 5.4.26 DSA 示左椎动脉开口处重度狭窄

（四）治疗过程

全麻下右股动脉置入 8F 动脉鞘，送入 260 cm 泥鳅导丝置于右颈内动脉，交换置入 70 cm 长鞘。沿长鞘送入 6F Navien 导管（115 cm）至右颈内动脉海绵窦段，送入 Transend 微导丝（0.014 in，300 cm）＋ Echelon-10 微导管，路径图下将微导丝送至 M3 段（图 5.4.28），沿微导丝送入 Gateway 球囊（2.0 mm×9 mm），加压至 8 atm，扩张后造影显示残余狭窄率约 40%（图 5.4.29），撤出球囊系统，送入 Wingspan 支架（2.5 mm×9 mm），释

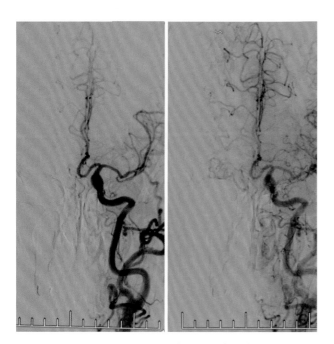

图 5.4.25 DSA 示前交通动脉开放

偿不足。高分辨率 MRI 提示管腔狭窄系动脉粥样硬化斑块所致，在口服双联抗血小板治疗下仍有反复 TIA，考虑药物治疗效果欠佳，有介入治疗指征。右颈动脉造影提示入路迂曲（图 5.4.27），拟使用 7F 长鞘结合 6F Navien 导引导管降低迂曲路径所致技术难度。治疗风险包括穿支闭塞、高灌注、支架内急性或亚急性血栓形成等。

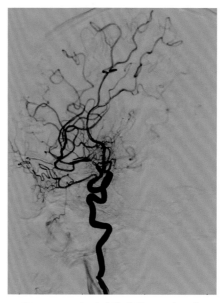

图 5.4.27 右颈动脉造影示入路迂曲

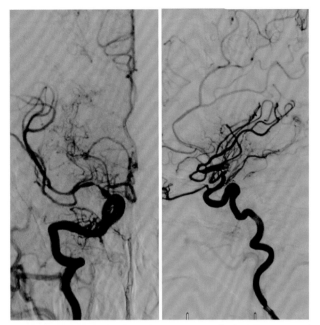

Fig. 5.4.24 DSA results showed severe stenoses in the M1 segment of the right MCA and the A1 segment of the right anterior cerebral artery (ACA). The territory of the right MCA was compensated by the right ACA and posterior cerebral artery (PCA), through the pial collaterals

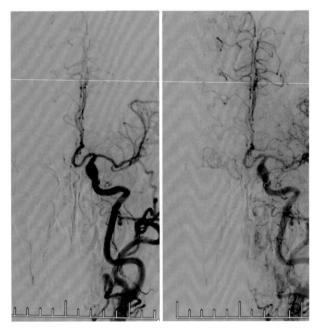

Fig. 5.4.25 DSA showed the anterior communicating artery was patent

MCA was a result of atherosclerotic plaque formation. Despite receiving aggressive medical treatment, the symptom of weakness in his left upper limb continued to recur. Consequently, endovascular treatment was prescribed for the patient. Treatment approach: the angiogram revealed tortuosity at the proximal access of the right carotid artery (Fig. 5.4.27). A 7F long sheath (70 cm) was employed in combination with a 6F Navien guide catheter (115 cm) to enhance the support force to the balloon and stent system. Potential risks associated with the procedure included occlusion of the perforating artery, hyperperfusion syndrome, and acute/subacute in-stent thrombosis.

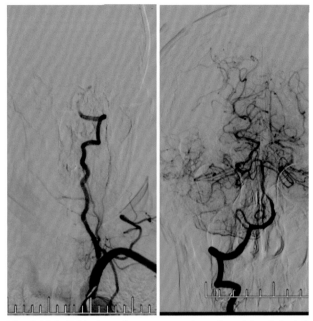

Fig. 5.4.26 DSA showed severe stenosis at the origin of the left vertebral artery

4. Treatment

Under general anesthesia, an 8F sheath was inserted into the right femoral artery. A 260 cm loach guide wire was navigated to the right internal carotid artery (ICA), after which the long sheath (70 cm) was positioned at the C1 segment of the right ICA. A 6F Navien catheter (115 cm) was advanced to the cavernous segment of the right ICA through the long sheath. The Echelon- 10 microcatheter and the Transend microwire (0.014 in, 300 cm) coaxially passed through the lesion to the M3 segment of the right MCA (Fig. 5.4.28). A 2.0 mm×9 mm Gateway balloon was pre-dilated the lesion, while a post-dilation angiogram showed a residual stenosis of 40% (Fig. 5.4.29). Then a 2.5 mm×9 mm

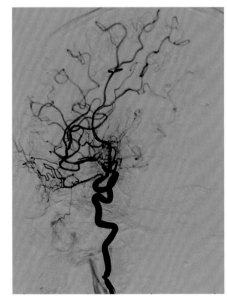

Fig. 5.4.27 The angiogram revealed tortuosity at the proximal access of the right carotid artery

放支架后造影显示残余狭窄率约 10%，前向血流 mTICI 分级 3 级（图 5.4.30）。患者左椎动脉开口处狭窄同期也一并予以处理（图 5.4.31）。

（五）讨论

柔顺的导引导管、更高的导管位置，能解决路径迂曲、微导丝支撑性不足的问题。但在具体操作时要充分考虑到器械长度问题，若想要常用的 130 ～

135 cm 的颅内专用扩张球囊或者支架系统顺利到位，选择 Navien 导管就不能过长（一般 115 cm 为佳），否则会造成球囊及支架系统出不了 Navien 导管头端。此外，具体操作过程中也要充分考虑到 Navien 导管及其外撑的长鞘或者 8F 导引导管前进位置过高时血管损伤（夹层、血管破裂等）的风险亦会增加。

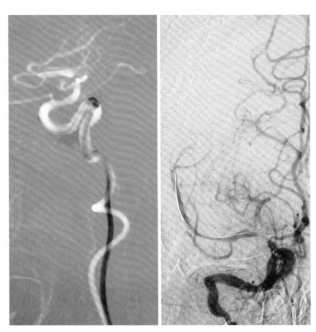

图 5.4.28　将 Transend 微导丝送至右大脑中动脉 M3 段

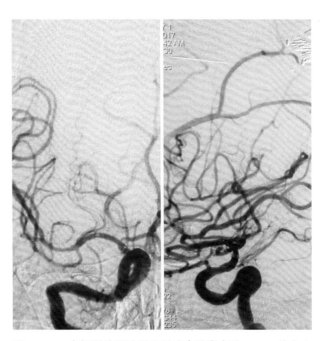

图 5.4.30　支架释放后造影显示残余狭窄率约 10%，前向血流 mTICI 分级 3 级

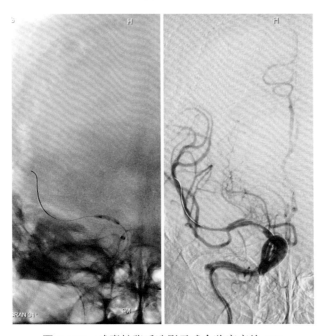

图 5.4.29　球囊扩张后造影示残余狭窄率约 40%

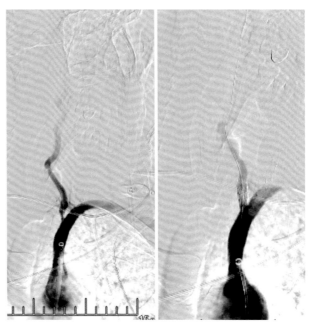

图 5.4.31　左椎动脉开口处狭窄置入支架

（马宁）

Wingspan stent was employed to fully cover the lesion. Post-stent implantation angiogram revealed a residual stenosis of 10%, along with a grade 3 antegrade blood flow (Fig. 5.4.30). Additionally, a stent was placed at the origin of the left vertebral artery (Fig. 5.4.31).

5. Comments

In cases of intracranial stenosis with proximal tortuous anatomy, the use of a flexible guide catheter is necessary to address the inadequate support force of the microwire. Additionally, to further improve the support force, a high guide catheter position is placed to access the lesion. When selecting the device, it is important to consider its length. A 115 cm Navien catheter is ideal for a 130–135 cm intracranial balloon or stent system to be properly positioned. If a longer Navien catheter is used, the balloon and stent system may not extend beyond the catheter tip. However, elevating the device to a higher position may increase the potential risk of arterial injury, such as dissection and vascular rupture.

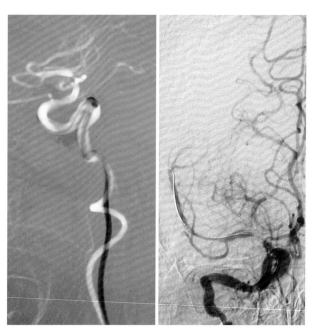

Fig. 5.4.28 The Echelon- 10 microcatheter and the Transend microwire (0.014 in, 300 cm) coaxially passed through the lesion to the M3 segment of the right MCA

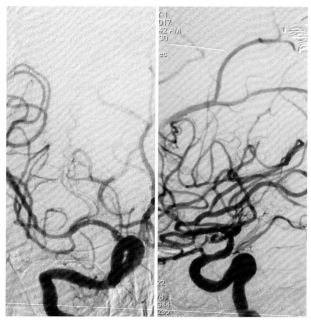

Fig. 5.4.30 Post-stent implantation angiogram revealed a residual stenosis of 10%, along with a grade 3 antegrade blood flow

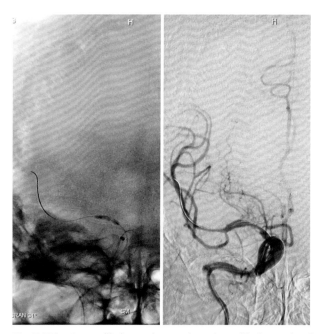

Fig. 5.4.29 A post-dilation angiogram showed a residual stenosis of 40%

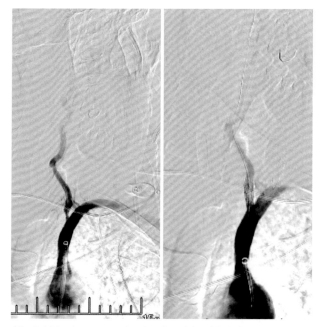

Fig. 5.4.31 A stent was placed at the origin of the left vertebral artery

(Translated by Rongrong Cui, Revised by Zhikai Hou)

第五节　远端着陆区解剖结构复杂

病例 20　着陆区复杂的基底动脉重度狭窄

（一）临床病史及影像分析

患者，女性，51 岁，主因"反复头晕伴行走不稳 2 月余"入院。

当地医院头部 MRI 示脑桥右侧急性梗死灶（图 5.5.1 A 和 B），MRA 示基底动脉近端重度狭窄，双侧大脑后动脉为胚胎型大脑后动脉（图 5.5.1 C 和 D）。给予双联抗血小板及降脂治疗后仍有头晕症状，并偶感视物重影，为行介入治疗收入我院。

既往史：2 型糖尿病 20 余年，高血压 8 年；嗜铬细胞瘤术后。

查体：神经系统查体无明显异常。

入院后 CTP：后循环供血区域低灌注（图 5.5.2）。

高分辨率 MRI：基底动脉次全闭塞，闭塞长度约 5 mm（图 5.5.3 A ～ C），增强扫描可见斑块明显强化（图 5.5.3 D ～ F），考虑溃疡性斑块。

DSA：左椎动脉优势，基底动脉近端次全闭塞，闭塞处存在两个腔道且病变局部迂曲成角，双侧大脑后动脉为胚胎型大脑后动脉；前循环未见明显向后循环供血区域代偿（图 5.5.4）。

入院后予以双联抗血小板（阿司匹林 100 mg 1 次 / 日＋氯吡格雷 75 mg 1 次 / 日）、降脂（阿托伐他汀 20 mg 1 次 / 日）等治疗。

（二）诊断

着陆区复杂的症状性基底动脉重度狭窄。

（三）术前讨论

患者基底动脉系本次责任血管，内科药物治疗后仍有症状反复，有血管内介入治疗指征。考虑到狭窄毗邻双侧 AICA，拟采用稍小直径球囊预扩张，再放置尺寸匹配的自膨式支架。相关风险包括穿支事件、动脉夹层、支架内急性或亚急性血栓形成、高灌注等。

（四）治疗过程

全麻下右股动脉穿刺入路，常规泥鳅导丝携 6F 导引导管经左椎动脉置于 V2 段中段，三维造影提示基底动脉近端次全闭塞（图 5.5.5 A）。将 Synchro-2 微导丝（0.014 in，200 cm）在 SL-10 微导管的辅

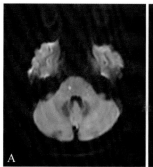
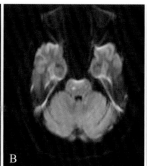
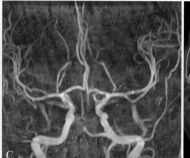
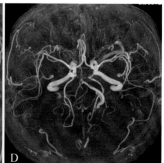

图 5.5.1　头部 MRI 示脑桥右侧急性梗死灶（**A** 和 **B**），MRA 示基底动脉近端重度狭窄，双侧大脑后动脉为胚胎型大脑后动脉（**C** 和 **D**）

Section 5 Complex Distal Landing Zones

Case 20 Severe stenosis of the basilar artery with a complex landing zone

1. Clinical presentation and radiological studies

A 51-year-old woman was admitted to the hospital due to paroxysmal dizziness and unsteady walking lasting over two months.

The MRI results indicated an acute cerebral infarction on the right side of the pontine (Fig. 5.5.1 A, B). The magnetic resonance angiography (MRA) revealed severe stenosis of the proximal basilar artery and bilateral fetal-type posterior cerebral arteries (Fig. 5.5.1 C, D). Despite dual antiplatelet therapy and intensive risk factor control, the patient continued to experience recurrent episodes of dizziness.

The patient has a medical history of diabetes for more than 20 years, hypertension for 8 years, and has undergone surgery for pheochromocytoma.

She was neurologically intact on admission.

CT perfusion revealed hypoperfusion in the posterior circulation (Fig. 5.5.2).

The high-resolution MRI revealed a subtotal occlusion of the basilar artery with a 5 mm occlusion lesion (Fig. 5.5.3 A–C). The contrast-enhanced scan showed significant intraplaque enhancement (Fig. 5.5.3 D–F), indicating an ulcerated plaque.

DSA demonstrated a dominant left vertebral artery, a two-cavity and tortuous lesion of subtotal occlusion at the proximal basilar artery, and fetal-type bilateral posterior cerebral arteries. Furthermore, there was no significant collateralization from the anterior circulation to the posterior circulation system (Fig. 5.5.4).

Following admission, she was prescribed a dual antiplatelet regimen consisting of daily doses of Aspirin at 100 mg and Clopidogrel at 75 mg, as well as a daily dose of Atorvastatin at 20 mg.

2. Diagnosis

Symptomatic severe stenosis of the basilar artery with a complex landing zone.

3. Treatment schedule

This case describes an individual who experienced acute pontine infarction due to symptomatic severe basilar artery stenosis. As the patient continued to experience recurrent dizziness symptoms under aggressive medical treatment, endovascular treatment was warranted. Given the stenosis lesion's proximity to the bilateral AICA, our treatment approach was to pre-dilate the stenosis lesion using a small-sized balloon and subsequently implant a self-expanding stent. Potential procedural risks included occlusion of the perforating artery, arterial dissection, in-stent thrombosis, and hyperperfusion syndrome.

4. Treatment

Under general anesthesia, a 6F guiding catheter was inserted at the V2 segment of the left vertebral artery. An angiogram confirmed a subtotal occlusion at the proximal segment of the basilar artery (Fig. 5.5.5 A). The Synchro-2 microwire (0.014 in, 200 cm) and SL-10 microcatheter

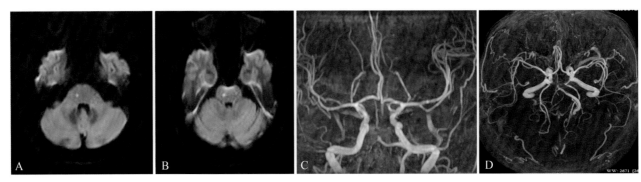

Fig. 5.5.1 The MRI showed acute cerebral infarction on the right side of the pontine (**A, B**). The MRA revealed severe stenosis of the proximal basilar artery and bilateral fetal-type posterior cerebral arteries (**C, D**)

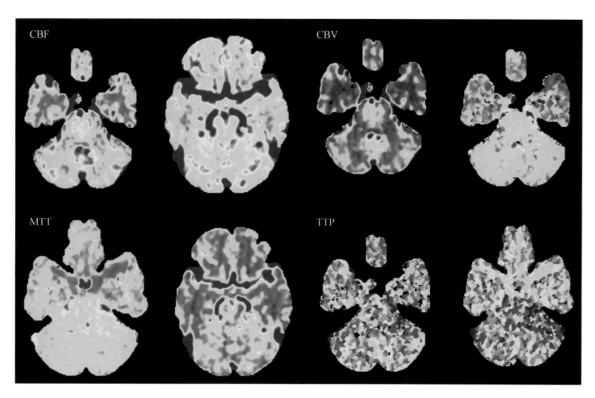

图 5.5.2 CTP 示后循环区域低灌注

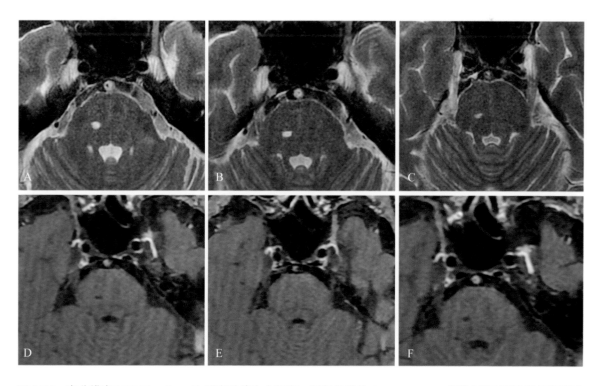

图 5.5.3 高分辨率 MRI 示：**A ～ C**. 基底动脉次全闭塞，闭塞长度约 5 mm；**D ～ F**. 增强扫描可见斑块明显强化

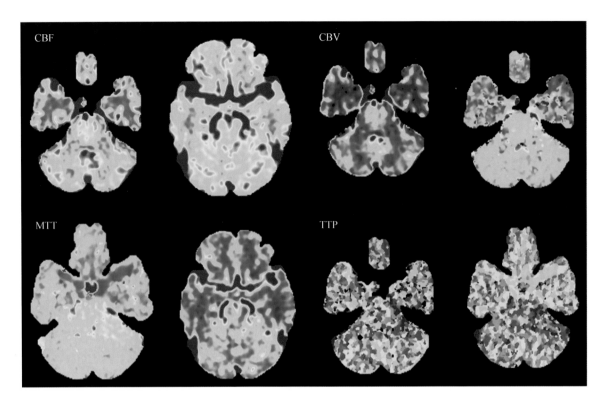

Fig. 5.5.2   CT perfusion revealed hypoperfusion in the posterior circulation

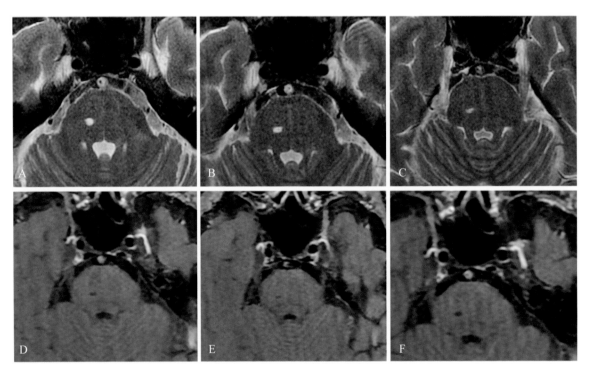

Fig. 5.5.3   HRMRI showed a subtotal occlusion of the basilar artery with a 5 mm occlusion lesion (**A**−**C**). The contrast-enhanced scan showed significant intra-plaque enhancement (**D**−**F**)

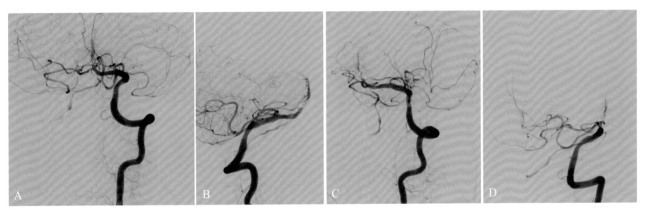

图 5.5.4　DSA 示左椎动脉优势，基底动脉近端次全闭塞，闭塞处存在两个腔道且病变局部迂曲成角，双侧大脑后动脉为胚胎型大脑后动脉；前循环未见明显向后循环供血区域代偿

助下，顺利通过病变段，到达左小脑上动脉（图 5.5.5 B），撤出 Synchro-2 微导丝，更换为 Transend 微导丝（0.014 in，300 cm），送入 Gateway 球囊（1.5 mm×9 mm）扩张病变（图 5.5.5 C 和 D）。撤出球囊，经微导丝送入 XT-27 微导管，经其送入

Neuroform EZ 自膨式支架（2.5 mm×15 mm）至基底动脉狭窄段释放，造影显示前向血流良好，mTICI 分级 3 级，残余狭窄率约为 20%（图 5.5.5 E 和 F）。观察 10 min，术后颅内动脉三维 DSA 提示基底动脉支架术后血流通畅（图 5.5.5 G）。

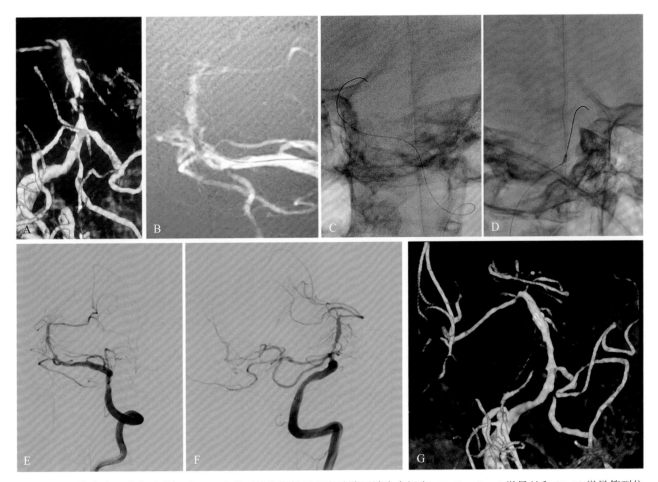

图 5.5.5　血管内介入治疗过程如下：**A**. 术前三维造影提示基底动脉近端次全闭塞；**B**. Synchro-2 微导丝和 SL-10 微导管到位于左小脑上动脉；**C** 和 **D**. Gateway 球囊扩张病变；**E** 和 **F**. 支架置入后造影示 mTICI 分级 3 级，残余狭窄率约 20%；**G**. 术后三维 DSA 示基底动脉支架术后血流通畅

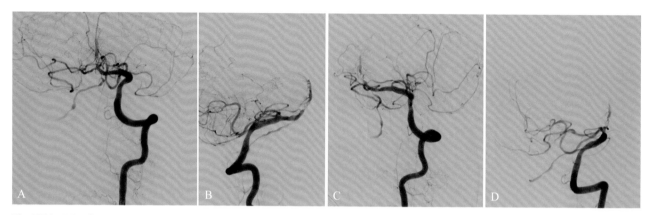

Fig. 5.5.4 DSA demonstrated a dominant left vertebral artery, a two-cavity and tortuous lesion of subtotal occlusion at the proximal basilar artery, and fetal-type bilateral posterior cerebral arteries. Furthermore, there was no significant collateralization from the anterior circulation to the posterior circulation system

coaxially traverse through the lesion to the left superior cerebellar artery (Fig. 5.5.5 B). The Synchro-2 microwire was withdrawn and replaced with the Transend microwire (0.014 in, 300 cm). The lesion was pre-dilated with a Gateway balloon (1.5 mm×9 mm) (Fig. 5.5.5 C, D). Subsequently, a 2.5 mm×15 mm Neuroform EZ stent was released to cover the lesion. After the stent implantation, an angiogram displayed a residual stenosis of 20%, with a grade 3 of antegrade blood flow (Fig. 5.5.5 E, F). After monitoring for around ten minutes, a post-procedural three- dimensional angiogram indicated the stent in the basilar artery was patent (Fig. 5.5.5 G).

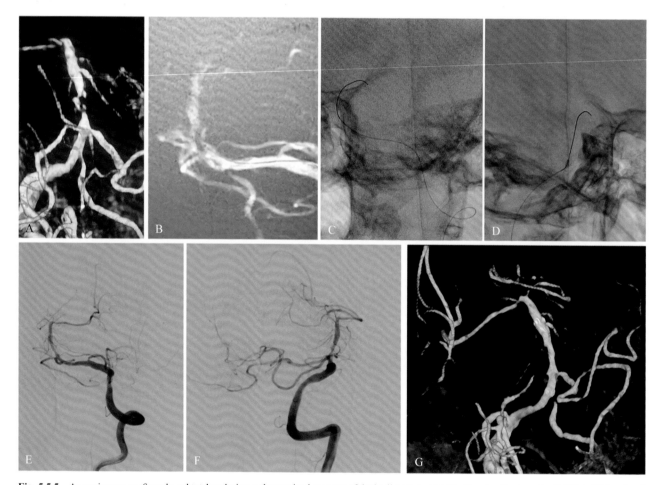

Fig. 5.5.5 An angiogram confirmed a subtotal occlusion at the proximal segment of the basilar artery (**A**). The Synchro-2 microwire (0.014 in, 200 cm) and SL-10 microcatheter coaxially traverse through the lesion to the left superior cerebellar artery (**B**). The lesion was pre-dilated with a Gateway balloon (1.5 mm×9 mm) (**C, D**). A 2.5 mm×15 mm Neuroform EZ stent was released to cover the lesion. After the stent implantation, an angiogram displayed a residual stenosis of 20%, with a grade 3 of antegrade blood flow (**E, F**). A three-dimensional DSA revealed the stent in the basilar artery was patent (**G**)

术后 CT 未见出血及梗死。患者无特殊不适。

（五）讨论

本例基底动脉次全闭塞，病变周围可见大量新生血管，血管内治疗穿支事件风险极大。同时术前 DSA 提示闭塞存在两个腔道且病变局部迂曲成角，另一方面基底动脉的顶端结构不完全，双侧大脑后动脉为胚胎型且右小脑上动脉未见显示，为导丝着陆带来困难。高分辨率 MRI 显示斑块为溃疡性斑块，右侧腔道应为通向远端的通道，这与导丝通过病变的路径一致。本例病变采用稍小直径球囊扩张病变并放置 off-label 自膨式支架，以减少术后穿支卒中风险。

（徐子奇　陈涵丰　俞妮妮　马宁）

病例 21　着陆区复杂的基底动脉重度狭窄

（一）临床病史及影像分析

患者，女，52 岁，主因"间断发作头晕 9 个月"入院。

当地医院头部 MRI 提示无新发梗死病灶（图 5.5.6）。头部 MRA 提示基底动脉重度狭窄（图 5.5.7）。予以双联抗血小板及他汀类药物治疗后仍有头晕反复发作，为行血管内介入治疗来我院就诊。

既往史：高血压及糖尿病病史 5 年。

查体：神经系统查体未见明显异常。

入院后 CTP：后循环区域低灌注（图 5.5.8）。

DSA：左椎动脉 V4 段闭塞，左 PICA 起始部重度狭窄（图 5.5.9 A 和 B），基底动脉中段重度狭

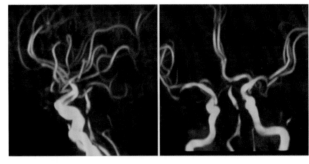

图 5.5.7　头部 MRA 示基底动脉重度狭窄

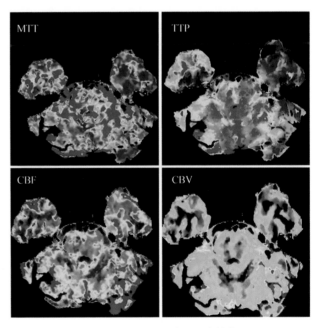

MTT　　TTP

CBF　　CBV

图 5.5.8　CTP 示后循环区域低灌注

窄，左侧胚胎型大脑后动脉，右大脑后动脉 P1 段中-重度狭窄（图 5.5.9 C 和 D）。

入院后给予双联抗血小板（阿司匹林 100 mg 1 次 / 日＋氯吡格雷 75 mg 1 次 / 日）、降脂（阿托伐他汀 10 mg 1 次 / 日）等治疗。

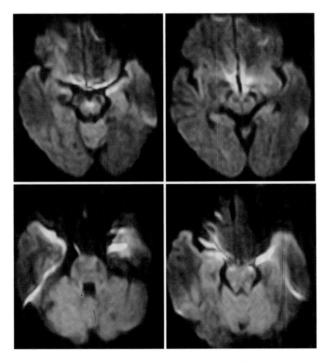

图 5.5.6　头部 MRI 未见新发梗死灶

The CT scan performed after the procedure indicated the absence of any cerebral hemorrhage or infarction.

5. Comments

This particular case involved an individual with subtotal occlusion and significant new vessel formation, which posed a considerable risk of perforating artery occlusion during endovascular treatment. The pre-procedural angiogram showed a tortuous two-cavity lesion of subtotal occlusion at the proximal basilar artery, along with an incomplete anatomical structure of the basilar artery, making it challenging to land the microwire. The high-resolution MRI depicted an ulcerated plaque on the basilar artery, with the right cavity leading to the distal segment of the basilar artery, which was also in line with the path taken by the microwire. To mitigate the risk of perforating artery occlusion following the procedure, a smallsized balloon was used to pre-dilate the stenotic lesion before implanting a self-expanding stent.

(Translated by Rongrong Cui, Revised by Zhikai Hou)

Case 21　Severe stenosis of the basilar artery with a complex landing zone

1. Clinical presentation and radiological studies

A 52-year-old woman was admitted to the hospital due to paroxysmal dizziness for 9 months.

The MRI result showed the absence of acute cerebral infarction (Fig. 5.5.6). The MRA indicated severe stenosis of the basilar artery (Fig. 5.5.7). Despite dual antiplatelet therapy and intensive risk factor control, the patient continued to experience recurrent episodes of dizziness.

Her medical history included hypertension and diabetes.

She was neurologically intact on admission.

CT perfusion revealed hypoperfusion in the posterior circulation territory (Fig. 5.5.8).

DSA revealed various medical conditions, including occlusion of the V4 segment of the left vertebral artery, severe stenosis at the origin of the left posterior inferior cerebellar artery (Fig. 5.5.9 A, B), severe stenosis of the mid-

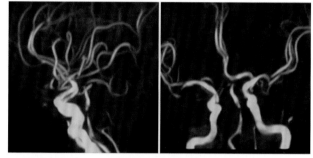

Fig. 5.5.7　The MRA showed severe stenosis of the basilar artery

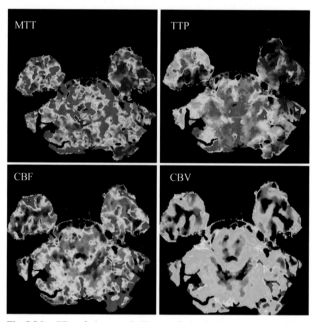

Fig. 5.5.8　CT perfusion revealed hypoperfusion in the posterior circulation territory

basilar artery, a fetal-type left posterior cerebral artery, and moderate to severe stenosis of the P1 segment of the right posterior cerebral artery (Fig. 5.5.9 C, D)

Upon admission, the patient was prescribed a dual antiplatelet regimen consisting of daily doses of Aspirin at 100 mg and Clopidogrel at 75 mg, as well as statin therapy with Atorvastatin at a daily dose of 10 mg.

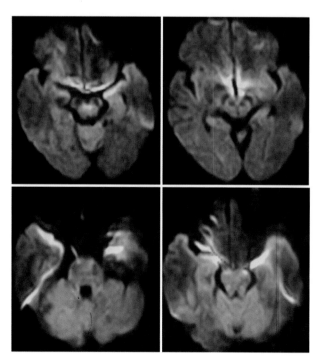

Fig. 5.5.6　The MRI showed no acute cerebral infarction

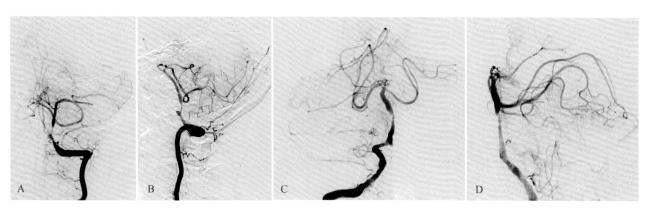

图 5.5.9　DSA 示：**A** 和 **B**. 左椎动脉 V4 段闭塞，左 PICA 起始部重度狭窄；**C** 和 **D**. 基底动脉中段重度狭窄，左侧胚胎型大脑后动脉，右大脑后动脉 P1 段中-重度狭窄

（二）诊断

着陆区复杂的症状性基底动脉重度狭窄。

（三）术前讨论

患者近期反复后循环缺血发作，规律内科药物治疗下效果欠佳，考虑基底动脉中段重度狭窄为责任病变，有血管内介入治疗指征。因右大脑后动脉 P1 段有中-重度狭窄，左大脑后动脉为胚胎型，术中拟选择小脑上动脉为微导丝着陆区。微导丝到位后先用小球囊预扩张，然后再放置自膨式支架。相关风险包括穿支闭塞、动脉夹层、急性或亚急性血栓形成等。

（四）治疗过程

全麻下右股动脉入路，将 6F 导引导管放置于右椎动脉 V2 段中段。路径图下将 Transend 微导丝（0.014 in，300 cm）越过狭窄段，导丝头端放置于左小脑上动脉中段（图 5.5.10 A）。沿微导丝送入 Gateway 球囊（2.0 mm×9 mm）准确定位于基底动脉狭窄处预扩张（图 5.5.10 B）。撤出球囊导管，送入 XT-27 微导管，将微导管的头端置于基底动脉顶端。将 Neuroform EZ 自膨式支架（3.0 mm×15 mm）头端导丝剪除（图 5.5.10 C），沿微导管送至基底动脉，完全覆盖病变后释放支架（图 5.5.10 D 和 E），造影显示前向血流良好，mTICI 分级 3 级，残余狭

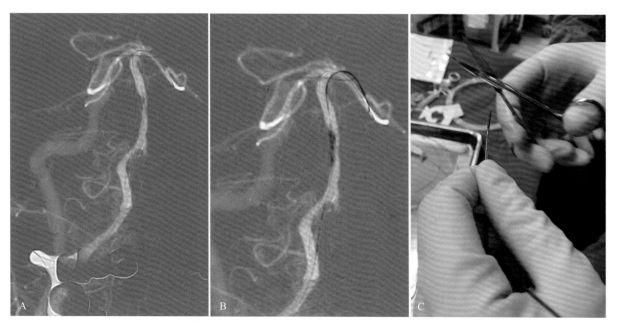

图 5.5.10　血管内介入治疗过程如下：**A**. Transend 微导丝到位于左小脑上动脉中段；**B**. Gateway 球囊预扩张病变；**C**. 剪除 Neuroform EZ 支架头端导丝

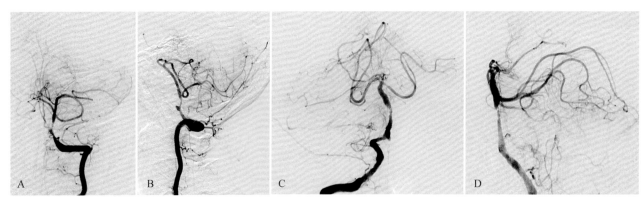

Fig. 5.5.9 DSA revealed an occlusion of the V4 segment of the left vertebral artery, severe stenosis at the origin of the left posterior inferior cerebellar artery (**A**, **B**), severe stenosis of the mid-basilar artery, a fetal-type left posterior cerebral artery, and moderate to severe stenosis of the P1 segment of the right posterior cerebral artery (**C**, **D**)

2. Diagnosis

Symptomatic severe stenosis of the basilar artery with a complex landing zone.

3. Treatment schedule

This case involved a patient with recurrent posterior circulation ischemia due to severe stenosis of the basilar artery. Despite undergoing dual antiplatelet therapy and intensive management of risk factors, the patient suffered from recurrent episodes of dizziness. As such, endovascular treatment was indicated. Treatment approach: given the patient's moderate-to-severe stenosis in the P1 segment of the right posterior cerebral artery and the presence of a fetal-type left posterior cerebral artery, it was decided that the superior cerebellar artery would serve as the optimal landing zone for the procedure. A small-sized balloon was used to pre-dilate the stenotic lesion, following which a self-expanding stent

was implanted. Potential risks associated with the procedure included occlusion of perforating arteries, arterial dissection, and in-stent thrombosis.

4. Treatment

Under general anesthesia, a 6F guiding catheter was positioned at the V2 segment of the right vertebral artery. A Transend microwire (0.014 in, 300 cm) was then navigated through the stenotic segment and advanced to the middle segment of the left superior cerebellar artery (Fig. 5.5.10 A). Subsequently, a 2.0 mm×9 mm Gateway balloon was utilized to dilate the lesion (Fig. 5.5.10 B). Following an exchange technique, an XT-27 microcatheter was delivered and its tip was placed at the distal segment of the basilar artery. A 3.0 mm×15 mm Neuroform EZ stent, with its tip clipped off (Fig. 5.5.10 C), was then deployed to fully cover the lesion (Fig. 5.5.10 D, E). Post-stent implantation angiogram revealed a residual stenosis of 25%, with a grade

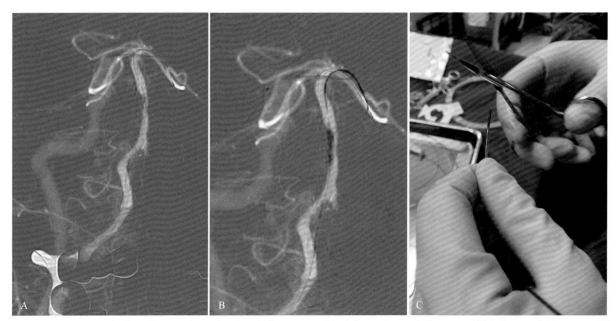

Fig. 5.5.10 (**A**) A Transend microwire was advanced to the middle segment of the left superior cerebellar artery. (**B**) A Gateway balloon was utilized to dilate the lesion. (**C**) The tip of the Neuroform EZ stent was clipped off

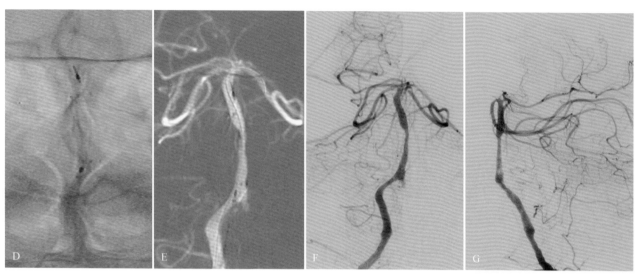

图 5.5.10 续。**D** 和 **E**.完全覆盖病变后释放支架；**F** 和 **G**.释放支架后造影

窄率约 25%（图 5.5.10 F 和 G）。观察 10 min 血流无变化后结束治疗。

术后查体同前。

术后即刻头部 CT 未见出血（图 5.5.11）。术后头部 CTA 示基底动脉支架内通畅（图 5.5.12）。

（五）讨论

本例基底动脉重度狭窄，因远端着陆区不佳（右大脑后动脉 P1 段狭窄，左大脑后动脉胚胎型，双侧小脑上动脉与基底动脉主干夹角较大），故支架释放导管仅能放置在基底动脉远段。考虑 XT-27 微导管头端距支架释放位置的解剖距离较近（约 10 mm），故术中决定剪除 Neuroform EZ 支架头端导丝，避免释放支架过程中头端导丝损伤血管。在此种情况下释放支架，须避免前推导丝，以免尖锐的支架头端致血管穿孔。本例残余狭窄稍重，与选择球囊直径稍小有关，考虑穿支闭塞风险未行球囊后扩张治疗。

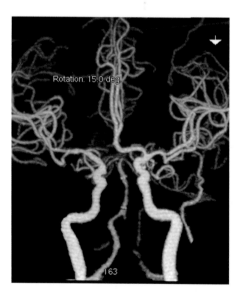

图 5.5.12 术后头部 CTA 提示基底动脉支架内通畅

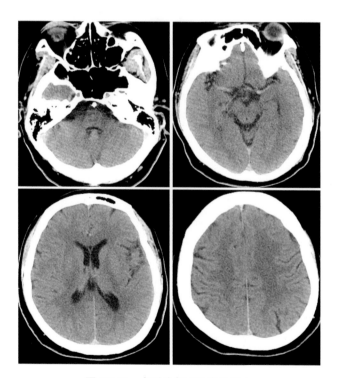

图 5.5.11 术后头部 CT 未见出血

（崔凯 张义森 姜鹏 马宁）

5.5 手术操作视频
（病例 21）

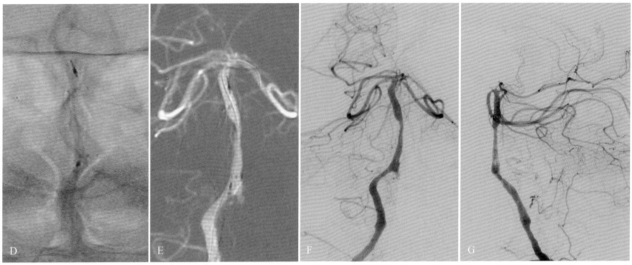

Fig. 5.5.10 Continued. (**D, E**) The Neuroform EZ stent was deployed to cover the lesion. (**F, G**) The angiogram after the stent implantation

3 for antegrade blood flow (Fig. 5.5.10 F, G). Following an observation period of ten minutes, an angiogram indicated that the stent in the basilar artery was patent.

CT scan performed after the procedure revealed no signs of cerebral hemorrhage (Fig. 5.5.11). Postprocedural CT angiography showed the basilar artery stent was patent (Fig. 5.5.12).

5. Comments

In this case, we reported a patient with severe basilar artery stenosis with a complex landing zone. the patient had moderate-to-severe stenosis in the right P1 segment and a fetaltype left posterior cerebral artery, with a large angle between the bilateral superior cerebellar artery and the trunk of the basilar artery. The stent release catheter was placed at the distal segment of the basilar artery during the procedure. Due to the relatively short anatomical distance (approximately 10 mm) between the XT-27 microcatheter tip and the stent release site, the stent tip was clipped off to avoid iatrogenic artery injury. In order to avoid perforation of the blood vessels by the sharp edges of the stent, it is recommended that the delivery wire not be pushed forward during stent deployment. The presence of significant residual stenosis after stent implantation may be related to the use of a small-sized balloon during pre-dilation. Due to the risk of occlusion of the perforating artery, post-dilation was not performed.

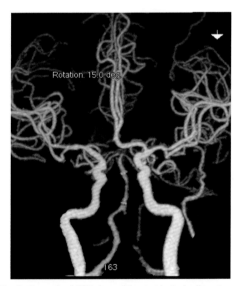

Fig. 5.5.12 Postprocedural CTA showed the stent in the basilar artery was patent

Fig. 5.5.11 Postprocedural CT showed no signs of cerebral hemorrhage

(Translated by Rongrong Cui, Revised by Zhikai Hou)

5.5 Video of endovascular therapy (Case 21)

第六节 狭窄合并动脉瘤

病例 22 症状性基底动脉狭窄合并远端动脉瘤

（一）临床病史及影像分析

患者，男性，60岁，主因"发作性意识丧失、四肢无力2月余"入院。

当地医院头部 MRI 提示左侧枕叶急性脑梗死（图5.6.1）。头部 MRA（图5.6.2）和头颈部 CTA（图5.6.3）提示基底动脉下段重度狭窄。给予双联抗血小板聚集和他汀类药物调脂等治疗后症状仍反复。为进一步诊治收入我院。

既往史：高血压病史15年，心肌梗死病史10年，2型糖尿病病史3年。吸烟40年，饮酒40年。

查体：神经系统查体未见明显异常。

术前改良 Rankin 量表评分1分。

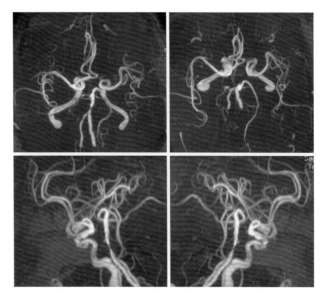

图5.6.2 头部 MRA 示基底动脉下段重度狭窄

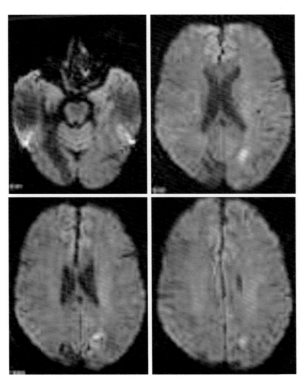

图5.6.1 头部 MRI 示左侧枕叶急性脑梗死

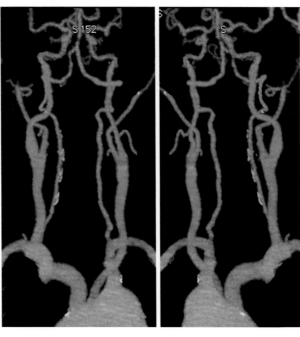

图5.6.3 头颈部 CTA 示基底动脉下段重度狭窄

Section 6   ICAS with Concurrent Aneurysm

Case 22   Symptomatic stenosis of the basilar artery concurrent with a terminal aneurysm

1. Clinical presentation and radiological studies

A 60-year-old male patient presented with episodes of sudden unconsciousness and weakness in all four limbs persisting for more than two months.

The MRI indicated acute cerebral infarcts in the left occipital lobe (Fig. 5.6.1). The result of the MRA (Fig. 5.6.2) and CTA (Fig. 5.6.3) identified severe stenosis at the lower segment of the basilar artery. Despite dual antiplatelet therapy and intensive risk factor control, the patient continued to experience recurrent episodes.

The patient had hypertension for 15 years, experienced a myocardial infarction 10 years ago, and was diagnosed with diabetes 3 years ago. Additionally, he had been smoking cigarettes and consuming alcohol for 40 years.

He was neurologically intact on admission.

The pre-procedural mRS score was 1.

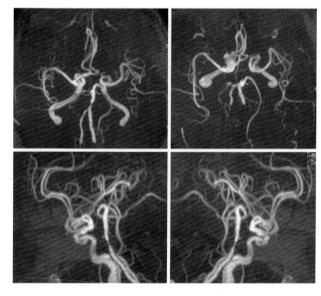

Fig. 5.6.2   The MRA showed severe stenosis at the proximal segment of the basilar artery

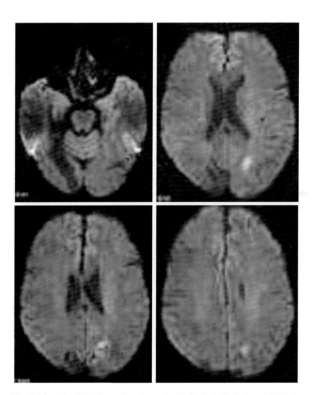

Fig. 5.6.1   The MRI showed acute cerebral infarcts in the left occipital lobe

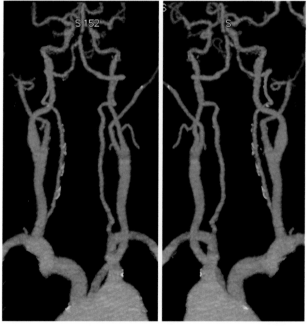

Fig. 5.6.3   The CTA showed severe stenosis at the proximal segment of the basilar artery

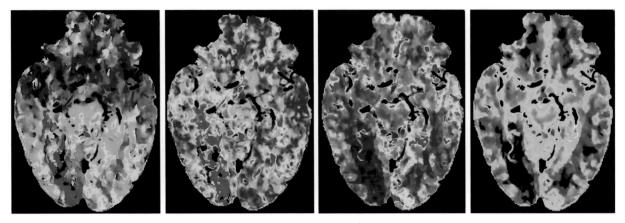

图 5.6.4　CTP 示右颞枕叶低灌注，MTT 和 TTP 延长，CBF 下降，CBV 正常

糖化血红蛋白 8.3%，低密度脂蛋白胆固醇（LDL-C）2.24 mmol/L。

血栓弹力图：AA 抑制率 98.3%，ADP 抑制率 20.6%。

CYP2C19 基因型：中等代谢型。

CTP：右颞枕叶低灌注，MTT 和 TTP 延长，CBF 下降，CBV 正常（图 5.6.4）。

头部 MRI：小脑多个点状急性梗死灶（图 5.6.5）。

高分辨率 MRI：基底动脉中下段斑块形成，斑块部分强化（图 5.6.6）。

DSA：前交通动脉开放，右后交通动脉纤细（图 5.6.7 A 和 B），左后交通动脉未开放（图 5.6.7 C 和 D），右椎动脉 V4 段以远显影浅淡（图 5.6.8），左椎动脉优势，基底动脉中下段重度狭窄，右大脑后动脉较为纤细，左大脑后动脉开口部成角明显（图 5.6.9），狭窄段左侧有 AICA 发出，但 AICA 较纤细，基底动脉狭窄远端见一约 1.5 mm×1.5 mm 动脉瘤，形态不规则（图 5.6.10）。

入院后给予双联抗血小板（阿司匹林 100 mg 1 次 / 日 + 氯吡格雷 75 mg 1 次 / 日）、强化降脂（阿托伐他汀 40 mg 1 次 / 日）等治疗。

（二）诊断

症状性基底动脉狭窄合并远端动脉瘤。

（三）术前讨论

患者有后循环脑梗死。MRA、CTA、DSA 均提示基底动脉重度狭窄，基底动脉为责任血管，且药物治疗效果欠佳，有介入治疗指征。基底动脉瘤形态不规则，有破裂风险，准备同期行动脉瘤栓塞术。基底动脉狭窄段较局限且直，拟放置球囊扩张式支架，支架释放后会覆盖动脉瘤的瘤颈，拟微导管钻支架网眼后栓塞动脉瘤。如果支架置入后，动脉瘤血液滞留，可考虑不予以栓塞。相关风险包括穿支动脉闭塞、动脉瘤破裂出血、急性或亚急性血栓形成。

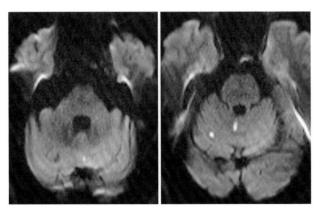

图 5.6.5　入院后头部 MRI 示小脑多个点状急性梗死灶

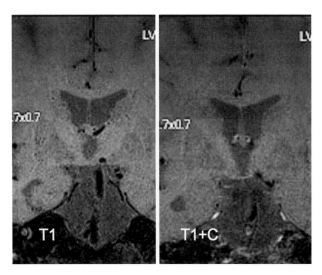

图 5.6.6　高分辨率 MRI 示基底动脉中下段斑块形成，斑块部分强化

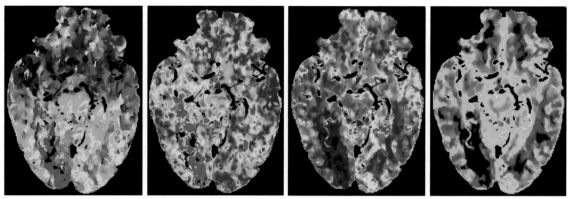

Fig. 5.6.4   CT perfusion revealed hypoperfusion in the right temporo-occipital lobe

The level of Glycosylated hemoglobin was 8.3%, and the concentration of LDL-C was at 2.24 mmol/L.

The thromboelastography test revealed a 98.3% inhibition of AA and a 20.6% inhibition of ADP. The individual's CYP2C19 genotype was that of an intermediate metabolizer.

The CT perfusion revealed hypoperfusion in the right temporo-occipital lobe, characterized by prolonged mean transit time (MTT) and time to peak (TTP), as well as reduced cerebral blood flow (CBF), while the cerebral blood volume (CBV) was normal (Fig. 5.6.4).

Subsequent MRI performed following admission showed multiple acute punctate infarctions in the cerebellum (Fig. 5.6.5).

High-resolution MRI demonstrated the existence of an atherosclerotic plaque at the middle to inferior segments of the basilar artery, exhibiting enhancement within the plaque on contrast-enhanced imaging (Fig. 5.6.6).

The DSA findings indicated that the anterior communicating artery was unobstructed, the right posterior communicating artery was tenuously patent (Fig. 5.6.7 A, B), and the left posterior communicating artery was not open (Fig. 5.6.7 C, D). Visualization of the distal segment to the V4 section of the right vertebral artery was suboptimal (Fig. 5.6.8). The left vertebral artery exhibited dominance, while the middle-inferior segments of the basilar artery displayed severe stenosis. The right posterior cerebral artery was also tenuously patent, and the origin of the left posterior cerebral artery was angulated (Fig. 5.6.9). Furthermore, a tenuous anterior inferior cerebellar artery originated from the left stenotic segment. An irregularly shaped aneurysm with a diameter of 1.5 mm was observed distal to the basilar artery stenosis (Fig. 5.6.10).

Following admission, he was prescribed a daily regimen of 100 mg of Aspirin, 75 mg of Clopidogrel, and 40 mg of Atorvastatin.

2. Diagnosis

Symptomatic stenosis of the basilar artery concurrent with a terminal aneurysm.

3. Treatment schedule

This case concerns a patient who suffered from posterior circulation infarction due to symptomatic basilar artery stenosis. Despite being on dual antiplatelet therapy and receiving intensive risk factor control, the patient continued to experience recurrent episodes. As a result, endovascular therapy was recommended. Additionally, the patient with severe basilar artery stenosis coexisted with an irregular aneurysm, which carried the inherent risk of rupture. To address this, we opted for a simultaneous aneurysm coiling procedure. Treatment approach: the stenotic lesion at the middle-inferior segment of the basilar artery was recognized to be relatively short and straight in nature. To address this, a balloon-expandable stent was utilized to cover the affected area. The neck of the aneurysm will be covered after the stent implantation. Subsequently, a microcatheter was navigated to the stent mesh for the purpose of embolizing the aneurysm. However, if there is stasis of blood within the aneurysm after the stent placement, coiling embolization may not be performed. Potential risks associated with the procedure included perforating artery occlusion, aneurysm rupture, and in-stent thrombosis.

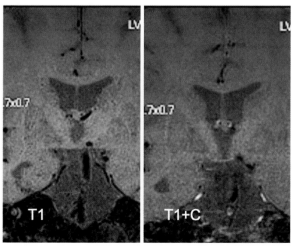

Fig. 5.6.6   HRMRI indicated the existence of an atherosclerotic plaque at the middle to inferior segments of the basilar artery, exhibiting enhancement within the plaque on contrast-enhanced imaging

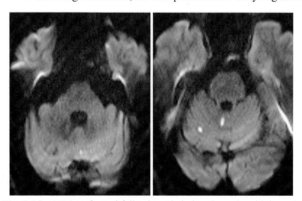

Fig. 5.6.5   MRI performed following admission showed multiple acute punctate infarctions in the cerebellum

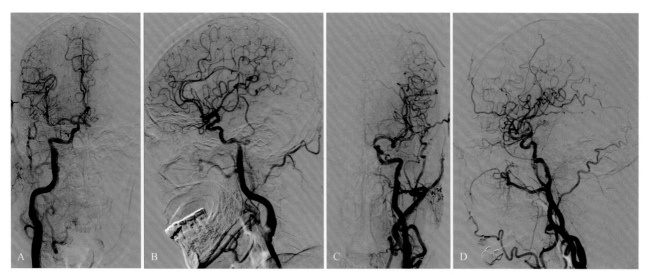

图 5.6.7 DSA 示前交通动脉开放，右后交通动脉纤细（**A** 和 **B**），左后交通动脉未开放（**C** 和 **D**）

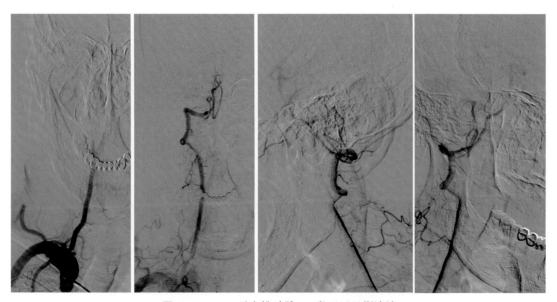

图 5.6.8 DSA 示右椎动脉 V4 段以远显影浅淡

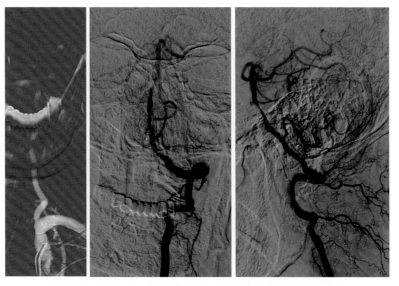

图 5.6.9 DSA 示左椎动脉优势，基底动脉中下段重度狭窄

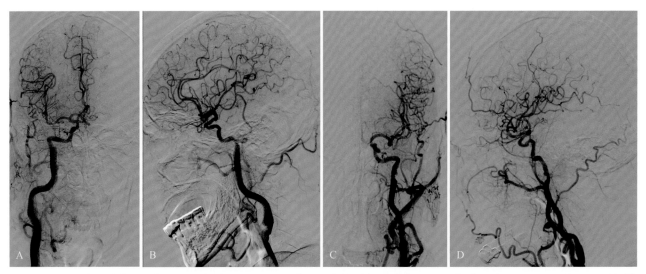

Fig. 5.6.7 DSA showed the anterior communicating artery was unobstructed, the right posterior communicating artery was tenuously patent (**A**, **B**), and the left posterior communicating artery was not open (**C**, **D**)

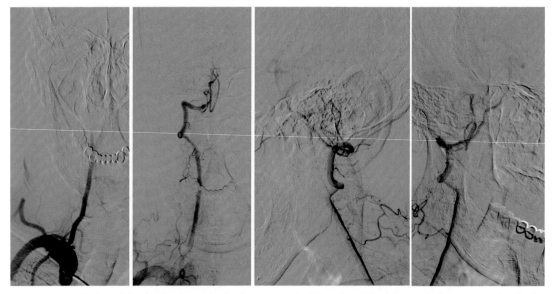

Fig. 5.6.8 DSA showed the visualization of the distal segment to the V4 section of the right vertebral artery was suboptimal

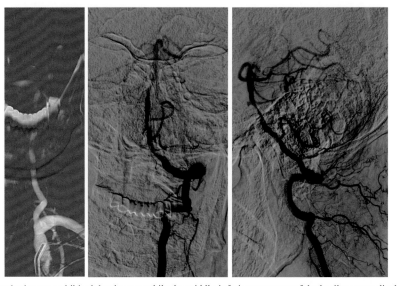

Fig. 5.6.9 The left vertebral artery exhibited dominance, while the middle-inferior segments of the basilar artery displayed severe stenosis

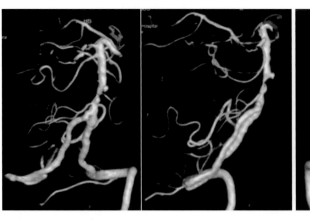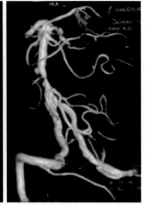

图 5.6.10　三维重建 DSA 示基底动脉狭窄段的左侧有 AICA 发出，但 AICA 较纤细，狭窄远端见一约 1.5 mm× 1.5 mm 动脉瘤，形态不规则

（四）治疗过程

　　全麻下右股动脉入路，6F 导引导管至左椎动脉 V2 段远端，造影示基底动脉重度狭窄（图 5.6.11）。路径图下沿导引导管送入 Transend 微导丝（0.014 in，300 cm）通过基底动脉狭窄段，至左大脑后动脉 P2 段以远，沿微导丝送入 Apollo 球囊扩张式支架（2.5 mm×13 mm），准确对位后加压球囊释放支架，撤出支架输送系统，造影提示支架贴壁良好，前向血流 mTICI 分级 3 级（图 5.6.12）。Echelon-10 微导管头端塑形后穿越支架放置在动脉瘤腔内，但微导管不能保持稳定，遂将微导管头端放置在瘤腔外，将弹簧圈（3D Axium 2 mm×2 cm 及 Axium 1.5 mm×2 cm）穿越支架后予以填塞。栓塞完毕后造影提示动脉瘤栓塞满意，血管通畅（图 5.6.13）。

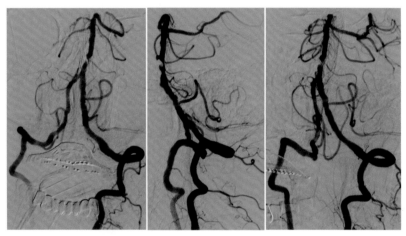

图 5.6.11　术前造影示基底动脉重度狭窄

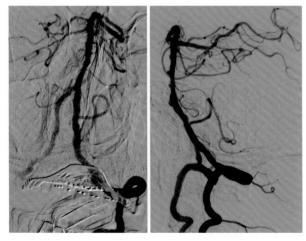

图 5.6.12　释放支架后造影示支架贴壁良好，前向血流 mTICI 分级 3 级

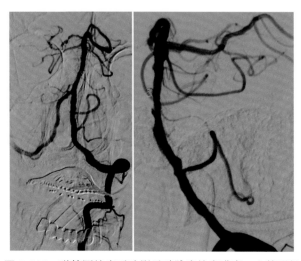

图 5.6.13　弹簧圈栓塞后造影示动脉瘤栓塞满意，血管通畅

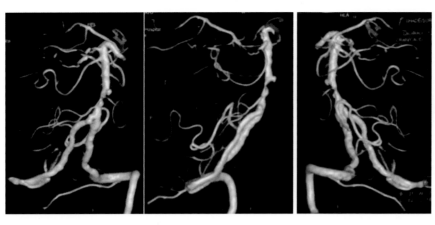

Fig. 5.6.10 DSA showed a tenuous anterior inferior cerebellar artery originating from the left stenotic segment. An irregularly shaped aneurysm with a diameter of 1.5 mm was observed distal to the basilar artery stenosis

4. Treatment

Under general anesthesia, a 6F guiding catheter was inserted into the V2 segment of the left vertebral artery. The angiogram confirmed the presence of severe stenosis of the basilar artery (Fig. 5.6.11). A Transend microwire (0.014 in, 300 cm) passed through the stenotic segment and was positioned at the distal P2 segment of the left posterior cerebral artery. Subsequently, a 2.5 mm×13 mm Apollo balloon-mounted stent was deployed to cover the lesion. The post-stent implantation angiogram exhibited exceptional stent wall apposition and a grade 3 of antegrade blood flow (Fig. 5.6.12). Efforts to insert the Echelon-10 microcatheter into the aneurysm cavity via the stent mesh proved unsuccessful, even after its tip was shaped accordingly. Consequently, the microcatheter tip was positioned outside the aneurysm cavity, and the coil (3D Axium 2 mm×2 cm and Axium 1.5 mm×2 cm) was inserted by crossing the stent. The post-coil embolization angiogram revealed full aneurysm embolization (Fig. 5.6.13).

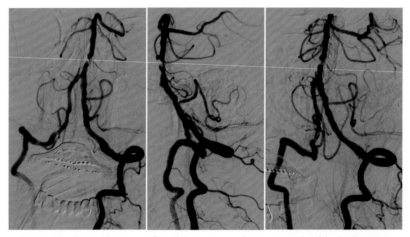

Fig. 5.6.11 The angiogram confirmed the presence of severe stenosis of the basilar artery

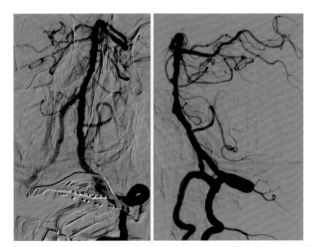

Fig. 5.6.12 The post-stent implantation angiogram exhibited exceptional stent wall apposition and a grade 3 of antegrade blood flow

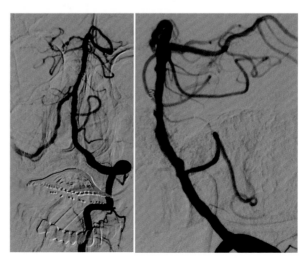

Fig. 5.6.13 The post-coil embolization angiogram revealed full aneurysm embolization

术后查体同前，复查头部CT未见出血（图5.6.14）。

术后CTA示基底动脉支架内通畅，动脉瘤栓塞满意（图5.6.15）。

术后CTP提示后循环低灌注较术前改善（图5.6.16）。

（五）讨论

本例未选择自膨式支架与大脑后动脉解剖有一定关系，右大脑后动脉较为纤细，左大脑后动脉开口部成角明显，都不太适合作为自膨式支架系统的着陆区。然而，放置球囊扩张式支架因不适合预先放置微导管，增加了后续动脉瘤栓塞的难度。

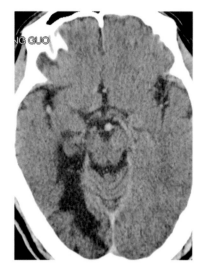

图5.6.14　术后头部CT未见出血

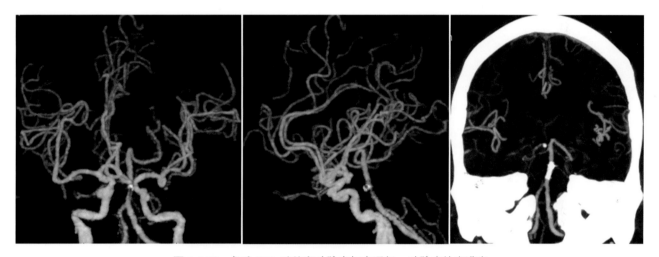

图5.6.15　术后CTA示基底动脉支架内通畅，动脉瘤栓塞满意

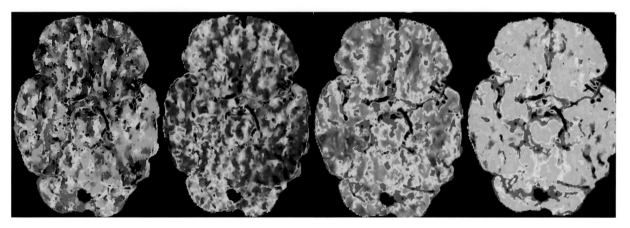

图5.6.16　术后CTP示后循环低灌注较术前改善

5.6　手术操作视频
（病例22）

（李新明　姚亮　邓一鸣　孙瑄　马宁　贺红卫　杨新健　缪中荣）

A Postprocedural CT scan revealed no evidence of cerebral hemorrhage (Fig. 5.6.14).

Postprocedural CT angiography showed the stent in the basilar artery was patent and that the aneurysm was completely embolized (Fig. 5.6.15).

Postprocedural CT perfusion showed an improvement in the hypoperfusion within the posterior circulation (Fig. 5.6.16).

5. Comments

The complex landing distal zone, characterized by a tenuous right posterior cerebral artery and a tortuous origin of the left posterior cerebral artery, presented a challenge for self-expandable stent release. As such, we opted for a balloon-mounted stent instead of a self-expandable stent for this case with symptomatic basilar artery stenosis. However, the implantation of balloon-expandable stents was unsuitable for the pre-placement of microcatheters, which increased the difficulty of subsequent aneurysm embolism.

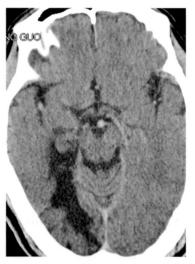

Fig. 5.6.14 Postprocedural CT scan revealed no evidence of cerebral hemorrhage

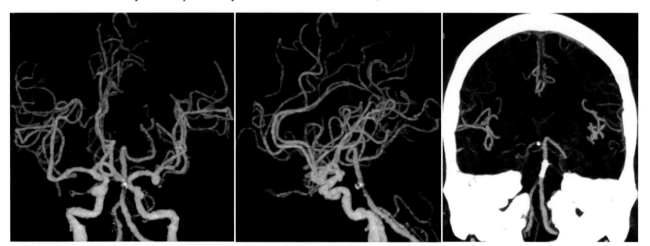

Fig. 5.6.15 Postprocedural CT angiography showed the stent in the basilar artery was patent and that the aneurysm was completely embolized

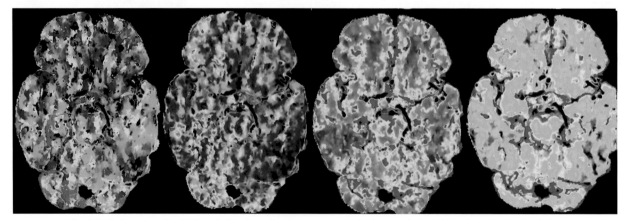

Fig. 5.6.16 Postprocedural CT perfusion showed an improvement in the hypoperfusion within the posterior circulation

5.6 Video of endovascular therapy (Case 22)

(Translated by Rongrong Cui, Revised by Zhikai Hou)

病例 23　基底动脉重度狭窄合并小脑前下动脉动脉瘤

（一）临床病史及影像分析

患者，女性，主因"发作性头晕半月余"入院。

当地医院头部 MRI 示右侧小脑多发点状梗死灶（图 5.6.17 A 和 B）。头部 MRA 示基底动脉下段重度狭窄（图 5.6.17 C 和 D）。为进一步治疗收入我院。

既往史：高血压和冠心病病史。

查体：神经系统查体无阳性体征。

DSA：双侧后交通动脉发育不全，左颈内动脉 C4 段中度狭窄（图 5.6.18）。右椎动脉优势，基底动脉下段重度狭窄，左小脑前下动脉起始部动脉瘤（图 5.6.19 A 和 B），左椎动脉发育不良，通过肌支和颈深动脉代偿供血（图 5.6.19 C 和 D）。

高分辨率 MRI：左椎动脉 V4 段完全闭塞（图 5.6.20 A），基底动脉下段偏心性重度狭窄，斑块偏

右侧壁（图 5.6.20 B）。

病后口服阿司匹林（100 mg 1 次 / 日）、替格瑞洛（90 mg 2 次 / 日）、瑞舒伐他汀（10 mg 1 次 / 日）治疗。

（二）诊断

症状性基底动脉重度狭窄合并小脑前下动脉动脉瘤。

（三）术前讨论

结合患者病史及相关影像学检查，基底动脉重度狭窄为责任病变，小脑前下动脉起始部动脉瘤未破裂，拟行基底动脉狭窄血管内介入治疗。相关风险包括医源性夹层、动脉瘤破裂、穿支事件、急性血栓形成等。

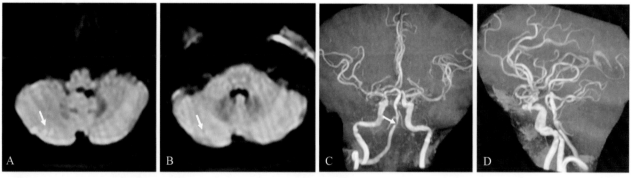

图 5.6.17　**A** 和 **B**. 头部磁共振 DWI 示右侧小脑多发点状梗死灶（箭头示）；**C** 和 **D**. 头部 MRA 示基底动脉下段重度狭窄（箭头示）

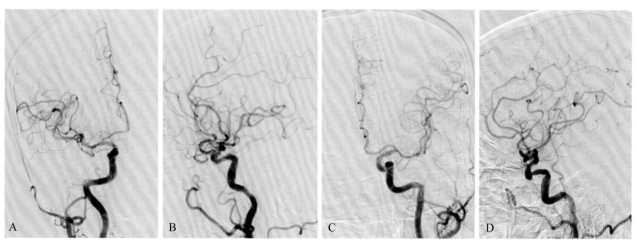

图 5.6.18　DSA 提示双侧后交通动脉发育不全，左颈内动脉 C4 段中度狭窄（**A ～ D**）

Case 23　Severe stenosis of the basilar artery concurrent with anterior inferior cerebellar artery aneurysm

1. Clinical presentation and radiological studies

A female patient presented with paroxysmal dizziness for about 15 days.

The MRI result indicated multiple punctate infarcts in the right cerebellar hemisphere (Fig. 5.6.17 A, B). The MRA suggested severe stenosis at the inferior segment of the basilar artery (Fig. 5.6.17 C, D).

She had a medical history of hypertension and coronary heart disease.

The physical examination indicated neurologically intact on admission.

The DSA examination revealed bilateral hypoplasia of the posterior communicating arteries. In addition, moderate stenosis was observed in the C4 segment of the left internal carotid artery (Fig. 5.6.18). And the right vertebral artery was dominant. A severe stenosis was located in the inferior segment of the basilar artery, along with an aneurysm at the origin of the left anterior inferior cerebellar artery (Fig. 5.6.19 A, B). Furthermore, the left vertebral artery was hypoplastic but compensated for by muscular branches and a deep cervical artery (Fig. 5.6.19 C, D).

High-resolution MRI indicated a complete occlusion of the V4 segment of the left vertebral artery (Fig. 5.6.20 A). Additionally, severe eccentric stenosis was found in the inferior segment of the basilar artery, with plaques predominantly located on the right-sided vessel wall (Fig. 5.6.20 B).

Since the onset of the symptoms, she has been on a regimen of dual antiplatelet therapy, consisting of Aspirin 100 mg daily and Ticagrelor 90mg twice daily, as well as statin therapy with Rosuvastatin 10mg daily.

2. Diagnosis

Symptomatic severe stenosis of the basilar artery concurrent with anterior inferior cerebellar artery aneurysm.

3. Treatment schedule

Based on the medical records and relevant radiological studies, it was determined that the severe stenosis in the basilar artery qualified for endovascular treatment. However, there were potential risks associated with the procedure, including iatrogenic dissection, aneurysm rupture, perforating artery occlusion, and in-stent thrombosis.

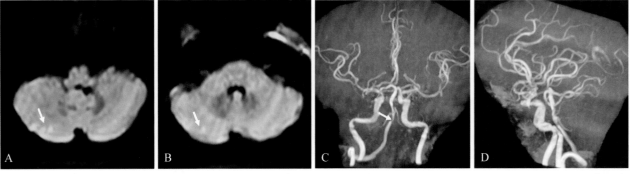

Fig. 5.6.17 MRI result indicated multiple punctate infarcts in the right cerebellar hemisphere (arrow) (**A, B**). MRA suggested severe stenosis at the inferior segment of the basilar artery (arrow) (**C, D**)

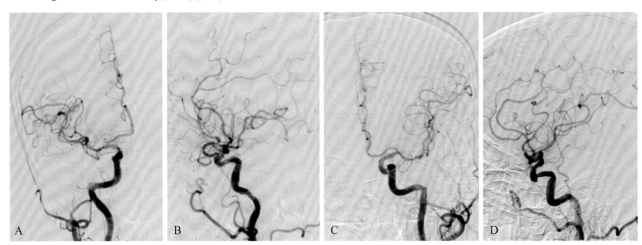

Fig. 5.6.18 DSA showed bilateral hypoplasia of the posterior communicating arteries and a moderate stenosis in the C4 segment of the left internal carotid artery (**A – D**)

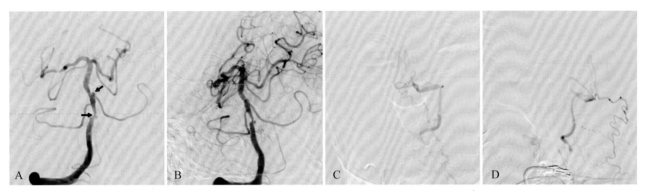

图 5.6.19 **A** 和 **B**. DSA 示右椎动脉优势，基底动脉下段重度狭窄，左小脑前下动脉起始部动脉瘤（箭头示）；**C** 和 **D**. 左椎动脉发育不良，通过肌支和颈深动脉代偿供血

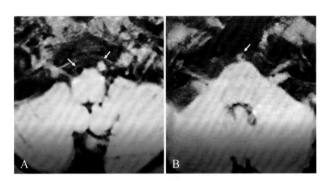

图 5.6.20 高分辨率 MRI 示：**A**. 左椎动脉 V4 段完全闭塞（箭头示）；**B**. 基底动脉下段偏心性重度狭窄（箭头示）

（四）治疗过程

全麻下右股动脉穿刺入路，置入 6F 鞘，将 6F 导引导管送至右椎动脉 V2 段，行右椎动脉颅内段造影，显示基底动脉下段重度狭窄，左小脑前下动脉动脉瘤（图 5.6.21 A）。在路径图下将 Transend 微导丝（0.014 in，300 cm）通过狭窄段送至右大脑后动脉 P1 段，沿微导丝送入 Gateway 球囊（2.5 mm×9 mm）至狭窄处，对位准确后充盈球囊（图 5.6.21 B），造影示狭窄明显改善（图 5.6.21 C），撤出球囊，沿微导丝送入 Wingspan 自膨式支架（3.5 mm×20 mm），支架远端置于小脑前下动脉开口远端，近端置于右椎动脉 V4 段完全覆盖狭窄病变，复查造影示支架贴壁良好，前向血流 mTICI 分级 3 级。观察 10 min 后，再次造影见支架内血流通畅，无急性血栓形成（图 5.6.21 D），结束手术。

（五）讨论

本例患者基底动脉重度狭窄合并左小脑前下动脉起始部动脉瘤，基底动脉重度狭窄为本次处理的主要病变，考虑动脉瘤较小并且形态规则，选择一枚能够同时覆盖狭窄病变和动脉瘤的支架，在解决狭窄的基础上给予动脉瘤血流导向的作用，待复查结果观察动脉瘤的变化。

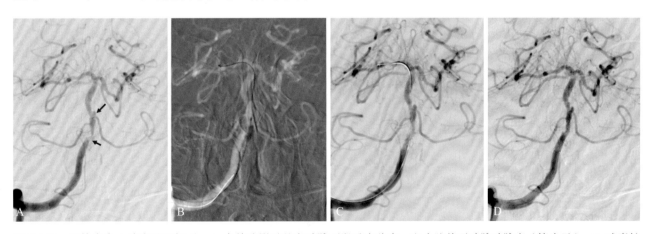

图 5.6.21 血管内介入治疗过程如下：**A**. 术前造影示基底动脉下段重度狭窄，左小脑前下动脉动脉瘤（箭头示）；**B**. 球囊扩张；**C**. 球囊扩张后造影；**D**. 支架术后再次造影显示支架内血流通畅

（宋佳 杨明 贾白雪 江裕华 马宁）

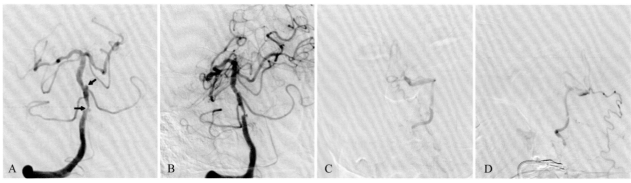

Fig. 5.6.19 DSA showed severe stenosis located in the inferior segment of the basilar artery, along with an aneurysm at the origin of the left anterior inferior cerebellar artery (arrow) (**A, B**). The left vertebral artery was hypoplastic but compensated for by muscular branches and a deep cervical artery (**C, D**)

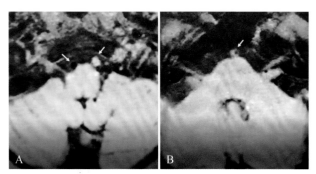

Fig. 5.6.20 HRMRI indicated a complete occlusion of the V4 segment of the left vertebral artery (arrow) (**A**). Additionally, severe eccentric stenosis was found in the inferior segment of the basilar artery, with plaques predominantly located on the right-sided vessel wall (arrow) (**B**)

4. Treatment

Under general anesthesia, a 6F guiding catheter was carefully positioned at the V2 segment of the right vertebral artery. The angiogram confirmed there was a severe stenosis in the inferior segment of the basilar artery as well as an aneurysm in the left anterior inferior cerebellar artery (Fig. 5.6.21 A). A Transend microwire (0.014 in, 300 cm) navigated through the stenotic segment and was placed at the P1 segment of the right posterior cerebral artery. A 2.5 mm×9 mm Gateway balloon was utilized to dilate the stenosis lesion (Fig. 5.6.21 B, C). Following that, A 3.5 mm ×20 mm Wingspan stent was implanted, with the distal end of the stent extending beyond the origin of the anterior inferior cerebellar artery and the proximal segment of the stent positioned at the V4 segment of the right vertebral artery to ensure that the lesion was completely covered. A post-stent implantation angiogram showed excellent stent wall apposition and a 3 grade of antegrade blood flow. Following a ten-minute observation period, a repeat angiogram revealed that the blood flow in the stent was found to be patent (Fig. 5.6.21 D).

5. Comments

This case describes a patient who presented with severe stenosis of the basilar artery along with an aneurysm at the origin of the left anterior inferior cerebellar artery. The primary objective of the endovascular treatment was to manage the stenosis lesion of the basilar artery. As for the small-sized and regular-shaped aneurysm in the origin of the anterior inferior cerebellar artery, a stent was selected to cover both the stenotic lesion and the aneurysm, thereby serving the dual purpose of improving the stenosis and providing blood flow guidance as well.

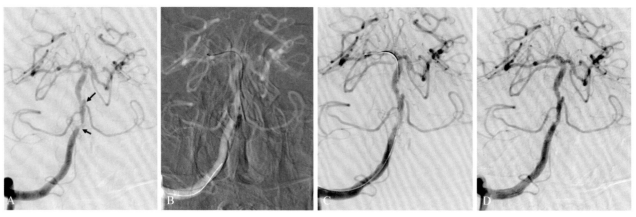

Fig. 5.6.21 The angiogram confirmed there was a severe stenosis in the inferior segment of the basilar artery as well as an aneurysm in the left anterior inferior cerebellar artery (arrow) (**A**). The lesion was dilated using a Gateway balloon (**B, C**). A repeat angiogram revealed that the blood flow in the stent was found to be patent (**D**)

(Translated by Rongrong Cui, Revised by Zhikai Hou)

第七节 串联病变

病例 24 右椎动脉 V1 段和 V4 段串联狭窄

（一）临床病史及影像分析

患者，男性，60 岁，主因"发作性头晕 3 个月"入院。

当地医院头颈部 CTA 示右椎动脉 V4 段重度狭窄，右椎动脉 V1 段中度狭窄，左椎动脉 V1 段重度狭窄（图 5.7.1）。给予药物治疗后仍有头晕反复发作，为行血管内治疗来我院就诊。

既往史：糖尿病和高脂血症病史 1 年。吸烟 30 年，未戒；饮酒 40 年，未戒。

查体：神经系统查体无阳性体征。

低密度脂蛋白胆固醇（LDL-C）：3.37 mmol/L。

血栓弹力图：AA 抑制率 100%，ADP 抑制率 33.9%。

头部 MRI：右胼胝体压部、右枕叶亚急性梗死灶（图 5.7.2 A）。

头部 MRA：右椎动脉 V4 段重度狭窄，左椎动脉 V4 段闭塞（图 5.7.2 B 和 C）。

高分辨率 MRI：右椎动脉颅内段管壁增厚强化（图 5.7.3）。

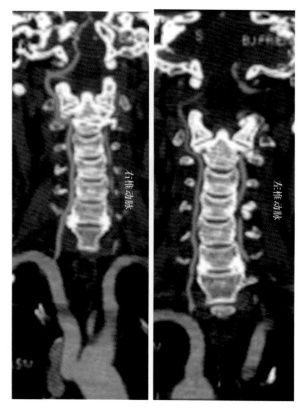

图 5.7.1 CTA 示右椎动脉 V4 段重度狭窄，右椎动脉 V1 段中度狭窄，左椎动脉 V1 段重度狭窄

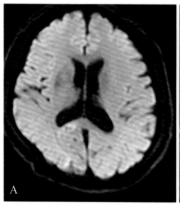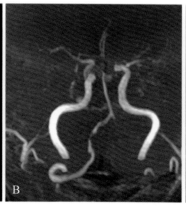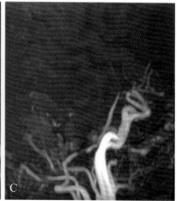

图 5.7.2 头部 MRI 示右胼胝体压部、右枕叶亚急性梗死灶（**A**）。MRA 示右椎动脉 V4 段重度狭窄，左椎动脉 V4 段闭塞（**B** 和 **C**）

Section 7 Tandem ICAS

Case 24 Tandem stenoses of the V1 and V4 segments of the right vertebral artery

1. Clinical presentation and radiological studies

A 60-year-old male patient presented with paroxysmal dizziness for three months.

The CT angiography revealed severe stenosis at the V4 segment of the right vertebral artery, along with moderate stenosis at the V1 segment of the right vertebral artery. Furthermore, severe stenosis was detected in the V1 segment of the left vertebral artery (Fig. 5.7.1). Despite undergoing dual antiplatelet and statin therapy, the patient's dizziness symptoms continued to recur.

The patient had a one-year history of diabetes and hyperlipidemia. Additionally, he had been a smoker for thirty years and a drinker for forty years.

The patient's physical examination upon admission indicated that he was neurologically intact.

The concentration of the LDL-C was 3.37 mmol/L.

The thromboelastography result indicated a 100% inhibition of AA and a 33.9% inhibition of ADP.

The MRI revealed subacute cerebral infarctions in the splenium of the right corpus callosum and the right occipital lobe (Fig. 5.7.2 A).

The MRA displayed severe stenosis of the V4 segment of the right vertebral artery and total occlusion of the V4 segment of the left vertebral artery (Fig. 5.7.2 B, C).

The high-resolution MRI exhibited that the vessel wall of the intracranial segment of the right vertebral artery was thickened and had significant enhancement on the contrast-enhanced scan (Fig. 5.7.3).

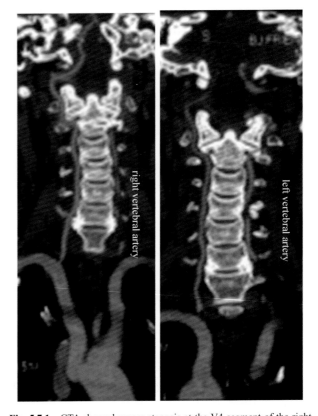

Fig. 5.7.1 CTA showed severe stenosis at the V4 segment of the right vertebral artery, along with moderate stenosis at the V1 segment of the right vertebral artery. Furthermore, severe stenosis was detected in the V1 segment of the left vertebral artery

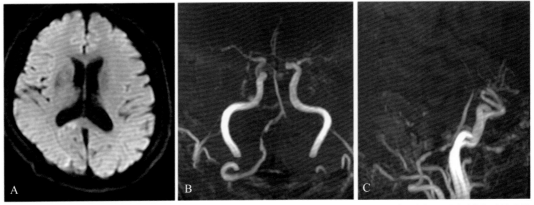

Fig. 5.7.2 MRI revealed subacute cerebral infarctions in the splenium of the right corpus callosum and the right occipital lobe (**A**). MRA displayed severe stenosis of the V4 segment of the right vertebral artery and total occlusion of the V4 segment of the left vertebral artery (**B, C**)

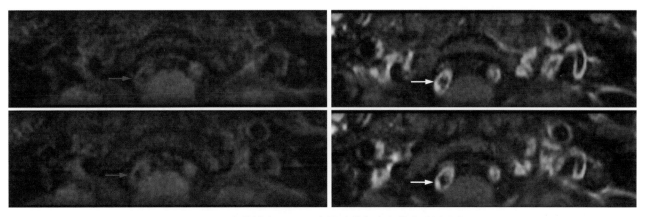

图 5.7.3 高分辨率 MRI 示右椎动脉颅内段管壁增厚强化

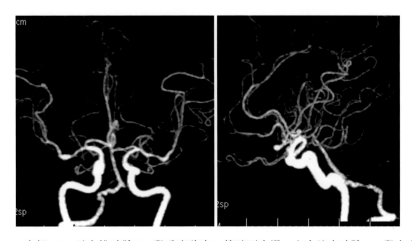

图 5.7.4 头部 CTA 示右椎动脉 V4 段重度狭窄，管壁不光滑，左大脑中动脉 M1 段中度狭窄

头部 CTA：右椎动脉 V4 段重度狭窄，管壁不光滑，左大脑中动脉 M1 段中度狭窄（图 5.7.4）。

头部 CTP：后循环区域低灌注（图 5.7.5）。

DSA：右侧后交通动脉开放（图 5.7.6），左大脑中动脉 M1 段轻度狭窄（图 5.7.7），右椎动脉 V1 段中度狭窄，右椎动脉 V4 段重度狭窄，管壁不光滑，局部有扩张（图 5.7.8），左椎动脉起始段重度狭窄，全程较细，止于小脑后下动脉（图 5.7.9）。

入院后给予双联抗血小板（阿司匹林 100 mg 1 次 / 日＋氯吡格雷 75 mg 1 次 / 日）及降脂（阿托伐他汀 40 mg 1 次 / 日）等治疗。

（二）诊断

症状性右椎动脉 V1、V4 段串联狭窄。

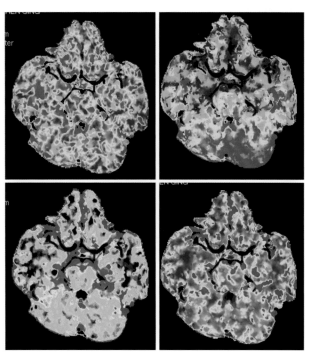

图 5.7.5 头部 CTP 示后循环区域低灌注

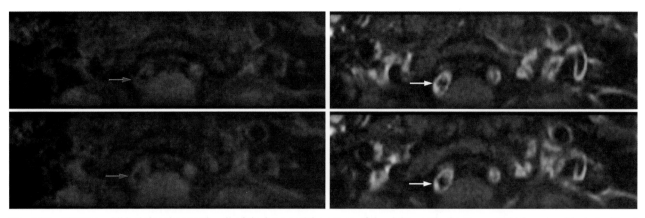

Fig. 5.7.3 HRMRI exhibited that the vessel wall of the intracranial segment of the right vertebral artery was thickened and had significant enhancement on the contrast-enhanced scan

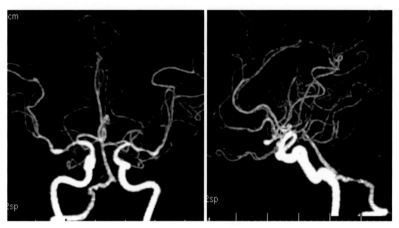

Fig. 5.7.4 CT angiography disclosed a severe stenosis at the V4 segment of the right vertebral artery and a moderate stenosis in the M1 segment of the left middle cerebral artery

The intracranial CT angiography disclosed a severe stenosis at the V4 segment of the right vertebral artery and a moderate narrowing in the M1 segment of the left middle cerebral artery (Fig. 5.7.4).

CT perfusion indicated hypoperfusion in the posterior circulation area (Fig. 5.7.5).

The DSA result showed the right posterior communicating artery was patent (Fig. 5.7.6) while the M1 segment of the left middle cerebral artery showed mild stenosis (Fig. 5.7.7). A moderate stenosis was detected at the V1 segment of the right vertebral artery, along with severe stenosis at the V4 segment of the right vertebral artery and focal vascular dilatation (Fig. 5.7.8). Furthermore, the left vertebral artery displayed severe stenosis at its origin, and it was tenuous along its entire course, eventually terminating at the posterior inferior cerebellar artery (Fig. 5.7.9).

After admission, he was prescribed a dual antiplatelet regimen consisting of daily doses of Aspirin (100 mg) and Clopidogrel (75 mg), as well as statin therapy with daily doses of Atorvastatin (40 mg).

2. Diagnosis

Symptomatic tandem stenoses of the V1 and V4 segments of the right vertebral artery.

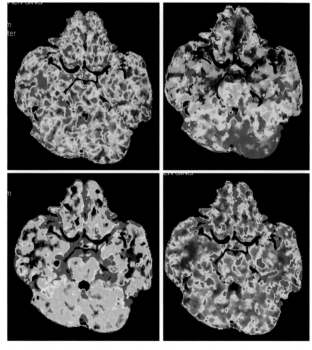

Fig. 5.7.5 CT perfusion indicated hypoperfusion in the posterior circulation area

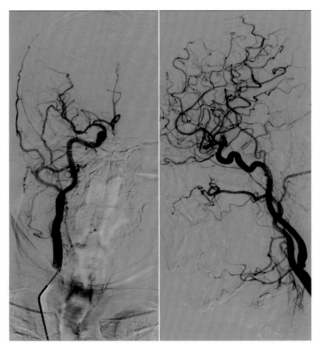

图 **5.7.6**　DSA 示右侧后交通动脉开放

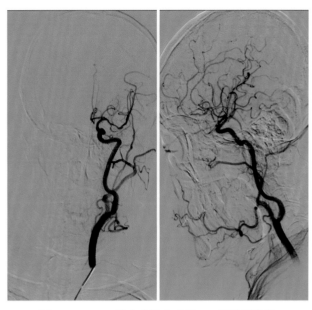

图 **5.7.7**　DSA 示左大脑中动脉 M1 段轻度狭窄

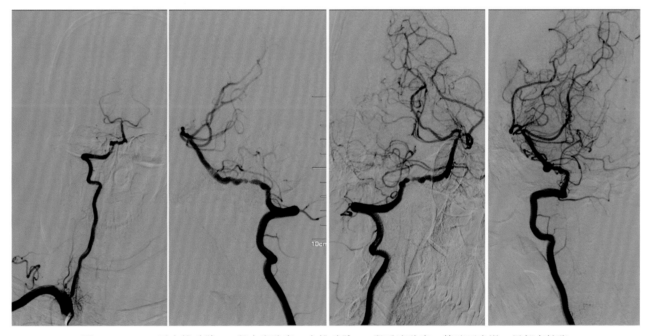

图 **5.7.8**　DSA 示右椎动脉 V1 段中度狭窄，右椎动脉 V4 段重度狭窄，管壁不光滑，局部有扩张

（三）术前讨论

　　患者右椎动脉 V4 段及左椎动脉 V1 段重度狭窄，近 3 个月反复发作后循环缺血症状，药物治疗效果差，有介入治疗指征。右椎动脉 V1 段中度狭窄，如果导引导管能顺利越过右椎动脉 V1 段，可不处理右椎动脉开口部病变，否则先处理近端病变

（单纯球囊扩张或者置入支架），帮助导引导管到位后，再处理远端病变。

（四）治疗过程

　　全麻下右股动脉穿刺置入 8F 动脉鞘，左椎动脉起始处置入 Blue 支架（4 mm×15 mm）（图 5.7.10）。其后 6F 导引导管无法通过右椎动脉

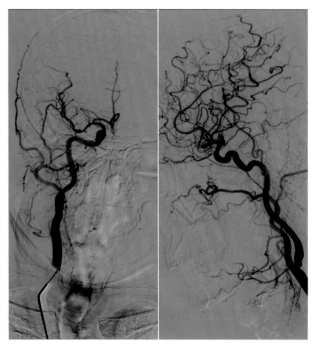

Fig. 5.7.6 DSA revealed the right posterior communicating artery was patent

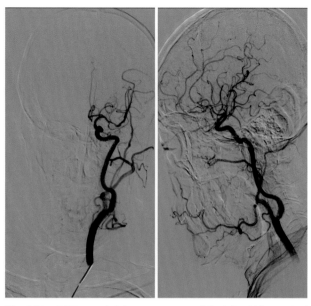

Fig. 5.7.7 DSA revealed the M1 segment of the left middle cerebral artery developed mild stenosis

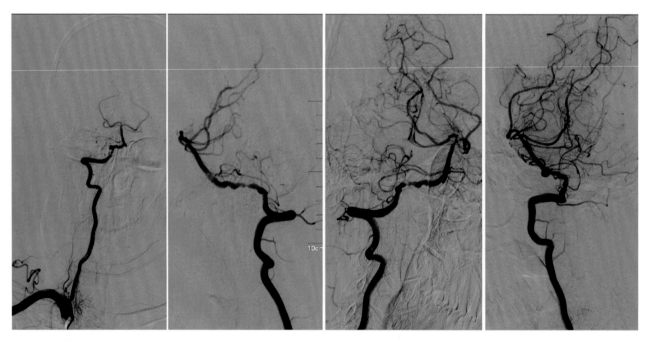

Fig. 5.7.8 DSA showed moderate stenosis of the V1 segment of the right vertebral artery, along with severe stenosis at the V4 segment of the right vertebral artery with focal vascular dilatation

3. Treatment schedule

The patient exhibited severe stenosis at the V4 segment of the right vertebral artery, along with severe stenosis at the V1 segment of the left vertebral artery. Despite receiving aggressive medical treatment, he continued to experience the symptom of dizziness. As a result, the patient was deemed a candidate for endovascular treatment of both the right V4 and left V1 segments. Treatment approach: if the guide catheter was unable to pass through the stenosis lesion located in the V1 of the right vertebral artery, primary balloon angioplasty, and/or stenting may be performed to recanalize the V1 segment of the right vertebral artery, thus facilitating appropriate positioning of the guide catheter.

4. Treatment

Under general anesthesia, a 4 mm×15 mm Blue stent was deployed at the origin of the left vertebral artery (Fig. 5.7.10).

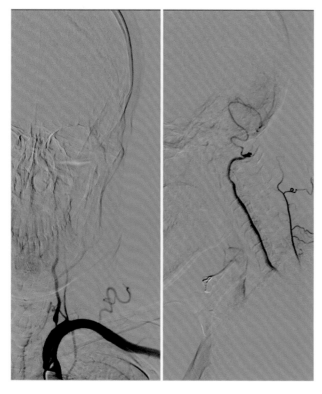

图 5.7.9　DSA 示左椎动脉起始段重度狭窄，全程较细，止于小脑后下动脉

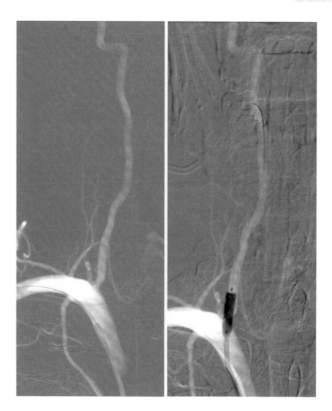

图 5.7.11　6F 导引导管无法通过右椎动脉 V1 段

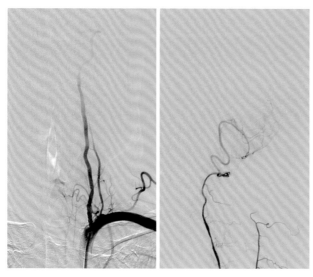

图 5.7.10　左椎动脉起始处置入一枚 Blue 支架

V1 段。遂经 6F 导引导管在右椎动脉 V1 段置入 Express 支架（5 mm×15 mm），其后使用球囊辅助技术，试图跟进 6 F 导引导管越过支架也未成功

（图 5.7.11）。更换 7F 长鞘（70 cm），经长鞘送入 5F Navien 导管至右椎动脉 V2 段，造影显示右椎动脉 V4 段重度狭窄（图 5.7.12）。送入 Transend 微导丝（0.014 in，300 cm）至左大脑后动脉 P2 段，沿微导丝送入赛诺球囊（2 mm×10 mm）预扩张右椎动脉 V4 段狭窄处（图 5.7.13 A 和 B）。球囊扩张后造影提示残余狭窄率约 50%（图 5.7.13 C 和 D）。撤出球囊，沿微导丝置入 Apollo 球囊扩张式支架（2.5 mm×8 mm），支架置入后造影显示残余狭窄率约为 10%（图 5.7.14）。观察 10 min 后造影同前无变化，遂结束手术。

术后查体同前，复查头部 CT 未见出血（图 5.7.15）。

术后头部 CTA：右椎动脉 V4 段支架内血流通畅（图 5.7.16）。

术后头部 CTP：后循环低灌注情况较术前改善（图 5.7.17）。

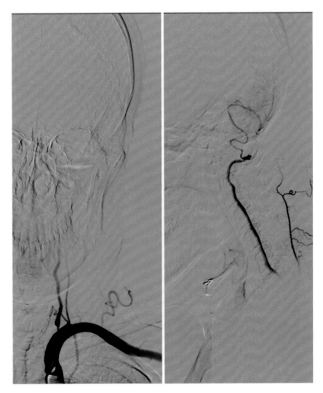

Fig. 5.7.9 DSA showed the left vertebral artery displayed severe stenosis at its origin, and it was tenuous along its entire course, eventually terminating at the posterior inferior cerebellar artery

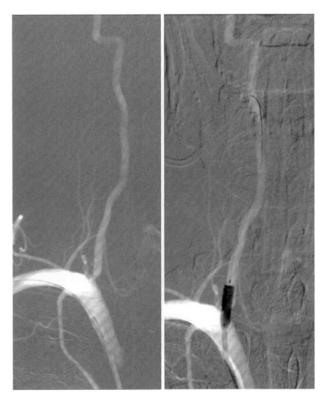

Fig. 5.7.11 The 6F guiding catheter was unable to pass through the V1 segment of the right vertebral artery

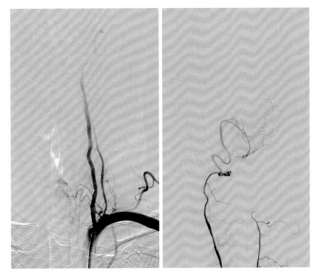

Fig. 5.7.10 A Blue stent was deployed at the origin of the left vertebral artery

The 6F guiding catheter was unable to pass through the V1 segment of the right vertebral artery. Therefore, an Express stent (5 mm×15 mm) was positioned at the V1 segment of the right vertebral artery through the 6F guiding catheter. The attempt to advance the 6F guide catheter through the right V1 segment utilizing the balloon-assisted technique was unsuccessful. (Fig. 5.7.11). A 7F long sheath (70 cm) was selected. The 5F Navien catheter was delivered through the 7F long sheath to the V2 segment of the right vertebral artery. The angiogram showed severe stenosis of the V4 segment of the right vertebral artery (Fig. 5.7.12). The Transend microwire (0.014, 300 cm) was delivered to the P2 segment of the left posterior cerebral artery. A Sino balloon (2 mm×10 mm) was used to pre-dilated the stenosis lesion of the V4 segment of the right vertebral artery (Fig. 5.7.13 A, B). The post-angiography angiogram revealed residual stenosis of 50% (Fig. 5.7.13 C, D). Subsequently, a 2.5 mm×8 mm Apollo stent was used to entirely cover the lesion. The post-stent implantation angiogram demonstrated residual stenosis of 10% (Fig. 5.7.14). After careful observation of 10 minutes, the final angiogram showed the stent in the right vertebral artery was patent.

The CT scan after the procedure indicated no signs of cerebral hemorrhage (Fig. 5.7.15).

The postprocedural CTA showed the V4 segment of the right vertebral artery was patent (Fig. 5.7.16).

The postprocedural CT perfusion displayed an amelioration in the hypoperfusion of the posterior circulation (Fig. 5.7.17).

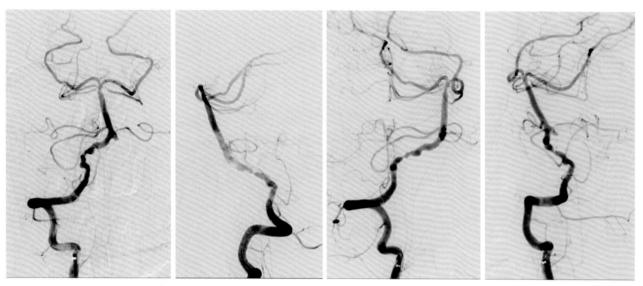

图 5.7.12　将 5F Navien 导管送至右椎动脉 V2 段后，造影显示右椎动脉 V4 段重度狭窄

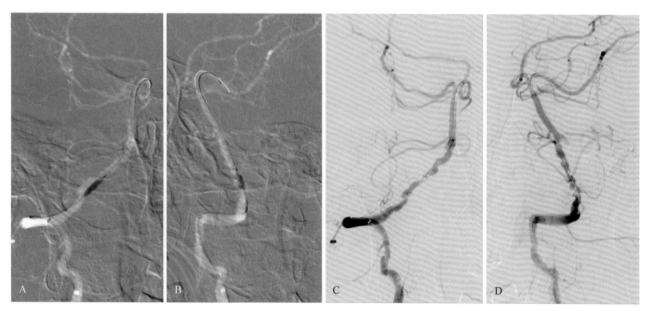

图 5.7.13　**A** 和 **B**.赛诺球囊预扩张右椎动脉 V4 段狭窄处；**C** 和 **D**.球囊扩张后造影示残余狭窄率约为 50%

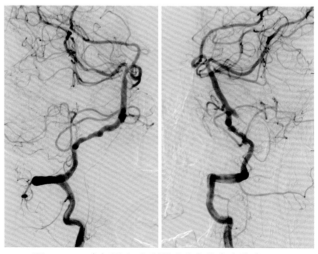

图 5.7.14　支架置入后造影示残余狭窄率约为 10%

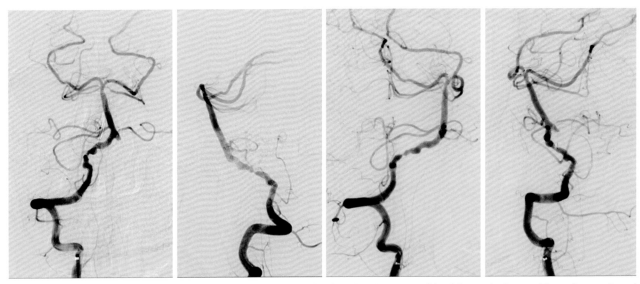

Fig. 5.7.12 The 5F Navien catheter was delivered through the 7F long sheath to the V2 segment of the right vertebral artery. The angiogram showed severe stenosis of the V4 segment of the right vertebral artery

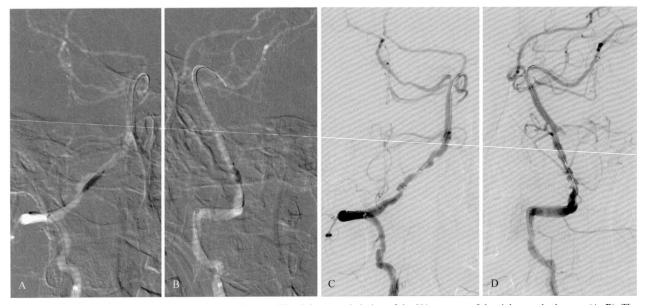

Fig. 5.7.13 A Sino balloon (2 mm × 10 mm) was used to pre-dilated the stenosis lesion of the V4 segment of the right vertebral artery (**A, B**). The post-angiography angiogram revealed residual stenosis of 50% (**C, D**)

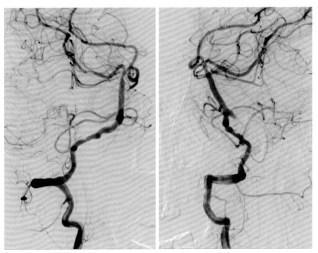

Fig. 5.7.14 The post-stent implantation angiogram demonstrated residual stenosis of 10%

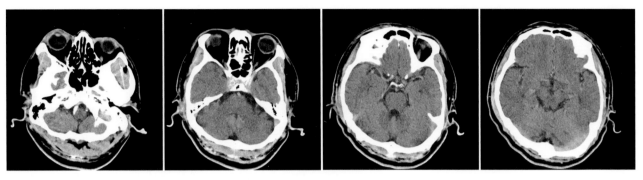

图 5.7.15 术后复查头部 CT 未见出血

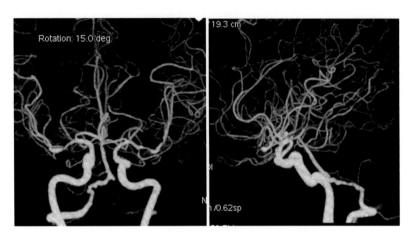

图 5.7.16 术后头部 CTA 示右椎动脉 V4 段支架内血流通畅

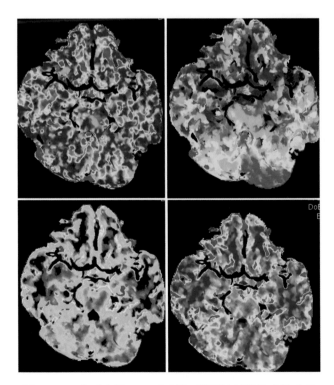

图 5.7.17 术后头部 CTP 示后循环低灌注情况较术前改善

（五）讨论

本例 6F 导引导管无法通过右椎动脉 V1 段，主要与主动脉角度过大，不能提供有效支撑有关，更换为 7F 长鞘后改善了支撑性，Navien 导管较为顺利地越过了支架。右椎动脉 V4 段狭窄，整体斑块较长，但由于放置较长的球囊扩张式支架或者自膨式支架发生穿支动脉闭塞的风险较大，故我们仅处理狭窄最重的节段。

（姚亮 邓一鸣 孙瑄 马宁）

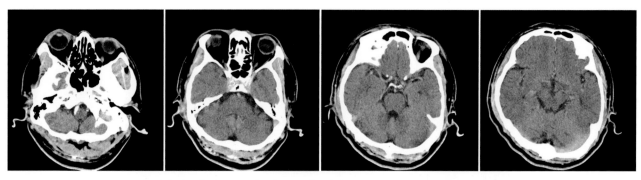

Fig. 5.7.15   The CT scan after the procedure indicated no signs of cerebral hemorrhage

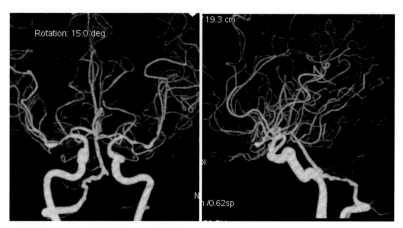

Fig. 5.7.16   The postprocedural CTA showed the V4 segment of the right vertebral artery was patent

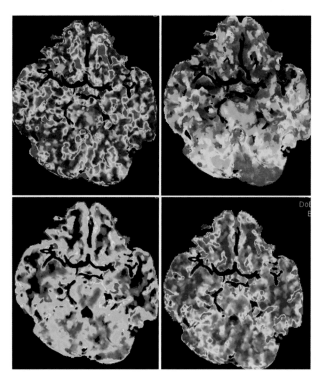

Fig. 5.7.17   The post-procedural CT perfusion displayed an amelioration in the hypoperfusion of the posterior circulation

5. Comments

During the procedure, the 6F guide catheter was unable to pass through the V1 segment of the right vertebral artery because of the inadequate support force. To advance the Navien catheter through the stent at the origin of the right V1 with sufficient support force, the 6F guide catheter was exchanged for a 7F long sheath. Moreover, in the V4 segment of the right vertebral artery, there were multiple stenoses and a longsegment atherosclerotic plaque. If a long-segment balloon-mounted stent or self-expandable stent were to be implanted, there would be a high risk of occluding the perforator arteries. Therefore, a short-segment balloon-mounted stent was deployed at the location with the most severe stenosis on the right V4.

(Translated by Rongrong Cui, Revised by Zhikai Hou)

病例 25　基底动脉多发狭窄

（一）临床病史及影像分析

患者，女性，主因"发作性头晕 5 月余"入院。

既往史：高血压病史 20 年，糖尿病及脑梗死病史 2 年。

查体：右侧肢体针刺觉减退。

头部 MRI：未见急性梗死灶（图 5.7.18 A 和 B）。

头部 MRA：基底动脉多发重度狭窄（图 5.7.18 C 和 D）。

DSA：双侧完全型胚胎型大脑后动脉（图 5.7.19），右椎动脉 V3 段重度狭窄（图 5.7.20 A 和 B），左椎动脉优势，基底动脉中远段见三处串联狭窄：近端狭窄程度重，长度最长，与双侧 AICA 解剖关系密切（特别是毗邻右侧 AICA）；中间狭窄程度稍轻；远端狭窄程度最重，长度较为局限，狭窄以远见局部血管扩张（图 5.7.20 C 和 D）。

高分辨率 MRI：基底动脉全程管壁增厚，管腔偏心性狭窄，局部可见管壁信号强度增加，T1 加权成像示基底动脉腹侧壁及右侧壁管腔局部高信号，考虑有斑块内出血（图 5.7.21）。

病后口服阿司匹林（100 mg 1 次 / 日）、氯吡格雷（75 mg 1 次 / 日）、阿托伐他汀（20 mg 1 次 / 日），并进行降压、降糖治疗。

（二）诊断

症状性基底动脉多发狭窄。

（三）术前讨论

根据 MRA 及 DSA 影像结果，患者双侧大脑后动脉系完全型胚胎型大脑后动脉，均未参与基底

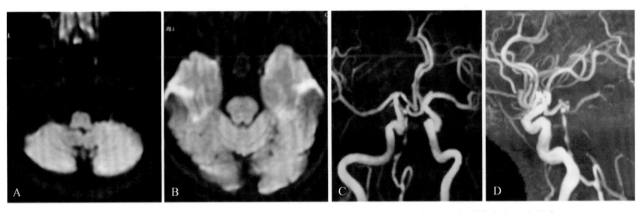

图 5.7.18　**A** 和 **B**. 头部 MRI 未见急性梗死灶；**C** 和 **D**. 头部 MRA 提示基底动脉多发重度狭窄

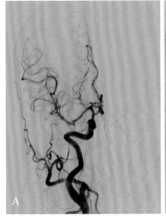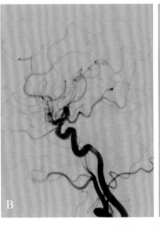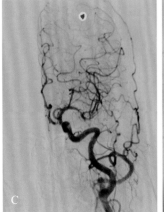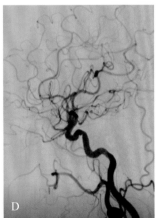

图 5.7.19　DSA 示双侧完全型胚胎型大脑后动脉（**A ～ D**）

Case 25　Multiple stenoses of the basilar artery

1. Clinical presentation and radiological studies

A female patient was admitted to the hospital due to recurrent episodes of dizziness over five months.

She had a 20-year medical history of hypertension, as well as diabetes mellitus and cerebral infarction for the past 2 years.

The physical examination revealed a decrease in pinprick sensation in the patient's right limbs.

The MRI did not reveal any acute cerebral infarction (Fig. 5.7.18 A, B).

The MRA showed the presence of multiple tandem and severe stenoses in the basilar artery (Fig. 5.7.18 C, D).

The DSA findings revealed bilateral posterior cerebral arteries developed full fetal-type (Fig. 5.7.19), a severe stenosis at the V3 segment of the right vertebral artery (Fig. 5.7.20 A, B), the existence of a dominant left vertebral artery. Multiple tandem stenoses at the middle-to-distal segments of the basilar artery. The severe stenosis located at the proximal segment was adjacent to the bilateral anterior inferior cerebellar arteries (AICAs), especially on the right side. The intermediate stenosis was relatively less severe in comparison. The distal stenosis was the most severe, with post-stenotic dilatation. (Fig. 5.7.20 C, D).

The high-resolution MRI scan revealed that the vessel wall of the entire course of the basilar artery was thickened, with a focal eccentric stenosis caused by an atherosclerotic plaque. T1-weighted imaging showed a focal hyperintensity on the ventral and right walls of the basilar artery, indicative of the presence of intraplaque hemorrhage (Fig. 5.7.21).

After admission, she was prescribed a dual antiplatelet regimen consisting of daily doses of Aspirin (100 mg) and Clopidogrel (75 mg), as well as statin therapy with daily doses of Atorvastatin (20 mg).

2. Diagnosis

Symptomatic multiple stenoses of the basilar artery.

3. Treatment schedule

The patient had multiple tandem stenoses in the basilar artery, which served as an isolated blood supply system. Radiological studies revealed that the bilateral posterior cerebral arteries had developed in a full fetal-type manner. Despite receiving aggressive medical treatment, the patient

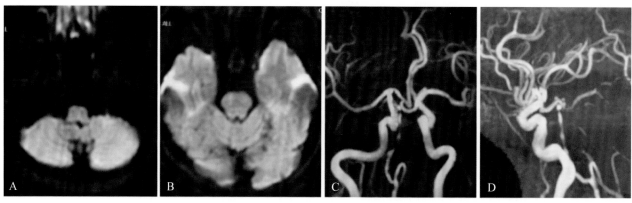

Fig. 5.7.18　The MRI did not reveal any acute cerebral infarction (**A**, **B**). The MRA showed the presence of multiple tandem stenoses in the basilar artery (**C**, **D**)

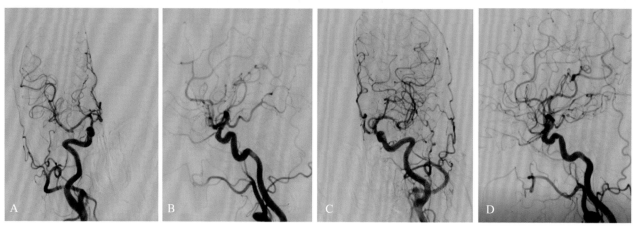

Fig. 5.7.19　DSA showed bilateral posterior cerebral arteries developed full fetal-type (**A**–**D**)

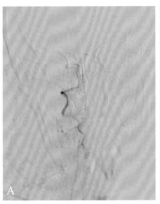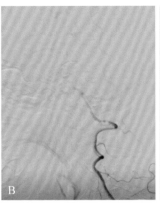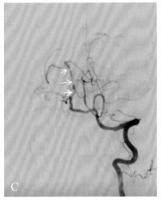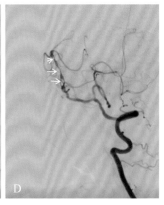

图 5.7.20　DSA 示右椎动脉 V3 段重度狭窄（**A** 和 **B**），左椎动脉优势，基底动脉中远段见三处串联狭窄：近端狭窄长度最长，与双侧 AICA 解剖关系密切（特别是右侧 AICA）；中间狭窄程度稍轻；远端狭窄程度最重，长度较为局限，狭窄远端局部血管扩张（箭头示）（**C** 和 **D**）

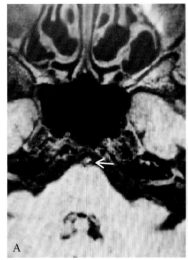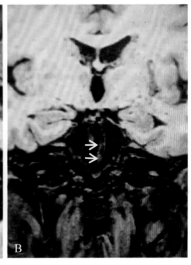

图 5.7.21　高分辨率 MRI 提示基底动脉全程管壁增厚，管腔偏心性狭窄，局部可见管壁信号强度增加，T1 加权成像示基底动脉腹侧壁及右侧壁管腔局部高信号，考虑有斑块内出血（箭头示）（**A** 和 **B**）

动脉尖的代偿供血，故患者近期反复头晕与基底动脉多发重度狭窄密切相关，拟行血管内介入治疗改善狭窄远端血供。相关风险包括穿支动脉损伤、医源性血管夹层、急性血栓形成等。

（四）治疗过程

全麻下右股动脉穿刺入路，将 6F 导引导管置于左椎动脉 V2 段。造影显示基底动脉多发狭窄，基底动脉尖膨大，考虑基底动脉尖动脉瘤（图 5.7.22 A 和 B）。在 SL-10 微导管辅助下将 Synchro 微导丝（0.014 in，300 cm）穿过狭窄段至基底动脉上段，但选入小脑上动脉困难，撤出微导管，保留微导丝。经微导丝送入 Gateway 球囊（1.5 mm×

9 mm）至基底动脉近端和中间狭窄处扩张（图 5.7.22 C 和 D），其中近端狭窄处扩张 2 次。扩张后造影显示近端狭窄程度明显改善，残余狭窄率约为 30%。中间狭窄程度略有改善，残余狭窄率约为 40%，前向血流 mTICI 分级 3 级（图 5.7.23）。观察 10 min 后造影显示血流通畅，病变扩张后无明显回缩，遂结束手术。

术后患者出现恶心、呕吐、构音障碍，伴左侧肢体力弱，最重时肌力 3 级。复查 MRI 显示脑桥右侧急性梗死（图 5.7.24 A）。MRA 显示基底动脉通畅，狭窄较术前明显改善（图 5.7.24 B 和 C）。

术后第 5 天出院，患者轻度构音障碍，左侧肢体肌力 4 级。患者自述头晕症状较术前改善。

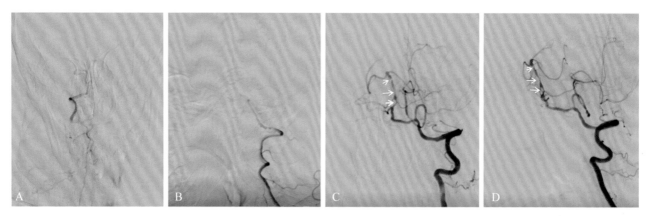

Fig. 5.7.20 DSA showed severe stenosis at the V3 segment of the right vertebral artery (**A**, **B**). The left vertebral artery was dominant. Multiple tandem stenoses at the middle-to-distal segments of the basilar artery. The severe stenosis located at the proximal segment was adjacent to the bilateral anterior inferior cerebellar arteries (AICAs), especially on the right side. The intermediate stenosis was relatively less severe in comparison. The distal stenosis was the most severe, with a post-stenotic dilatation (arrow) (**C**, **D**)

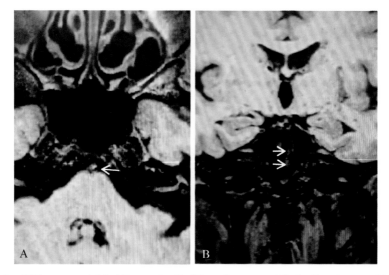

Fig. 5.7.21 The high-resolution MRI scan revealed that the vessel wall of the entire course of the basilar artery was thickened, with a focal eccentric stenosis caused by an atherosclerotic plaque. T1-weighted imaging showed a focal hyperintensity on the ventral and right walls of the basilar artery, indicative of the presence of intraplaque hemorrhage (arrow) (**A**, **B**)

continued to experience episodes of dizziness. Therefore, she was recommended to undergo endovascular treatment for her basilar artery. There are potential risks associated with this procedure, including occlusion of perforating arteries, iatrogenic dissection, and acute in-stent thrombosis.

4. Treatment

Under general anesthesia, a 6F guiding catheter was positioned at the V2 segment of the left vertebral artery. The angiogram confirmed the presence of multiple tandem stenoses of the basilar artery, along with an aneurysm located at the tip of the basilar artery (Fig. 5.7.22 A, B). A Synchro microwire (0.014 in, 300 cm) was used to navigate through the stenosis segment and was positioned at the superior segment of the basilar artery. A 1.5 mm×9 mm Gateway balloon was then used to sequentially pre-dilate the proximal and the intermediate stenoses (Fig. 5.7.22 C, D). The post-balloon dilation angiogram indicated a residual stenosis of

30% at the proximal stenosis, whilst the intermediate stenosis exhibited a residual stenosis of 40% accompanied by a grade 3 antegrade blood flow (Fig. 5.7.23). Following a ten-minute observation period, the final angiogram revealed that the basilar artery was patent, and significantly, there was no evidence of elastic recoil after the balloon angiography.

After the procedure, the patient presented with symptoms of nausea, vomiting, dysarthria, and weakness in the left limbs, with muscle strength graded at a maximum of 3 in the most severe condition. Repeated MRI scans displayed an acute infarct on the right side of the pons (Fig. 5.7.24 A), whilst the MRA demonstrated that the basilar artery remained patent, with a significant improvement in the degree of stenosis observed. (Fig. 5.7.24 B, C).

On discharge, the patient experienced mild dysarthria, with muscle strength graded at 4 in the left limbs. Additionally, there was partial relief from the patient's dizziness.

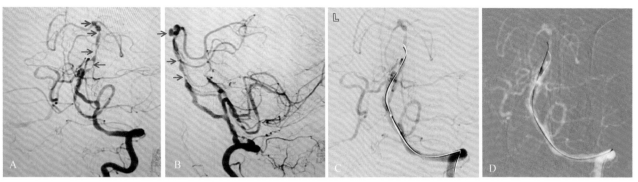

图 5.7.22　**A** 和 **B**. 术前造影显示基底动脉多发狭窄，基底动脉尖膨大，考虑基底动脉尖动脉瘤；**C** 和 **D**. Gateway 球囊扩张基底动脉近端和中间狭窄

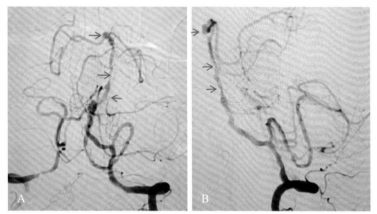

图 5.7.23　球囊扩张后造影显示近端狭窄程度明显改善，残余狭窄率约 30%。中间狭窄程度略有改善，残余狭窄率约 40%，前向血流 mTICI 分级 3 级

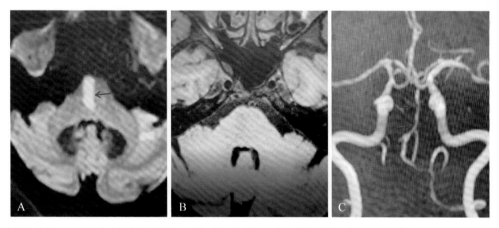

图 5.7.24　术后复查头部 MRI 提示脑桥右侧急性梗死灶（箭头示）（**A**），基底动脉通畅（**B**）；头部 MRA 显示狭窄明显改善（**C**）

（五）讨论

本例属基底动脉串联病变，斑块负荷重，虽用 1.5 mm 直径的小球囊扩张病变，术后仍发生穿支事件。患者基底动脉尖端膨隆，考虑动脉瘤，与狭窄远端血流动力学改变密切相关。对于基底动脉远端狭窄，因动脉瘤及远端微导丝着陆区的因素，未予以处理。本例后续需加强康复及高压氧治疗，以期尽快恢复。

（宋佳　杨明　贾白雪
江裕华　马宁）

5.7　手术操作视频（病例 25）

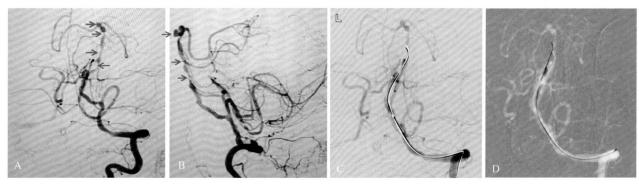

Fig. 5.7.22   The angiogram confirmed the presence of multiple tandem stenoses of the basilar artery, along with an aneurysm located at the tip of the basilar artery (**A, B**). A 1.5 mm×9 mm Gateway balloon was then used to pre-dilate the proximal and the intermediate stenoses in a sequential manner (**C, D**)

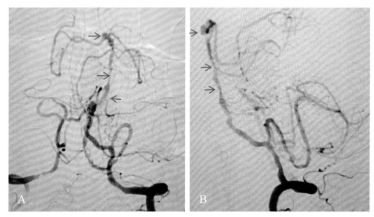

Fig. 5.7.23   The post-balloon dilation angiogram indicated a residual stenosis of 30% at the proximal stenosis, whilst the intermediate stenosis exhibited a residual stenosis of 40% accompanied by a grade 3 antegrade blood flow (**A, B**)

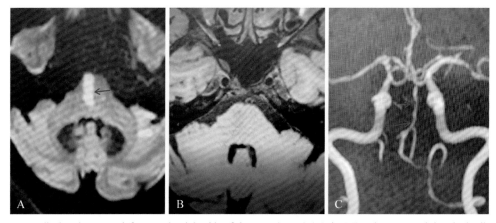

Fig. 5.7.24   MRI scans displayed an acute infarct on the right side of the pons (arrow) (**A**) the MRA demonstrated that the basilar artery remained patent, with a significant improvement in the degree of stenosis observed (**B, C**)

5. Comments

This case pertains to a patient with multiple tandem stenoses of the basilar artery, along with a high plaque burden. Despite undergoing submaximal angioplasty with a small-sized balloon (1.5 mm), the patient suffered an ischemic stroke due to perforating artery occlusion. The hemodynamic abnormality at the distal end of the basilar artery stenosis was closely related to an aneurysm at the tip of the basilar artery. Due to the challenges of the distal landing zone of the microwire and the presence of the aneurysm, angioplasty was not conducted on the distal basilar artery stenosis. Rehabilitation of the limbs and hyperbaric oxygen therapy could be beneficial for the patient's recovery.

(Translated by Rongrong Cui,
Revised by Zhikai Hou)

5.7   Video of endovascular therapy (Case 25)

病例 26　右颈内动脉 C4 段和 C7 段串联狭窄

（一）临床病史及影像分析

患者，男性，50 岁，主因"发作性左侧肢体无力 41 天"入院。

既往史：高血压和糖尿病病史。

查体：神经系统查体示左下肢肌力 5-级，左侧巴宾斯基征（＋）。

头部 MRI：右侧基底节区急性梗死灶（图 5.7.25 A 和 B）。

头部 MRA：右大脑中动脉血流信号浅淡，右颈内动脉 C7 段至大脑中动脉 M1 段近端重度狭窄（图 5.7.25 C）。

DSA：右颈内动脉 C7 段至大脑中动脉 M1 段近端重度狭窄，狭窄远端前向血流减慢，mTICI 分级 2a 级，右颈内动脉 C4 段中-重度狭窄，右胚胎型大脑后动脉（图 5.7.26）。

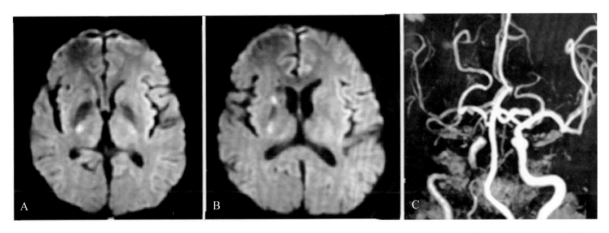

图 5.7.25　**A** 和 **B**.头部 MRI 示右侧基底节区急性梗死灶；**C**.头部 MRA 示右大脑中动脉血流信号浅淡，右颈内动脉 C7 段至大脑中动脉 M1 段近端重度狭窄

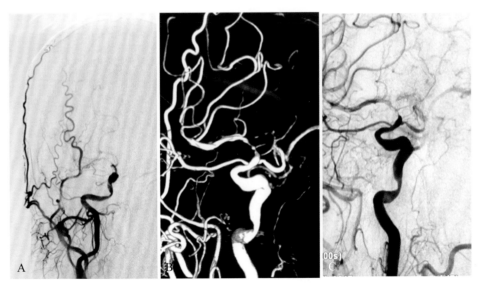

图 5.7.26　DSA 示右颈内动脉 C7 段至大脑中动脉 M1 段近端重度狭窄，右颈内动脉 C4 段中-重度狭窄，右胚胎型大脑后动脉（**A ～ C**）

Case 26　Tandem stenoses of the C4 and C7 segments of the right internal carotid artery

1. Clinical presentation and radiological studies

A 50-year-old male patient was admitted to the hospital due to paroxysmal weakness of the left limbs for forty-one days.

He had a history of diabetes and hypertension.

Physical examination showed the muscle strength in the left lower limb was grade 5-, and the left Babinski sign was positive.

The MRI result indicated acute infarction in the right basal ganglia (Fig. 5.7.25 A, B).

The MRA results disclosed severe stenosis from the C7 segment of the right internal carotid artery to the proximal M1 segment of the right middle cerebral artery (Fig. 5.7.25 C).

The DSA results displayed a severe stenosis extending from the right C7 segment to the right proximal M1 segment, accompanied by an impaired antegrade blood flow grade of 2a. In addition, moderate-to-severe stenosis was observed at the C4 segment. Furthermore, the right posterior cerebral artery exhibited a fetal-type pattern (Fig. 5.7.26).

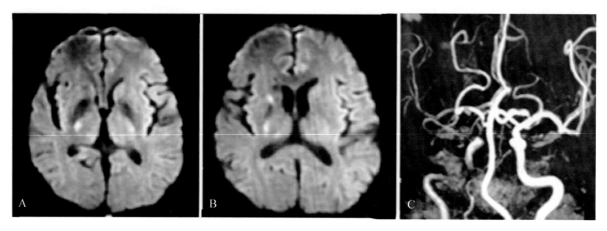

Fig. 5.7.25　The MRI result indicated acute infarction in the right basal ganglia (**A, B**). The MRA results disclosed severe stenosis from the C7 segment of the right internal carotid artery to the proximal M1 segment of the right middle cerebral artery (**C**)

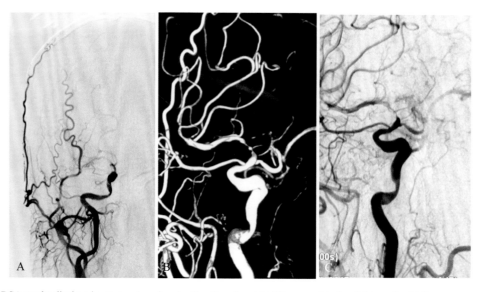

Fig. 5.7.26　The DSA results displayed a severe stenosis extending from the right C7 segment to the right proximal M1 segment, accompanied by an impaired antegrade blood flow grade of 2a. In addition, moderate-to-severe stenosis was observed at the C4 segment. Furthermore, the right posterior cerebral artery exhibited a fetal-type pattern

本次起病后患者一直接受双联抗血小板（阿司匹林 100 mg 1 次 / 日，氯吡格雷 75 mg 1 次 / 日）、他汀类药物调脂（阿托伐他汀 20 mg 1 次 / 日）治疗，以及控制危险因素相关治疗。

（二）诊断

右颈内动脉 C4 段和 C7 段症状性串联狭窄。

（三）术前讨论

患者右颈内动脉 C7 段重度狭窄，合并同侧颈内动脉 C4 段中 - 重度狭窄，其供血区域特别是大脑中动脉供血区域低灌注明显，虽经内科药物治疗仍有症状反复，有血管内介入治疗指征。拟先球囊扩张 C4 段，再球囊扩张 C7 段，必要时行支架置入术。相关风险包括动脉夹层、栓子脱落、穿支动脉闭塞、术后高灌注。

（四）治疗过程

全麻下右股动脉入路，8F 导引导管置于右颈总动脉末端，路径图下泥鳅导丝将 6F Navien 导管（115 cm）置于右颈内动脉 C2 段，造影示右颈内动脉 C4 段中 - 重度狭窄，右颈内动脉 C7 段重度狭窄（图 5.7.27）。选用 Avigo 微导丝（0.014 in，200 cm）通过右颈内动脉 C4 段狭窄，沿微导丝送入赛诺球囊（3 mm×10 mm），6 atm 压力扩张球囊，扩张后造影显示残余狭窄率约为 30%，跟进 Navien 导管接近 C4 段病变。将 Transend 微导丝（0.014 in，300 cm）携带 TREK 球囊（2.5 mm×8 mm）同轴，将微导丝头端置于右大脑中动脉 M2 段（图 5.7.28 A），跟进球囊至 C7 段狭窄处扩张（图 5.7.28 B 和 C）。撤出球囊送入 XT-27 微导管，经微导管释放 Neuroform EZ 自膨式支架（2.5 mm×15 mm）完全覆盖狭窄段（图 5.7.28 D）。撤出微导管释放支架，复查造影提示右颈内动脉末端及大脑中动脉近端残余狭窄率小于 10%，同侧大脑前动脉可见顺行显影，前向血流 mTICI 分级 3 级，右颈内动脉 C4 段残余狭窄率约 30%，无明显弹性回缩，不予以置入支架（图 5.7.29），遂结束治疗。

（五）讨论

本例右颈内动脉 C4 段及 C7 段（波及大脑中动脉 M1 段近端）狭窄，先球囊扩张近端病变，再跟进中间导管，以增加处理远端病变时的支撑力。由于较低的血流灌注，大脑中动脉 M1 段及其远端分支血管床塌陷，选用经导管释放的自膨式支架会较其他类型支架更容易到位和释放。另外，近端病变（C4 段）球囊扩张后血管无明显回缩，且残余狭窄率约为 30%，遂未予支架置入。

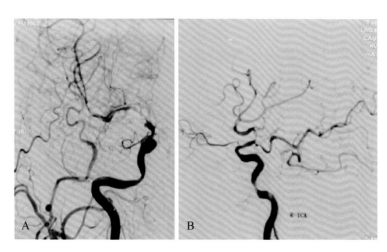

图 5.7.27　术前造影示右颈内动脉 C4 段中 - 重度狭窄，右颈内动脉 C7 段重度狭窄（**A** 和 **B**）

Since the onset of symptoms, he has been prescribed a dual antiplatelet regimen consisting of daily doses of 100 mg of Aspirin and 75mg of Clopidogrel. In addition, he has also been taking a daily dose of 20mg of Atorvastatin.

2. Diagnosis

Symptomatic tandem stenoses of the C4 and C7 segments of the right internal carotid artery.

3. Treatment schedule

The patient was found to have a severe stenosis of the right C7 segment and a moderate-to-severe stenosis at the C4 segment of the ipsilateral internal carotid artery. The DSA results showed significant hypoperfusion in its territory, particularly in the middle cerebral artery territory. Although receiving aggressive medical treatment, the patient experienced recurrent symptoms and thus was indicated for endovascular treatment. Treatment approach: Successive primary balloon angioplasty was performed on the C4 and C7 segments of the right internal carotid artery, followed by stent implantation if needed. Potential risks included artery dissection, embolus dislodgment, the occlusion of perforating arteries, and hyperperfusion syndrome.

4. Treatment

Under general anesthesia, an 8 French guide catheter was inserted through the right femoral artery and positioned at the end of the right carotid common artery. A 6F Navien catheter (115 cm) was then positioned at the C2 segment of the right internal carotid artery. The angiogram results confirmed the presence of a moderate-to-severe stenosis at the C4 segment of the right internal carotid artery, as well as a severe stenosis at the C7 segment of the right internal carotid artery (Fig. 5.7.27). An Avigo microwire (0.014 in, 200 cm) navigated through the C4 segment of the right internal carotid artery. Then a 3 mm×10 mm Sino balloon was utilized to dilate the C4 lesion. The post-dilation angiogram showed residual stenosis was 30%. Additionally, a Transend microwire (0.014 in, 300 cm) was placed at the M2 segment of the right middle cerebral artery (Fig. 5.7.28 A) and a 2.5 mm×8 mm TREK balloon was utilized to dilate the stenosis at the right C7 segment (Fig. 5.7.28 B, C). Next, an XT-27 microcatheter was used to release a 2.5 mm× 15 mm Neuroform EZ stent, which successfully covered the entire C7 segment (Fig. 5.7.28 D). A post-stent implantation angiogram revealed a residual stenosis of less than 10% for the right C7 segment, accompanied by antegrade blood flow of grade 3. As for the residual stenosis at the right C4 segment, it remained at 30% without any significant elastic recoil, which is why we decided not to implant a stent in this segment. (Fig. 5.7.29).

5. Comments

The patient in this case presented with tandem stenoses affecting both the C4 and C7 segments of the right internal carotid artery, as well as involving the proximal M1 segment of the middle cerebral artery. To address this issue during the procedure, we first performed primary balloon angioplasty on the proximal lesion and subsequently used an intermediate catheter to increase support force for treating the distal lesion. Due to hypoperfusion of blood flow, the vascular bed of the right M1 segment and its distal branches collapsed, making a self-expanding stent, released via microcatheter, a more appropriate choice than other types of stents. Additionally, because there was no significant elastic recoil and only a residual stenosis of 30% for the proximal lesion after the balloon angioplasty, we decided against performing stent implantation.

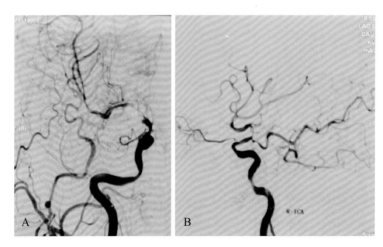

Fig. 5.7.27   The angiogram results confirmed the presence of a moderate-to-severe stenosis at the C4 segment of the right internal carotid artery, as well as severe stenosis at the C7 segment of the right internal carotid artery (**A, B**)

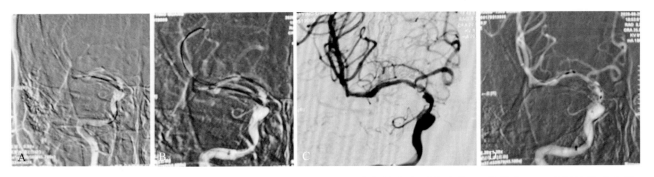

图 5.7.28 **A**. Transend 微导丝置于右大脑中动脉 M2 段；**B**. TREK 球囊扩张右颈内动脉 C7 段狭窄；**C**. 球囊扩张后造影；**D**. 释放 Neuroform EZ 支架完全覆盖狭窄段

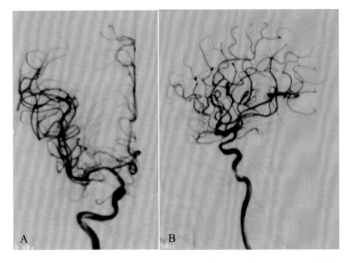

图 5.7.29 释放支架后造影提示右颈内动脉末端及大脑中动脉近端残余狭窄率小于 10%，前向血流 mTICI 分级 3 级，右颈内动脉 C4 段残余狭窄率约 30%，无明显弹性回缩

（蒯东　成涛　胡琼　何勇）

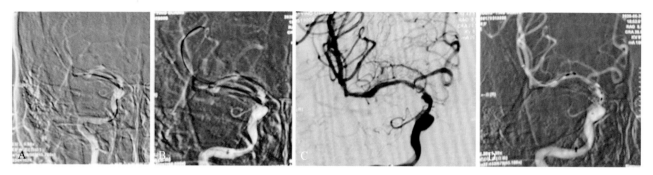

Fig. 5.7.28 A Transend microwire was placed at the M2 segment of the right middle cerebral artery (**A**), a TREK balloon was utilized to dilate the C7 segment of the right internal carotid artery (**B**, **C**). Then a Neuroform EZ stent was used to cover the stenosis at the right C7 segment (**D**)

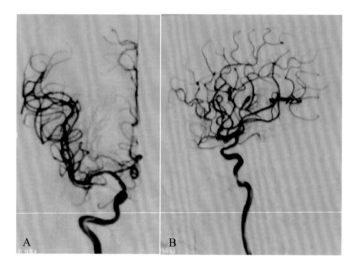

Fig. 5.7.29 A post-stent implantation angiogram revealed residual stenosis of less than 10% for the right C7 segment, accompanied by antegrade blood flow of grade 3. As for the residual stenosis at the right C4 segment, it remained at 30% without any significant elastic recoil

(Translated by Rongrong Cui, Revised by Zhikai Hou)

第八节　狭窄毗邻重要穿支动脉（边支保护技术）

病例 27　左椎基底动脉交界区狭窄毗邻穿支动脉

（一）临床病史及影像分析

患者，男性，53 岁，主因"发作性双眼视物模糊 50 天，视物重影 1 周"入院。

当地医院头部 MRI 示左侧侧脑室旁、右枕叶多发急性梗死灶（图 5.8.1）。磁共振 SWI 序列示左颞叶陈旧性脑出血，双额顶叶、脑桥及左小脑半球多发微出血灶（图 5.8.2）。

头部 MRA 示右椎动脉 V4 段闭塞，左椎动脉 V4 段和基底动脉交界区重度狭窄（图 5.8.3）。弓上 CTA 示双椎动脉 V4 段和基底动脉交界区重度狭窄（图 5.8.4）。

予以双联抗血小板、他汀类药物治疗后患者症状好转。1 周前患者出现双眼视物成双，持续时间 5 s 至 5 min 不等，每天发作 2 ～ 3 次。为进一步行血管内治疗收入我院。

既往史：高血压及脑出血病史 5 年。吸烟 25 年。
查体：神经系统查体无阳性体征。

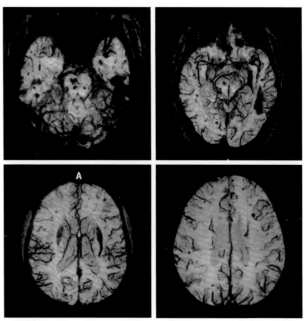

图 5.8.2　SWI 序列示左颞叶陈旧性脑出血，双额顶叶、脑桥及左小脑半球多发微出血灶

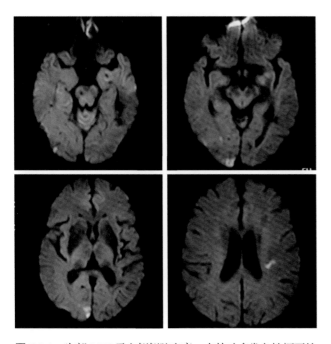

图 5.8.1　头部 MRI 示左侧侧脑室旁、右枕叶多发急性梗死灶

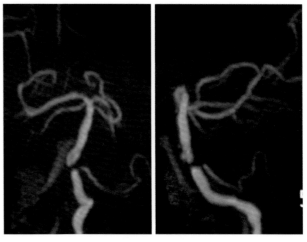

图 5.8.3　头部 MRA 示右椎动脉 V4 段闭塞，左椎动脉 V4 段和基底动脉交界区重度狭窄

Section 8   ICAS adjacent to Perforating Artery (Side–branch protection technique)

Case 27   The left vertebro-basilar artery junction stenosis adjacent to perforating arteries

1. Clinical presentation and radiological studies

A 53-year-old male patient was admitted to the hospital due to paroxysmal blurred vision in both eyes for fifty days, as well as diplopia for the past week.

The MRI results showed multiple acute infarctions in the left periventricular area and the right occipital lobe (Fig. 5.8.1). Additionally, susceptibility-weighted imaging (SWI) revealed the presence of old cerebral hemorrhage in the temporal lobe of the left side, as well as multiple microbleed lesions in the frontal and parietal lobes on both sides, the pons, and the left hemisphere of the cerebellum (Fig. 5.8.2).

The MRA results indicated the occlusion at the V4 segment of the right vertebral artery, as well as severe stenosis at the junction of the left vertebro-basilar artery (Fig. 5.8.3). Additionally, CT angiography demonstrated the presence of severe stenosis at the junction of the vertebro-basilar arteries (Fig. 5.8.4).

The patient's symptoms showed improvement following aggressive medical treatment. However, the patient began experiencing diplopia one week ago, with each episode lasting between 5 seconds to 5 minutes, and occurring 2–3 times per day.

The patient has a 5-year history of hypertension and cerebral hemorrhage, as well as a 25-year history of smoking. A neurological examination yielded negative results.

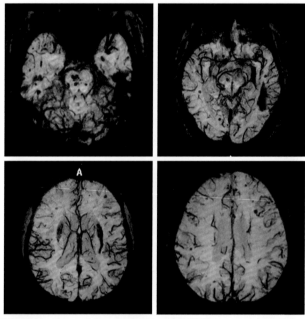

Fig. 5.8.2   Susceptibility-weighted imaging (SWI) revealed the presence of old cerebral hemorrhage in the temporal lobe of the left side, as well as multiple microbleed lesions in the frontal and parietal lobes on both sides, the pons, and the left hemisphere of the cerebellum

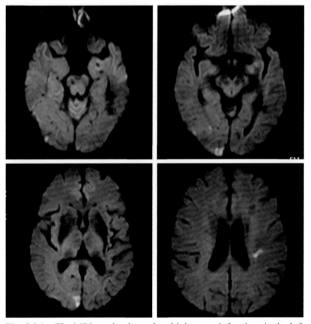

Fig. 5.8.1   The MRI results showed multiple acute infarctions in the left periventricular area and the right occipital lobe

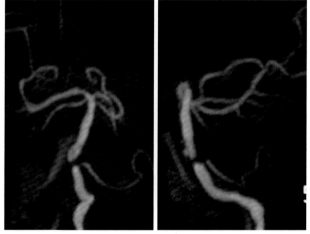

Fig. 5.8.3   The MRA results indicated the occlusion at the V4 segment of the right vertebral artery, as well as severe stenosis at the junction of the left vertebro-basilar artery

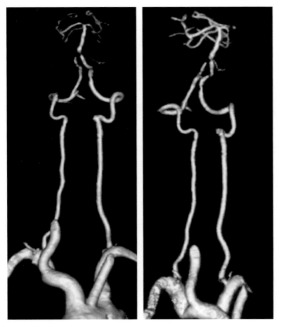

图 5.8.4 弓上 CTA 示双椎动脉 V4 段和基底动脉交界区重度狭窄

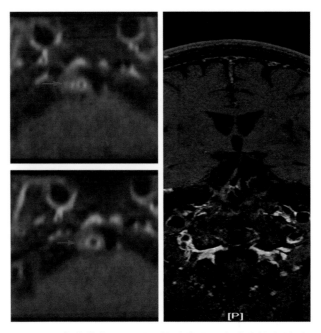

图 5.8.6 高分辨率 MRI 示双椎动脉及基底动脉管壁增厚，多发斑块，部分斑块内出血

LDL-C：2 mmol/L。

血栓弹力图：AA 抑制率 98.6%，ADP 抑制率 29.6%。

头部 CT：脑内多发陈旧性缺血灶（图 5.8.5）。

高分辨率 MRI：双椎动脉、基底动脉管壁增厚，多发斑块，部分斑块内出血（图 5.8.6）。

DSA：右后交通动脉未开放（图 5.8.7 A 和 B），左后交通动脉开放（图 5.8.7 C 和 D），右椎动脉

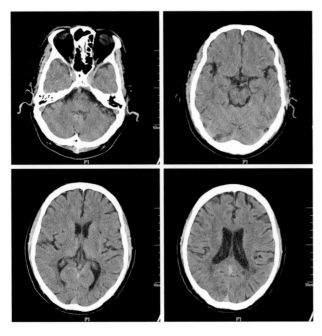

图 5.8.5 头部 CT 示脑内多发陈旧性缺血灶

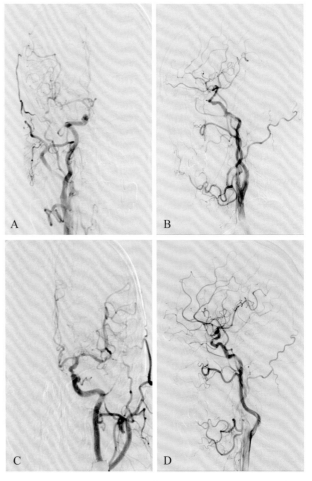

图 5.8.7 DSA 示右后交通动脉未开放（**A** 和 **B**），左后交通动脉开放（**C** 和 **D**）

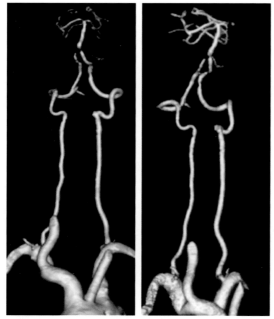

Fig. 5.8.4   CTA demonstrated the presence of severe stenosis at the junction of the vertebro-basilar arteries

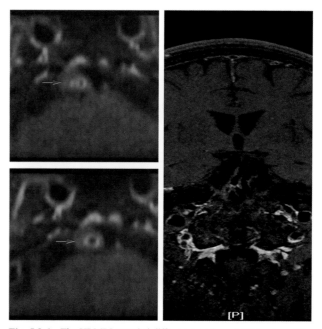

Fig. 5.8.6   The HRMRI revealed diffuse eccentric wall thickening of the intracranial vertebral and basilar arteries, with a focal vessel wall appearing hyperintense, indicating the presence of intraplaque hemorrhage

The concentration of LDL-C was measured at 2 mmol/L.

The Thromboelastography result indicated a 98.6% inhibition of AA and a 29.6% inhibition of ADP.

The noncontrast CT indicated multiple old cerebral infarcts (Fig. 5.8.5).

The high-resolution MRI (HRMRI) revealed diffuse eccentric wall thickening of the intracranial vertebral and basilar arteries, with a focal vessel wall appearing hyperintense, indicating the presence of intraplaque hemorrhage (Fig 5.8.6).

The DSA result showed that the right posterior communicating artery was occluded (Fig. 5.8.7 A, B), while the left posterior communicating artery was patent (Fig. 5.8.7 C, D). Moreover, there was an occlusion of the V4 segment of the right

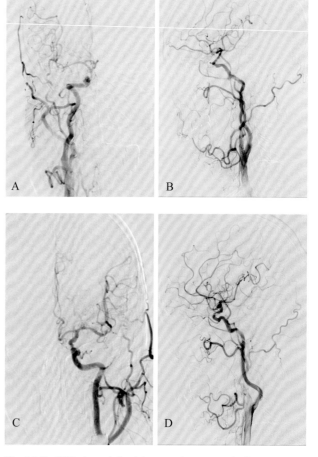

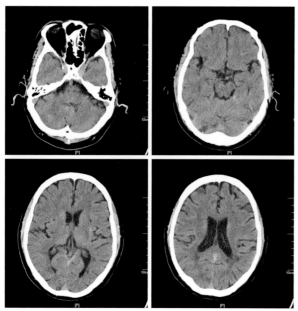

Fig. 5.8.5   The non-contrast CT indicated multiple old cerebral infarcts

Fig. 5.8.7   DSA showed the right posterior communicating artery was occluded (**A, B**), while the left posterior communicating artery was patent (**C, D**)

V4 段发出 PICA 后闭塞，PICA 供应双侧小脑半球（图 5.8.8 A 和 B），左椎动脉 V4 段和基底动脉交界区重度狭窄，狭窄处有左 AICA 发出（图 5.8.8 C 和 D）。

入院后给予双联抗血小板（阿司匹林 100 mg 1 次 / 日 ＋ 氯吡格雷 75 mg 1 次 / 日）、降脂（阿托伐他汀 20 mg 1 次 / 日）及降压等治疗。

（二）诊断

症状性左椎基底动脉交界区狭窄。

（三）术前讨论

患者右椎动脉 V4 段闭塞，左椎动脉 V4 段与基底动脉交界区重度狭窄，并伴有反复后循环缺血症状，高分辨率 MRI 提示系动脉粥样硬化性斑块所致，抗血小板聚集治疗后症状仍反复发作，有介入治疗指征。病变处有重要的左 AICA 发出，拟先球

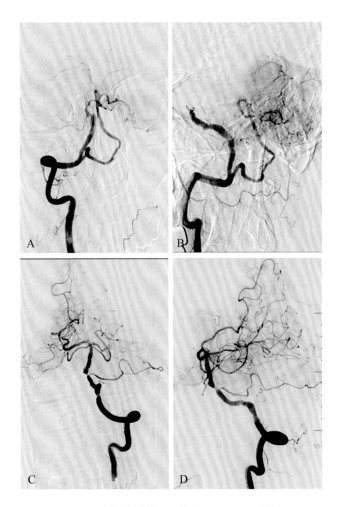

图 5.8.8　DSA 示右椎动脉 V4 段发出 PICA 后闭塞，PICA 供应双侧小脑半球（**A** 和 **B**）；左椎动脉 V4 段和基底动脉交界区重度狭窄，狭窄处有左 AICA 发出（**C** 和 **D**）

囊扩张，再放置自膨式支架。拟在球囊扩张过程中采用边支保护技术。相关风险包括穿支动脉闭塞、急性或亚急性血栓形成等。

（四）治疗过程

全麻下右股动脉入路，送入 6F 导引导管至左椎动脉 V2 段远端，术前造影示左椎动脉 V4 段和基底动脉交界区重度狭窄（图 5.8.9）。

路径图下送入 Synchro 微导丝（0.014 in，300 cm），在 Echelon-10 微导管支持下置于左 AICA 内。撤出微导管，保留微导丝（图 5.8.10 A 和 B）。将 Transend 微导丝（0.014 in，300 cm）送至右大脑后动脉 P2 段（图 5.8.10 C）。沿 Transend 微导丝送入 Gateway 球囊（2.75 mm×9 mm）至狭窄处预扩张（图 5.8.10 D 和 E），撤出球囊后造影显示狭窄明显改善（图 5.8.10 F）。撤出左 AICA 内 Synchro 微导丝，沿 Transend 微导丝送入 Wingspan 自膨式支架（3.5 mm× 15 mm）至病变处并释放（图 5.8.11 A 和 B），造影显示支架贴壁良好，前向血流 mTICI 分级 3 级（图 5.8.11 C 和 D）。术后查体同前。

术后立即复查头部 CT 未见出血或梗死（图 5.8.12）。术后复查头部 CTA 示左椎动脉 V4 段与基底动脉交界区支架内通畅（图 5.8.13）。

（五）讨论

本例因左 AICA 毗邻狭窄段，故采用边支保护技术，以减少边支受损概率。因微导丝头端位于

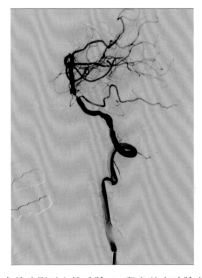

图 5.8.9　术前造影示左椎动脉 V4 段和基底动脉交界区重度狭窄

vertebral artery distal to the PICA, which supplied the bilateral cerebellar hemispheres (Fig. 5.8.8 A, B), as well as severe stenosis of the junction between the left vertebral and basilar arteries, with the left anterior inferior cerebellar artery (AICA) arising from the stenotic segment (Fig. 5.8.8 C, D).

Upon admission, a dual antiplatelet regimen comprising a daily dosage of 100 mg of Aspirin and 75 mg of Clopidogrel, as well as a daily dose of 20 mg of Atorvastatin, was prescribed to him.

2. Diagnosis

Symptomatic stenosis of the left vertebro-basilar artery junction.

3. Treatment schedule

The patient presented with occlusion of the V4 segment of the right vertebral artery and severe stenosis of the left vertebro-basilar artery junction. He continued to experience symptoms of posterior circulation ischemia, even after receiving aggressive medical therapy. As a result, endovascular treatment was deemed necessary to alleviate his symptoms. As the left AICA

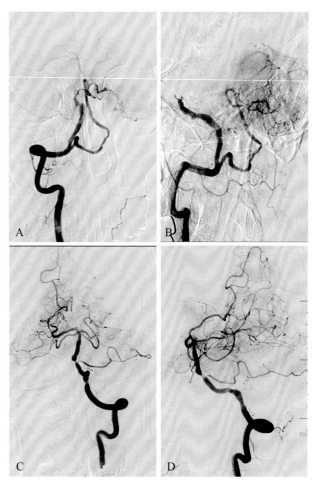

Fig. 5.8.8 There was an occlusion of the V4 segment of the right vertebral artery distal to the PICA, which supplied the bilateral cerebellar hemispheres (**A, B**), as well as severe stenosis of the junction between the left vertebral and basilar arteries, with the left anterior inferior cerebellar artery (AICA) arising from the stenotic segment (**C, D**)

was originating from the stenotic lesion, the lesion was predilated and followed by the implantation of a self-expanding stent. A side-branch protection technique will be implemented during balloon dilatation. However, the procedure may also carry potential risks such as occlusion of perforating arteries and acute/subacute in-stent thrombosis.

4. Treatment

Under general anesthesia, a 6F guiding catheter was inserted through the right femoral access and advanced into the V2 segment of the left vertebral artery. The angiogram confirmed the presence of severe stenosis at the junction of the left vertebro-basilar artery. (Fig. 5.8.9).

With the assistance of the Echelon-10 microcatheter, a Synchro microwire (0.014 in, 300 cm) was positioned at the left AICA (Fig. 5.8.10 A, B). A Transend microwire (0.014 in, 300 cm) was placed at the P2 segment of the right posterior cerebral artery (Fig. 5.8.10 C). Subsequently, a Gateway balloon (2.75 mm×9 mm) was delivered to pre-dilate the lesion (Fig. 5.8.10 D, E). A post-dilation angiogram showed significant improvement in the degree of stenosis at the left vertebro-basilar junction (Fig. 5.8.10 F). Thereafter, the Synchro microwire in the left AICA was withdrawn and a 3.5 mm×15 mm Wingspan stent was deployed to cover the lesion (Fig. 5.8.11 A, B). After the stent implantation, the final angiogram showed excellent stent wall attachment and a grade 3 of the antegrade blood flow (Fig. 5.8.11 C, D).

The non-contrast CT scan performed after the procedure indicated no evidence of cerebral hemorrhage or infarction (Fig. 5.8.12).

Postprocedural CTA showed the stent in the left vertebro-basilar junction was patent (Fig. 5.8.13).

5. Comments

Given the proximity of the stenotic lesion to the left AICA, we employed the side-branch protection technique to

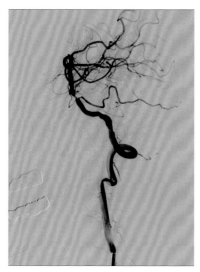

Fig. 5.8.9 The angiogram confirmed the presence of severe stenosis at the junction of the left vertebro-basilar artery

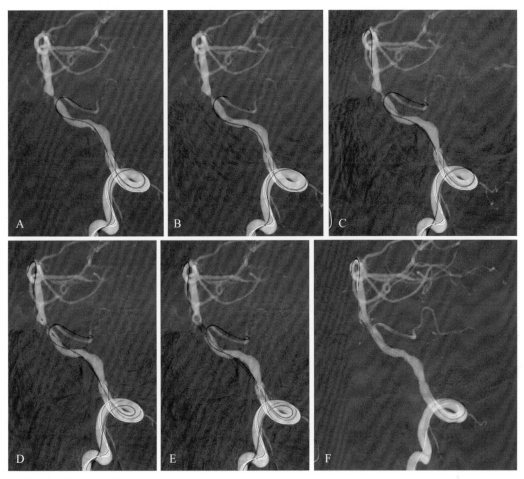

图 5.8.10　血管内介入治疗过程如下：**A** 和 **B**. 将 Synchro 微导丝置于左 AICA 内；**C**. 将 Transend 微导丝置于右大脑后动脉 P2 段；**D** 和 **E**. Gateway 球囊扩张狭窄病变；**F**. 球囊扩张后造影显示狭窄明显改善

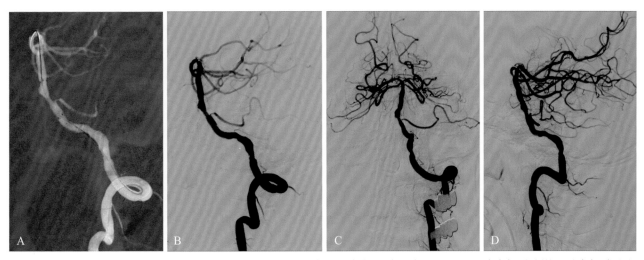

图 5.8.11　**A** 和 **B**. 沿 Transend 微导丝送入 Wingspan 自膨式支架至病变处并释放；**C** 和 **D**. 释放支架后造影显示支架贴壁良好，前向血流 mTICI 分级 3 级

AICA 远端，从另一微导丝推送装置时要更为谨慎，避免 AICA 内微导丝的剧烈位置变动导致血管损伤。此外，边支与血管主干角度过大会导致超选困难，如果评估边支闭塞后存在侧支代偿，适时放弃保护也是一种临床选择。

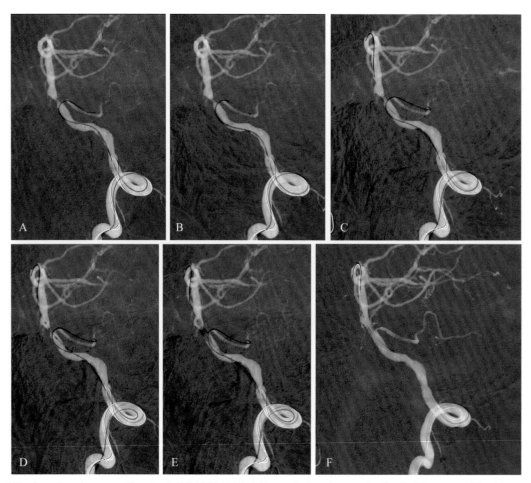

Fig. 5.8.10 A Synchro microwire was positioned at the left AICA (**A, B**). A Transend microwire was placed at the P2 segment of the right posterior cerebral artery (**C**), a Gateway balloon was delivered to pre-dilate the lesion (**D, E**), a post-dilation angiogram showed significant improvement in the degree of stenosis at the left vertebro-basilar junction (**F**)

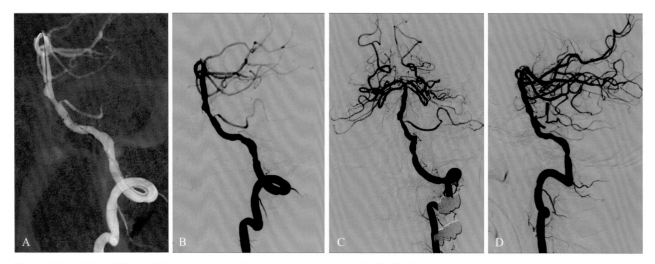

Fig. 5.8.11 A 3.5 mm×15 mm Wingspan stent was deployed to cover the lesion (**A, B**). The final angiogram showed excellent stent wall attachment and a grade 3 of the antegrade blood flow (**C, D**)

safeguard the left AICA throughout the procedure. To prevent potential vascular injury resulting from microwire migration in the AICA, it is prudent to exercise caution pushing forward the device while using the microwire in the right P2 segment. Furthermore, the excessive angle between the branch artery and parent trunk may pose challenges to implementing the side-branch protection technique. In cases where there is adequate collateral compensation following occlusion of the branch artery, timely discontinuation of side-branch artery protection is also a viable option.

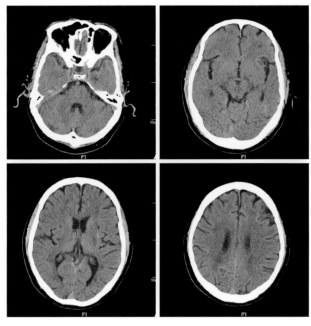

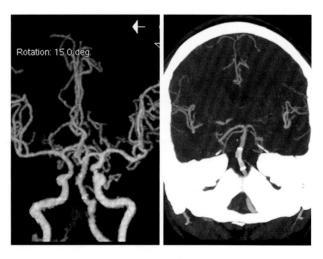

图 5.8.13　术后复查头部 CTA 示左椎动脉 V4 段与基底动脉交界区支架内通畅

图 5.8.12　术后复查头部 CT 未见出血或梗死

5.8　手术操作视频
（病例 27）

（王天保　宋立刚　马宁）

病例 28　左大脑中动脉分叉部重度狭窄

（一）临床病史及影像分析

患者，女性，62 岁，主因"发作性言语不利、右侧肢体活动不利 1 年"入院。

当地医院头部 MRI 示左侧颞叶、顶叶多发急性梗死灶（图 5.8.14 A ~ C）。头部 MRA 示左大脑中动脉 M1 段重度狭窄（图 5.8.14 D）。给予双联抗血小板、他汀类药物调脂等治疗后症状仍反复。为进一步治疗收入我院。

既往史：吸烟 30 年。

查体：神经系统查体无阳性体征。

血栓弹力图：AA 抑制率 96.3%，ADP 抑制率 31%。

头部 CTA：左大脑中动脉水平段（M1 段）近分叉处重度狭窄（图 5.8.15 A）。

头部 CTP：左大脑中动脉供血区域低灌注（图 5.8.15 B）。

DSA：右颈内动脉系统未见明显异常（图 5.8.16 A）。左大脑中动脉早分叉，近分叉处大脑中动脉上干及下干起始处重度狭窄，同侧大脑前动脉及后循环向左大脑中动脉供血区域代偿欠佳（图 5.8.16 B 和 C）。

高分辨率 MRI：左大脑中动脉 M1 段管壁增厚，局部管腔重度狭窄近乎闭塞，局部管壁有强化（图 5.8.17）。

入院后给予双联抗血小板（阿司匹林 100 mg 1 次 / 日＋氯吡格雷 75 mg 1 次 / 日）、降脂（阿托伐他汀 20 mg 1 次 / 日）治疗。

（二）诊断

症状性左大脑中动脉分叉部重度狭窄。

（三）术前讨论

患者反复出现局灶性神经功能缺损症状，内科

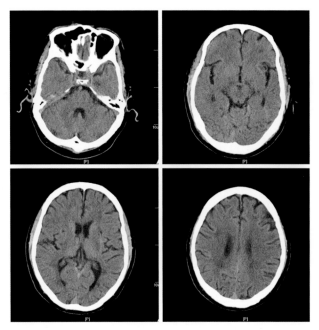

Fig. 5.8.12 Postprocedural CT indicated no evidence of cerebral hemorrhage or infarction

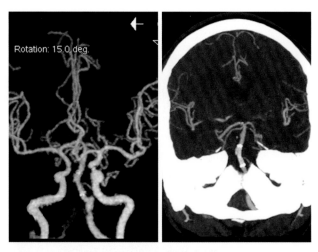

Fig. 5.8.13 Postprocedural brain CTA showed the stent in the left vertebro-basilar junction was patent

(Translated by Rongrong Cui, Revised by Zhikai Hou)

5.8 Video of endovascular therapy (Case 27)

Case 28　Severe stenosis of the left middle cerebral artery bifurcation

1. Clinical presentation and radiological studies

A 62-year-old female patient presented with paroxysmal dysarthria and weakness of the right limbs for one year.

The MRI results showed multiple acute infarctions in the left temporal and parietal lobes (Fig. 5.8.14 A–C). The MRA revealed severe stenosis in the M1 segment of the left middle cerebral artery (Fig. 5.8.14 D). Despite receiving aggressive medical treatment, the patient continued to experience recurrent episodes of symptoms.

She had a 30-year history of smoking.

She had no neurological deficits on admission.

The thromboelastography result indicated a 96.3% inhibition of AA and a 31% inhibition of ADP.

The CT angiography exhibited significant stenosis located adjacent to the bifurcation of the M1 segment of the left middle cerebral artery (Fig. 5.8.15 A).

The CT perfusion indicated hypoperfusion in the territory of the left middle cerebral artery (Fig. 5.8.15 B).

According to the DSA results, no remarkable abnormality was detected in the right internal carotid artery system (Fig. 5.8.16 A). A severe stenosis was observed in the bifurcation of the left middle cerebral artery, with the upper and lower divisions involved. Additionally, there was inadequate compensation from the ipsilateral anterior cerebral artery and the posterior circulation system to the territory of the left middle cerebral artery (Fig. 5.8.16 B, C).

The high-resolution MRI (HRMRI) revealed thickening of the wall of the left middle cerebral artery, resulting in severe stenosis at the left M1 segment. Additionally, the contrast-enhancement sequence demonstrated strong intraplaque enhancement (Fig. 5.8.17).

Upon admission, she has prescribed a dual antiplatelet regimen comprising a daily dose of 100 mg Aspirin and 75mg Clopidogrel, alongside a daily dose of 20 mg Atorvastatin.

2. Diagnosis

Symptomatic stenosis of the left middle cerebral artery bifurcation.

3. Treatment schedule

Despite receiving aggressive medical treatment, the patient persisted in experiencing recurrent episodes of deficits in focal neurological function. Based on the clinical manifestation and radiological studies, the stenosis located adjacent to the bifurcation of the left middle cerebral artery was identified as the culprit lesion. The patient was indicated undergoing

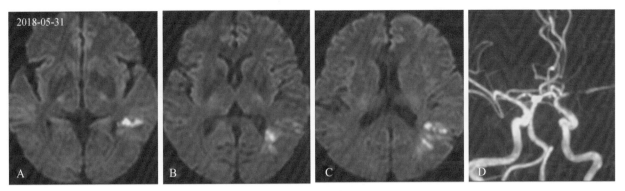

图 5.8.14　头部 MRI 提示左侧颞叶、顶叶多发急性梗死灶（**A ～ C**），MRA 提示左大脑中动脉 M1 段重度狭窄（**D**）

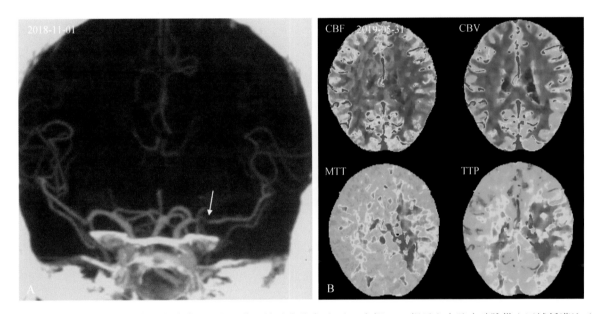

图 5.8.15　头部 CTA 提示左大脑中动脉 M1 段近分叉处重度狭窄（**A**），头部 CTP 提示左大脑中动脉供血区域低灌注（**B**）

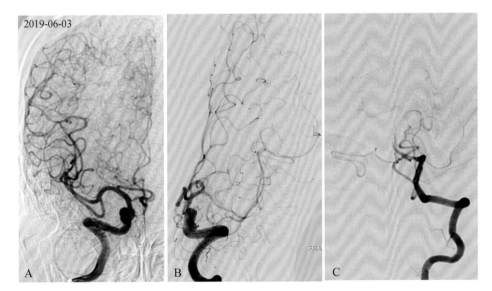

图 5.8.16　DSA 示右颈内动脉系统未见明显异常（**A**）；左大脑中动脉早分叉，近分叉处大脑中动脉上干及下干起始处重度狭窄，同侧大脑前动脉及后循环向左大脑中动脉供血区域代偿欠佳（**B 和 C**）

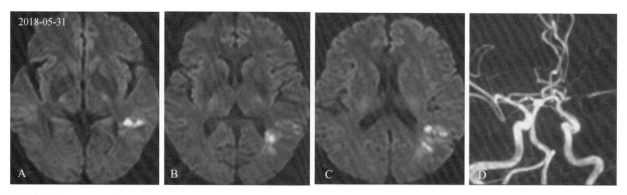

Fig. 5.8.14 The MRI results showed multiple acute infarctions in the left temporal and parietal lobes (**A–C**). The MRA revealed severe stenosis in the M1 segment of the left middle cerebral artery (**D**)

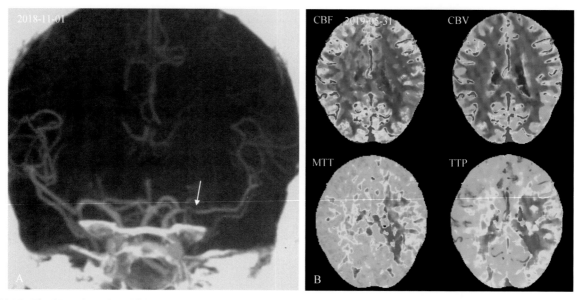

Fig. 5.8.15 The CT angiography exhibited significant stenosis located adjacent to the bifurcation of the M1 segment of the left middle cerebral artery (**A**). CT perfusion indicated hypoperfusion in the territory of the left middle cerebral artery (**B**)

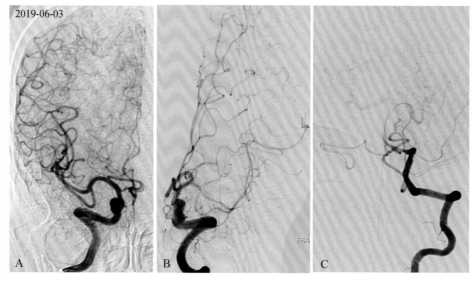

Fig. 5.8.16 DSA results showed no remarkable abnormality was detected in the right internal carotid artery system (**A**), a severe stenosis was observed in the bifurcation of the left middle cerebral artery, with the upper and lower divisions involvement. Additionally, there was inadequate compensation from the ipsilateral anterior cerebral artery and the posterior circulation system to the territory of the left middle cerebral artery (**B, C**)

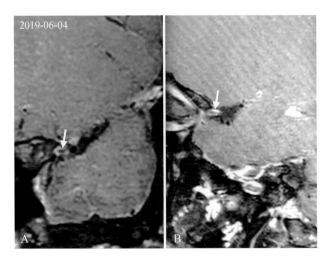

图 5.8.17　高分辨率 MRI 示左大脑中动脉 M1 段管壁增厚，局部管腔重度狭窄近乎闭塞，局部管壁有强化（箭头示）

治疗效果欠佳，结合临床症状与影像学检查考虑左大脑中动脉 M1 段为责任血管，且 CTP 提示相应区域低灌注，有介入治疗指征。左大脑中动脉早分叉，分叉处上干及下干起始处均有狭窄。拟在上、下干分别置入双微导丝，分别行小球囊扩张同时保护分支。再酌情放置支架，必要时放置 Y 型双支架。手术风险包括穿支动脉卒中、动脉夹层、急性或亚急性支架内血栓形成、术后高灌注综合征等。

（四）治疗过程

全麻下右股动脉入路，将 6F 导引导管头端置于左颈内动脉 C2 段。术前造影显示左大脑中动脉 M1 段分叉处重度狭窄，累及上、下干起始处（图 5.8.18 A）。

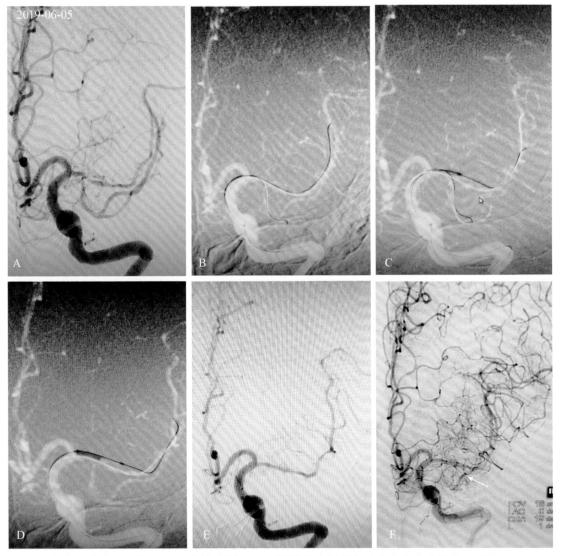

图 5.8.18　血管内介入治疗过程如下：**A**. 术前造影；**B**. 双微导丝分别到位于左大脑中动脉上、下干；**C**. Gateway 球囊（1.5 mm×9 mm）扩张上干病变；**D**. Gateway 球囊（2.0 mm×9 mm）再次扩张上干病变；**E**. Neuroform EZ 支架覆盖上干病变后，下干未显影；**F**. 观察 10 min 后动脉晚期可见闭塞下干由上干经软脑膜动脉代偿逆行显影（箭头示）

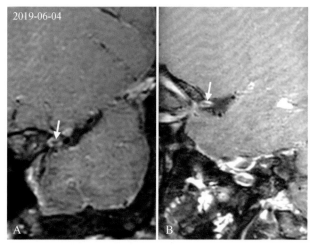

Fig. 5.8.17 HRMRI revealed thickening of the wall of the left middle cerebral artery, resulting in severe stenosis at the left M1 segment. Additionally, the contrast-enhancement sequence demonstrated strong intra-plaque enhancement (arrow)

endovascular therapy. The stenosis affected not only the bifurcation of the left middle cerebral artery but also involved both its upper and lower divisions. To protect the divisions of the left middle cerebral artery, the microwires were intended to be positioned separately at its upper and lower divisions during submaximal angioplasty. If needed, a Y-dual stent system could also be employed. Possible risks included occlusion of the perforating artery, iatrogenic artery dissection, acute/subacute in-stent thrombosis, and hyperperfusion syndrome.

4. Treatment

Under general anesthesia, a 6F guiding catheter was introduced via the right femoral artery and placed at the C2 segment of the left internal carotid artery. The angiogram revealed severe stenosis at the bifurcation of the left middle cerebral artery, which affected both its upper and lower divisions (Fig. 5.8.18 A).

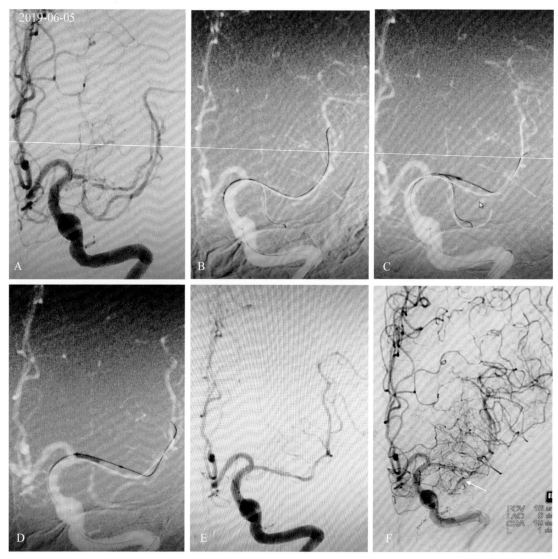

Fig. 5.8.18 (**A**) The angiogram before the procedure. (**B**) The microwires were positioned at the upper and lower division of the left middle cerebral artery, respectively. (**C**) A Gateway balloon (1.5 mm×9 mm) was used to dilate the stenosis of the upper division. (**D**) A Gateway balloon (2.0 mm×9 mm) was sent to the upper division for the second balloon dilation. (**E**) The angiogram demonstrated that the residual stenosis in the upper division was approximately 10%, with an enhanced antegrade blood flow. The lower division was not observed (**F**) In the late arterial phase, the lower division was visualized through the pial artery of the upper trunk (arrow)

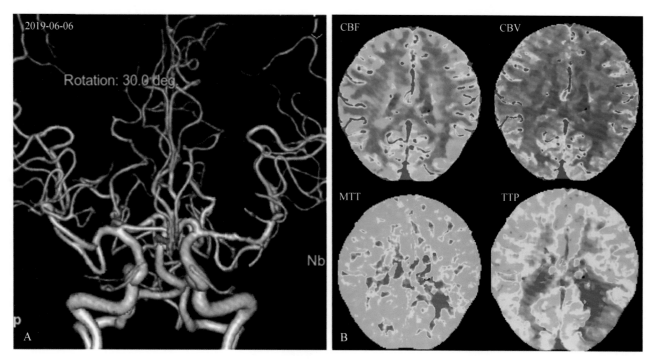

图 5.8.19　**A**. 术后 CTA 示左大脑中动脉支架术后管腔通畅，下干显影良好；**B**. 术后 CTP 示左侧大脑半球低灌注较术前明显好转

路径图引导下沿导引导管送入 Synchro 微导丝（0.014 in，300 cm）携 SL-10 微导管通过左大脑中动脉近分叉处狭窄，分别送至上、下干（图 5.8.18 B）。尝试送入 Gateway 球囊（1.5 mm×9 mm）至下干，但球囊到位困难，遂撤出球囊，再次送入球囊至上干狭窄处进行扩张（图 5.8.18 C）。第一次球囊扩张后造影显示残余狭窄明显，撤出下干微导丝，经上干微导丝送入 Gateway 球囊（2.0 mm×9 mm）再次进行扩张（图 5.8.18 D）。撤出球囊，经微导丝送入 Neuroform EZ 支架（3.0 mm×15 mm）释放。造影显示支架覆盖上干狭窄段，残余狭窄率约 10%，血流明显改善，远端血管较前显影改善，但下干未显影（图 5.8.18 E）。观察 10 min 无改变，考虑穿支架网眼开通下干风险大，动脉晚期可见闭塞下干由上干经软脑膜动脉代偿逆行显影，遂结束手术（图 5.8.18 F）。

术后立即复查头部 CT 未见出血。

术后复查头部 CTA ＋ CTP：左大脑中动脉支架术后管腔通畅，下干显影良好（图 5.8.19 A）。左侧大脑半球低灌注较术前明显好转（图 5.8.19 B）。

（五）讨论

本例左大脑中动脉 M1 段分叉部病变，累及分叉部近端及上、下干开口，我们术前拟行上、下干双导丝保护技术，由于下干与主干成角过大，球囊不能到位，未按计划使用小球囊扩张下干。上干扩张后，拟放置支架于主干至上干，因担心输送导管致下干导丝移位，故提前撤出下干微导丝。释放支架后下干闭塞，考虑再次开通下干困难，不得已结束手术。所幸支架释放后增加了上干血流，闭塞下干远端经侧支有逆行显影。术后第 2 天复查 CTA，下干又幸运再通。本例显示，对于颅内分叉部病变，如主干与分支血管角度过大且开口处存在狭窄，实施微导丝保护技术即可。如行开口处成形扩张，有球囊不能到位的可能。

（苗春芝　王坤　姜鹏　马宁）

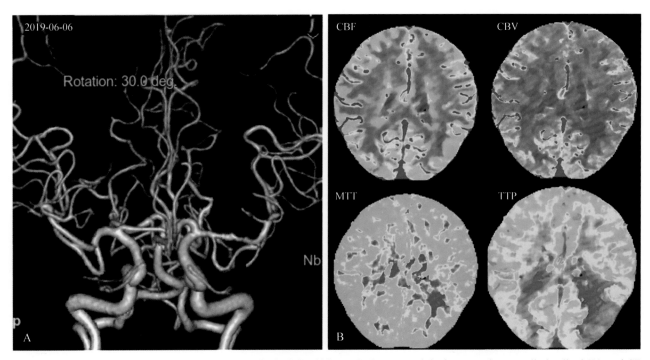

Fig. 5.8.19 Postprocedural CTA revealed a patent stent in the left middle cerebral artery, and the lower trunk was well visualized (**A**), and CT perfusion exhibited an amelioration in left cerebral hemisphere hypoperfusion (**B**)

Under the roadmap, the Synchro microwire (0.014 in, 300 cm) and SL-10 microcatheter were coaxially advanced through the stenosis lesion. The microwires were positioned at the upper and lower division of the left middle cerebral artery, respectively (Fig. 5.8.18 B). A Gateway balloon (1.5 mm×9 mm) could not be advanced through the stenotic lesion of the lower division. The balloon was retracted and instead delivered into the upper division where it was used to gradually dilate the stenotic lesion of the upper division (Fig. 5.8.18 C). The post-balloon dilation angiogram revealed that there was still significant residual stenosis. Consequently, the microwire was withdrawn from the lower division and a Gateway balloon (2.0 mm×9 mm) was introduced into the upper division for a second balloon dilation (Fig. 5.8.18 D). Subsequently, a 3.0 mm×15 mm Neuroform EZ stent was employed to enclose the stenosis in the upper division. The angiogram demonstrated that the residual stenosis in the upper division was approximately 10%, with an enhanced antegrade blood flow. Regrettably, the lower division was not observed (Fig. 5.8.18 E). This posed a challenge in the recanalization of the lower division through the stent mesh. In the late arterial phase, the lower division was visualized through the pial artery of the upper trunk (Fig. 5.8.18 F). Consequently, the procedure was terminated. The CT performed after the procedure revealed no evidence of cerebral hemorrhage.

After the procedure, the CTA revealed a patent stent in the left middle cerebral artery, and the lower trunk was well visualized (Fig. 5.8.19 A). The CT perfusion exhibited an amelioration in left cerebral hemisphere hypoperfusion (Fig. 5.8.19 B).

5. Comments

In this particular case, the patient exhibited a stenosis at the bifurcation of the left middle cerebral artery, involving both the origins of the upper and lower divisions. While performing the procedure, a double microwire side-branch protection technique was designated to safeguard the divisions. Nonetheless, owing to an extreme angle between the lower division and the main trunk, the balloon could not be placed to dilate the lower division as intended. Following the balloon dilation of the upper division, it was determined that a Neuroform EZ stent would be needed to cover the stenosis, extending from the main trunk to the upper division. As a precaution against potential microwire migration when delivering the microcatheter, the microwire in the lower division was carefully retracted. However, it proved challenging to recanalize the occluded lower division after stent deployment. Despite this setback, there was a silver lining: the antegrade blood flow in the upper division improved following stent implantation. This improvement in blood flow effectively compensated for the distal segment of the lower division through collateral circulation. Following the procedure, a repeated CTA demonstrated successful recanalization of the lower division. Endovascular treatment for intracranial stenosis at the bifurcation may require the implementation of the microwire protection technique, particularly in cases where an extreme angle exists between the lower division and the main trunk. It is worth noting that, in such cases, the balloon for dilating the branch origin may not be appropriately positioned.

(Translated by Rongrong Cui, Revised by Zhikai Hou)

第九节 球囊扩张困难

病例 29 基底动脉重度狭窄球囊扩张困难

（一）临床病史及影像分析

患者，男性，64 岁，主因"头晕 1 周"入院。
既往史：高血压、糖尿病和脂代谢紊乱病史。
查体：神经系统查体无阳性体征。
头颅 MRI：无新发脑梗死（图 5.9.1）。
头部 MRA：基底动脉中段重度狭窄（图 5.9.2）。
CTA：双颈内动脉 C1 段迂曲（图 5.9.3 A）。
左椎动脉优势，基底动脉中段重度狭窄（图 5.9.3
B～D）。

本次起病后患者行双联抗血小板（阿司匹林

100 mg 1 次 / 日，氯吡格雷 75 mg 1 次 / 日）及降
脂（阿托伐他汀 20 mg 1 次 / 日）治疗。

（二）诊断

症状性基底动脉中段重度狭窄。

（三）术前讨论

患者基底动脉中段重度狭窄，侧支循环代偿
差，考虑头晕系其供血区域低灌注所致，拟行血管
内干预治疗。准备球囊预扩张基础上再放置自膨式
支架。相关风险包括穿支卒中、术后高灌注等。

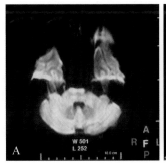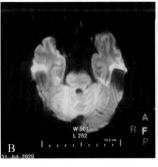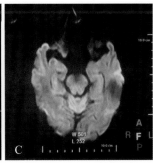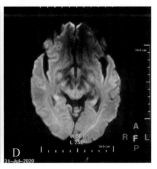

图 5.9.1 头颅 MRI 未见新发梗死（**A ～ D**）

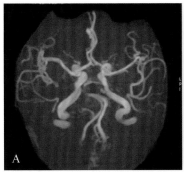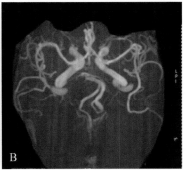

图 5.9.2 头部 MRA 提示基底动脉中段重度狭窄（**A 和 B**）

Section 9   ICAS with Failed Balloon Angioplasty

Case 29   Failed balloon angioplasty of severe stenosis of the basilar artery

1. Clinical presentation and radiological studies

A 64-year-old man was admitted to the hospital due to dizziness for one week.

The patient has a medical history of hypertension, diabetes, and lipoprotein metabolism disorders.

Upon admission, the patient's neurological status was intact.

The MRI showed the absence of acute infarction (Fig. 5.9.1).

The MRA revealed severe stenosis at the middle segment of the basilar artery (Fig. 5.9.2).

The CT angiography revealed that the C1 segments of the bilateral internal carotid arteries were tortuous (Fig. 5.9.3 A). The left vertebral artery was dominant and the middle segment of the basilar artery exhibited severe stenosis (Fig. 5.9.3 B–D).

He was prescribed a dual antiplatelet regimen consisting of daily doses of 100mg Aspirin and 75 mg Clopidogrel, along with statin therapy involving a daily dose of 20 mg of Atorvastatin from the onset of the disease.

2. Diagnosis

Symptomatic severe stenosis of the middle segment of the basilar artery.

3. Treatment schedule

This case features a patient with significant stenosis at the middle segment of the basilar artery, with inadequate collateral compensation. The recurrent dizziness symptoms were caused by hypoperfusion in the territory of the basilar artery due to severe stenosis. The treatment approach involved predilating the basilar artery stenosis using a balloon, followed by selfexpanding stent implantation. Potential risks associated with the procedure included the occlusion of perforating arteries and hyperperfusion syndrome.

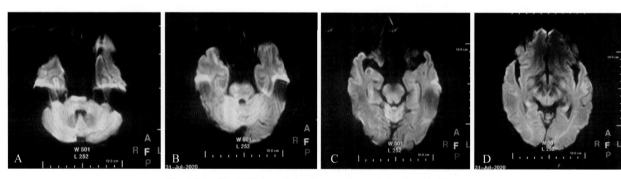

Fig. 5.9.1   The MRI showed the absence of acute infarction (**A–D**)

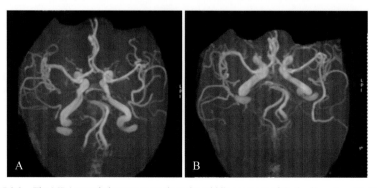

Fig. 5.9.2   The MRA revealed severe stenosis at the middle segment of the basilar artery (**A, B**)

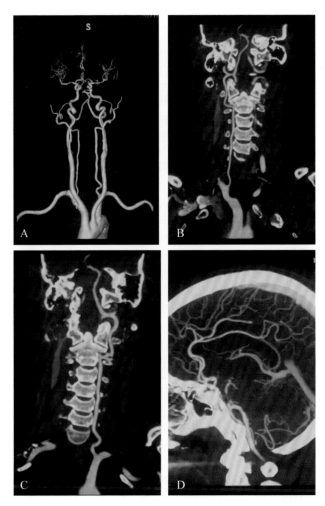

图 5.9.3　CTA 示双颈内动脉 C1 段迂曲（**A**），基底动脉中段重度狭窄（**B ～ D**）

（四）治疗过程

全麻下右股动脉穿刺入路，将 6F 导引导管置于左椎动脉 V2 段，造影显示基底动脉中段重度狭窄（图 5.9.4 A）。选择 Synchro 微导丝（0.014 in，300 cm）结合 SL-10 微导管越过病变至左大脑后动脉 P2 段。试图跟进微导管越过病变未获成功，撤出微导管，经微导丝送入 Gateway 球囊（1.5 mm×15 mm），但球囊也未能通过病变。撤出球囊，再次送入微导管到狭窄近端，将 Synchro 微导丝更换为 PT2 微导丝（0.014 in，300 cm），并将微导丝头端调整至左大脑后动脉 P2 段（图 5.9.4 B）。再次经微导丝送入球囊至病变，仍有较大阻力，最终球囊越过病变，以 10 atm 扩张，但球囊扩张欠佳，撤出球囊造影，见狭窄程度同前（图 5.9.4 C）。

撤出 1.5 mm 直径球囊，更换为 2.0 mm×15 mm Gateway 球囊扩张病变，扩张压力至 10 atm，见球囊远近端充盈可，但球囊中部"束腰征"明显（图 5.9.5 A）。此时造影显示，前向血流明显改善，但残余狭窄率大于 70%。考虑到病变处斑块较硬，对比扩张前影像，病变远端狭窄程度明显改善，病变近端弹性回缩明显（图 5.9.5 B 和 C）。我们未予以进一步球囊扩张和放置支架。观察 10 min 后造影，显示无改变，遂结束治疗。

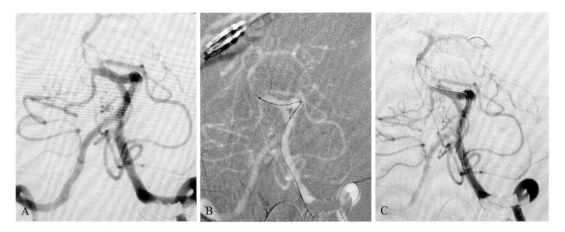

图 5.9.4　DSA 示基底动脉中段重度狭窄（**A**）。微导管及球囊均到位困难，更换微导丝，并将微导丝头端调整至左大脑后动脉 P2 段（**B**）。再次送入球囊，到位后扩张欠佳，病变狭窄程度同前（**C**）

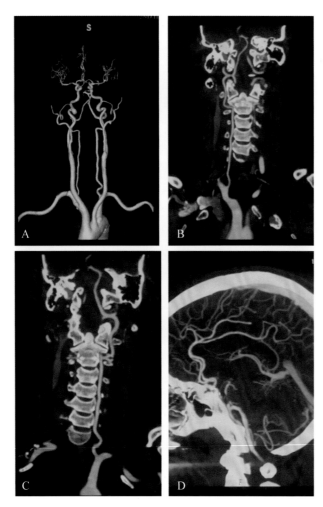

Fig. 5.9.3 The CT angiography revealed that the C1 segments of the bilateral internal carotid arteries were tortuous (**A**), the left vertebral artery was dominant and the middle segment of the basilar artery exhibited severe stenosis (**B–D**)

4. Treatment

Under general anesthesia, a 6F guiding catheter was inserted through the right femoral artery and positioned at the V2 segment of the left vertebral artery. An angiogram revealed significant stenosis at the middle segment of the basilar artery (Fig. 5.9.4 A). The Synchro microwire (0.014 in, 300 cm) and SL-10 microcatheter were intended to coaxially advance through the stenosis lesion and reached into the P2 segment of the left posterior cerebral artery. Unfortunately, the SL-10 microcatheter faced a challenge passing through the stenotic lesion and had to be retracted. Similarly, attempts to advance a Gateway balloon (1.5 mm × 15 mm) into the lesion were not successful, thus requiring its withdrawal. The SL-10 microcatheter was advanced to the proximal site of the stenotic lesion, and the Synchro microwire was replaced with a PT2 microwire (0.014 in, 300 cm) (Fig. 5.9.4 B). Despite several attempts, the Gateway balloon (1.5 mm × 15 mm) eventually crossed the lesion and pre-dilation was performed slowly at 10 atm pressure. The post-balloon angiography angiogram revealed obvious elastic recoil and significant stenosis, similar to the initial presentation (Fig. 5.9.4 C).

A Gateway balloon (2.0 mm × 15 mm) was employed to dilate the lesion at 10 atm pressure. While the distal and proximal sites of the balloon inflated well, the middle of the balloon showed a "girdle waist sign" (Fig. 5.9.5 A). The subsequent angiogram revealed a significant improvement in antegrade blood flow, but the residual stenosis remained greater than 70%. The plaque within the lesion was believed to be hardened. While the stenosis at the distal site of the lesion was significantly improved, obvious elastic recoil was observed at the proximal site of the lesion. (Fig. 5.9.5 B, C). Further balloon angioplasty and stent implantation were not performed. After a 10-minute observation period, the angiogram showed no change in the residual stenosis, thus concluding the procedure.

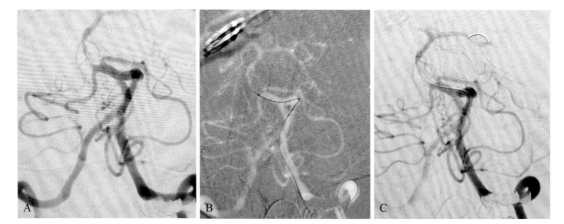

Fig. 5.9.4 DSA showed severe stenosis at the middle segment of the basilar artery (**A**). Both the microcatheter and Gateway balloon had difficulty in passing through the lesion, then the synchro microwire was replaced with a PT2 microwire (**B**). The Gateway balloon eventually crossed the lesion and pre-dilation was performed. The post-balloon angiography angiogram revealed obvious elastic recoil and significant stenosis (**C**)

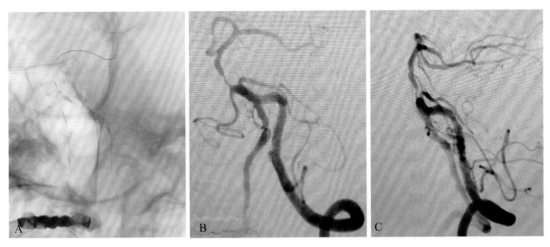

图 5.9.5　球囊中部"束腰征"（**A**）。DSA 示残余狭窄率大于 70%，病变远端狭窄程度明显改善，病变近端弹性回缩明显（**B**和**C**）

（五）讨论

本病例基底动脉中段重度狭窄，扩张球囊时压力明显大于命名压，病变近端仍未扩张开。此时可以选择更大扩张压力，或更大直径球囊扩张，或放置球囊扩张式支架，但考虑到潜在血管破裂及穿支动脉损伤的风险，未予以上述策略。预扩张不理想也不适宜于放置自膨式支架，会因支架贴壁不良而诱发血栓，此外还有支架系统不能顺利回撤的风险。本例患者术后临床症状虽有改善，但若近远期出现再狭窄如何处理，需充分权衡利弊后再定夺。

（于江华　马宁）

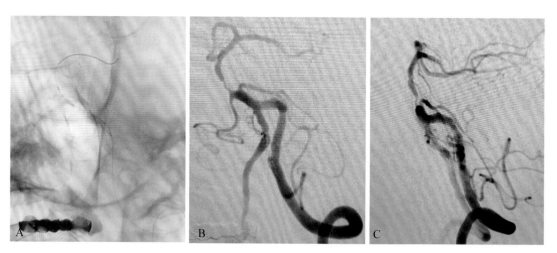

Fig. 5.9.5   The middle of the balloon showed a "girdle waist sign" (**A**). DSA showed the residual stenosis remained greater than 70%. While the stenosis at the distal site of the lesion was significantly improved, obvious elastic recoil was observed at the proximal site of the lesion (**B**, **C**)

5. Comments

We presented a case of a patient with severe stenosis in the middle segment of the basilar artery. Despite a higher dilation pressure than the specified nominal pressure, there was no marked improvement at the proximal site of the lesion. Alternative options such as angioplasty using a larger balloon or implantation of a balloon-expandable stent may have been considered, but these approaches entail potential risks of vascular rupture and perforator artery injury. Therefore, we refrained from utilizing such methods. Implanting a self-expanding stent after an unsatisfactory predilation may lead to thrombus formation due to poor stent apposition and the risk of a difficult stent retrieval. Although the patient's clinical symptoms partially improved after the procedure, careful consideration of the benefits and risks of deal with the short- and long-term restenosis should be conducted.

(Translated by Rongrong Cui, Revised by
Zechen Liu and Zhikai Hou)

第十节 溃疡性狭窄

病例 30 右大脑中动脉 M1 段溃疡性狭窄

（一）临床病史及影像分析

患者，男性，68 岁，主因"发作性左侧肢体无力 1 天"入院。

既往史：高血压 10 余年，肝内胆管结石 9 年，脑梗死 7 年，脂代谢紊乱病史 7 年。

查体：神经系统查体示左侧肢体肌力 5-级。

头颅 MRI ＋ MRA：右侧脑室旁新发梗死（图 5.10.1 A ～ C），右大脑中动脉 M1 段重度狭窄（图 5.10.1 D 和 E）。

DSA：右大脑中动脉 M1 段重度狭窄，狭窄偏下壁分布，远心端下壁见充盈缺损，狭窄后扩张，远心端上壁见豆纹动脉发出，未见明显同侧大脑前动脉经软脑膜动脉向大脑中动脉供血区域代偿（图 5.10.2 A）。右颈内动脉 C1 段远端迂曲（图 5.10.2 B），左颈内动脉系统未见明显狭窄（图 5.10.2 C 和 D）。左椎动脉优势，未见明显后循环向前循环代偿（图 5.10.2 E 和 F）。右椎动脉 V1 段轻度狭窄（图 5.10.2 G 和 H）。

入院后给予双联抗血小板（阿司匹林 100 mg 1 次 / 日＋氯吡格雷 75 mg 1 次 / 日）、降脂（阿托伐他汀 20 mg 1 次 / 日）、降压等治疗。

（二）诊断

症状性右大脑中动脉 M1 段溃疡性重度狭窄。

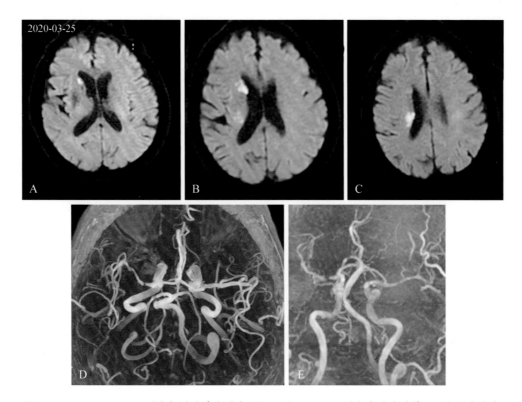

图 5.10.1 A ～ C. MRI 示右侧脑室旁新发梗死；**D 和 E.** MRA 示右大脑中动脉 M1 段重度狭窄

Section 10   Ulcerative Stenosis

Case 30   Ulcerative stenosis of the M1 segment of the right middle cerebral artery

1. Clinical presentation and radiological studies

A 68-year-old male patient was admitted to the hospital due to episodes of paroxysmal left-sided hemiplegia for one day.

The patient had a history of hypertension for over 10 years, intrahepatic bile duct stones for 9 years, and cerebral infarction and lipoprotein metabolism disorders for 7 years.

The neurological examination revealed that muscle strength in the left limb was at a grade 5 minus.

The MRI results showed acute infarction in the right periventricular area (Fig. 5.10.1 A–C). The MRA indicated severe stenosis in the M1 segment of the right middle cerebral artery (Fig. 5.10.1 D, E).

The DSA result demonstrated severe stenosis in the M1 segment of the right middle cerebral artery. Moreover, a filling defect was observed in the inferior wall of the distal stenosis segment, along with a post-stenotic arterial dilation. The lenticulostriate arteries originated from the upper wall of the distal stenosis segment, while any substantial compensation from the ipsilateral anterior cerebral artery to the middle cerebral artery was absent (Fig. 5.10.2 A). Additionally, the distal C1 segment of the right internal carotid artery exhibited tortuosity (Fig. 5.10.2 B). There was no significant stenosis detected in the left internal carotid artery system (Fig. 5.10.2 C, D). The angiogram of the posterior circulation displayed a dominant left vertebral artery, with no significant compensation from the posterior circulation to the anterior circulation (Fig. 5.10.2 E, F). Moreover, a mild stenosis was observed at the V1 segment of the right vertebral artery (Fig. 5.10.2 G, H).

Upon admission, a dual-antiplatelet regimen comprising a daily dosage of 100 mg of Aspirin and 75 mg of Clopidogrel was prescribed, in addition to a daily dosage of 20 mg of Atorvastatin and antihypertensive medications.

2. Diagnosis

Symptomatic ulcerative severe stenosis of the M1 segment of the right middle cerebral artery.

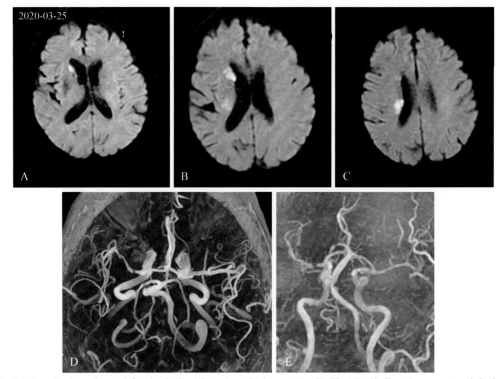

Fig. 5.10.1   The MRI results showed acute infarction in the right periventricular area (**A–C**). The MRA indicated severe stenosis in the M1 segment of the right middle cerebral artery (**D, E**)

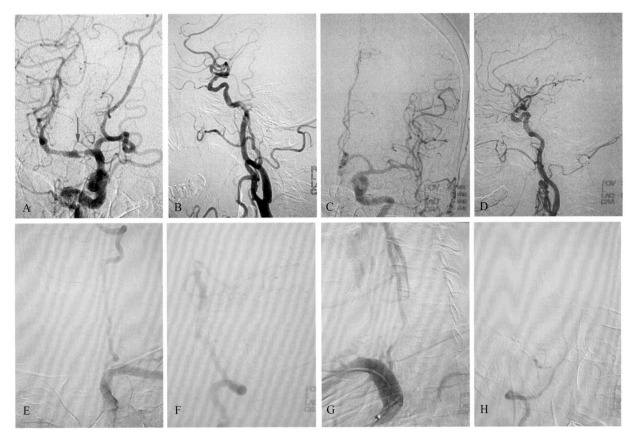

图 5.10.2　**A**. 右大脑中动脉 M1 段重度狭窄，狭窄偏下壁分布，远心端下壁见充盈缺损，狭窄后扩张，远心端上壁见豆纹动脉发出（箭头示），未见明显同侧大脑前动脉经软脑膜动脉向大脑中动脉供血区域代偿；**B**. 右颈内动脉 C1 段远端迂曲；**C** 和 **D**. 左颈内动脉系统未见明显狭窄；**E** 和 **F**. 左椎动脉优势，未见明显后循环向前循环代偿；**G** 和 **H**. 右椎动脉 V1 段轻度狭窄

（三）术前讨论

本例症状性右大脑中动脉 M1 段重度狭窄患者，血管造影时狭窄病变局部可见"充盈缺损"，提示斑块不稳定，且侧支代偿欠佳。遂予以血管内介入治疗。拟先球囊扩张，再酌情放置自膨式支架。相关风险包括穿支事件、动脉夹层、支架内急性或亚急性血栓形成等。

（四）治疗过程

全麻下右股动脉穿刺入路，将 6F 导引导管置于右颈内动脉 C1 段远端，造影显示右大脑中动脉 M1 段重度狭窄（图 5.10.3 A）。

Synchro 微导丝（0.014 in，300 cm）携 Echelon-10 微导管越过病变（图 5.10.3 B），将微导管置于 M2 段，通过交换技术更换为 Transend 微导丝（0.014 in，300 cm），经微导丝送入 Gateway 球囊（2.0 mm×9 mm）扩张病变（图 5.10.3 C 和 D），至球囊充盈

完全（图 5.10.3 E）。球囊扩张后造影显示血管有明显弹性回缩。撤出球囊，更换为 XT-27 微导管，于狭窄处释放 Neuroform EZ 支架（2.5 mm×15 mm）（图 5.10.3 F 和 G），但支架在最狭窄处仍未完全张开，残余狭窄率约 70%（图 5.10.3 H）。

因残余狭窄率重，遂再次将 Transend 微导丝在微导管帮助下越过支架，送入 Ultra-soft 球囊（2.5 mm×9 mm）至支架中段，扩张至球囊完全充盈（图 5.10.4 A），其后造影示残余狭窄率约 30%（图 5.10.4 B）。观察 10 min，支架远端和中段有少许附壁血栓（图 5.10.4 C），动脉内予以替罗非班 0.15 mg 缓慢注入后血栓溶解（图 5.10.4 D）。再次观察 10 min 无变化后结束治疗。

（五）讨论

本例病变应该属于血管内介入治疗挑战性病变。其形态较为少见，局部斑块掀起，斑块远端下

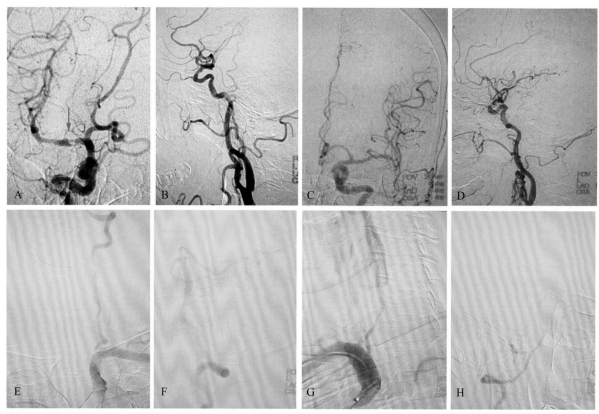

Fig. 5.10.2 DSA showed severe stenosis in the M1 segment of the right middle cerebral artery. Moreover, a filling defect was observed in the inferior wall of the distal stenosis segment, along with a post-stenotic arterial dilation. The lenticulostriate arteries originated from the upper wall of the distal stenosis segment (arrow). The substantial compensation from the ipsilateral anterior cerebral artery to the middle cerebral artery was absent (**A**). The distal C1 segment of the right internal carotid artery exhibited tortuosity (**B**). There was no significant stenosis detected in the left internal carotid artery system (**C, D**). The angiogram of the posterior circulation displayed a dominant left vertebral artery, with no significant compensation from the posterior circulation to the anterior circulation (**E, F**), a mild stenosis was observed at the V1 segment of the right vertebral artery (**G, H**)

3. Treatment schedule

The patient exhibited significant stenosis in the M1 segment of the right middle cerebral artery. The DSA results demonstrated a filling defect in the stenosis lesion, accompanied by inadequate collateral compensation. Therefore, it was deemed necessary for the patient to undergo endovascular therapy. Treatment approach: Primary balloon pre-dilation was performed, followed by self-expanding stent implantation. Potential procedure risks included the occlusion of the perforating arteries, arterial dissection, and acute/subacute in-stent thrombosis.

4. Treatment

Under general anesthesia, a 6F guiding catheter was inserted via the right femoral artery and placed at the C1 segment of the right internal carotid artery. The angiogram confirmed severe stenosis in the M1 segment of the right middle cerebral artery (Fig. 5.10.3 A).

The Synchro microwire (0.014 in, 300 cm) and Echelon-10 microcatheter were carefully advanced through the lesion, coaxially reaching the M2 segment of the right middle cerebral artery (Fig. 5.10.3 B). Subsequently, the Synchro microwire was substituted with a Transend microwire (0.014 in, 300 cm). A 2.0 mm×9 mm Gateway balloon was utilized to pre-dilate the stenosis lesion (Fig. 5.10.3 C, D). The

Gateway balloon was inflated to its full capacity (Fig.5.10.3 E). However, the post-balloon angioplasty angiogram revealed significant elastic recoil of the vessel wall. Consequently, the Gateway balloon was carefully withdrawn, and the Echelon-10 microcatheter was substituted with the XT-27 microcatheter. A 2.5 mm×15 mm Neuroform EZ self-expanding stent was employed to cover the lesion (Fig. 5.10.3 F, G). However, it did not fully expand at the narrowest location, resulting in a residual stenosis of approximately 70% (Fig. 5.10.3 H).

In light of the obvious residual stenosis, the Transend microwire was maneuvered through the stent with the assistance of the microcatheter. Subsequently, an Ultrasoft balloon (2.5 mm×9 mm) was delivered to postdilate the middle segment of the stent (Fig. 5.10.4 A). Following this procedure, the post-balloon angioplasty angiogram demonstrated a residual stenosis of approximately 30% (Fig. 5.10.4 B). Following a 10-minutes observation period, the presence of mural thrombus within the distal and middle segments of the stent was observed (Fig. 5.10.4 C). The thrombus underwent dissolution following the intra-arterial administration of 0.15 mg of tirofiban (Fig. 5.10.4 D).

5. Comments

The case presented a challenging instance of intracranial ulcerative stenosis for endovascular treatment. The rare

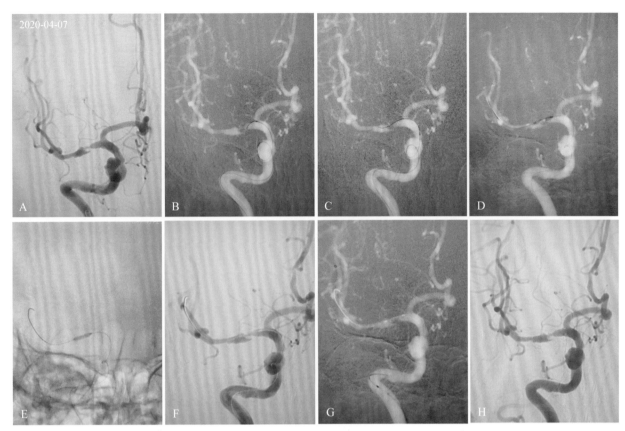

图5.10.3 **A**.术前造影示右大脑中动脉M1段重度狭窄；**B**.Synchro微导丝和Echelon-10微导管同轴越过病变；**C**和**D**.Gateway球囊（2.0 mm×9 mm）扩张病变；**E**.Gateway球囊完全充盈；**F**和**G**.释放Neuroform EZ支架（2.5 mm×15 mm）；**H**.释放支架后造影示残余狭窄率约70%

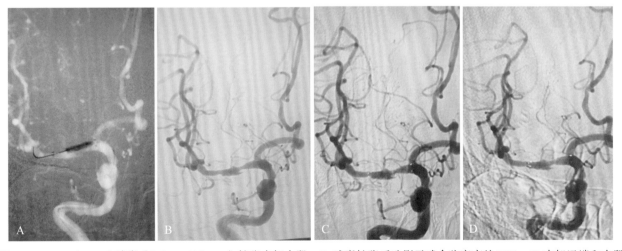

图5.10.4 **A**.Ultra-soft球囊（2.5 mm×9 mm）扩张支架中段；**B**.球囊扩张后造影示残余狭窄率约30%；**C**.支架远端和中段有少许附壁血栓形成；**D**.动脉内予以替罗非班0.15 mg后血栓溶解

壁见充盈缺损，我们考虑系斑块纤维帽破裂后，斑块内容物脱落所致。"斑块掀起样溃疡性斑块"需要与血管夹层相鉴别，后者在椎动脉颅内段更为常见，此外，夹层性狭窄一般较软，扩张不需要太多压力，扩张后放置支架也能取得较好的形态学结果。本例在治疗过程中，病变扩张后弹性回缩明显，其支架内急性血栓形成也与反复扩张有关。当然，选择具有更大扩张压力的大直径球囊，也许有更好的扩张效果，但考虑到病变远端存在狭窄后扩张，还是应选择略为保守的治疗策略。

（袁景林 杨海华 马宁）

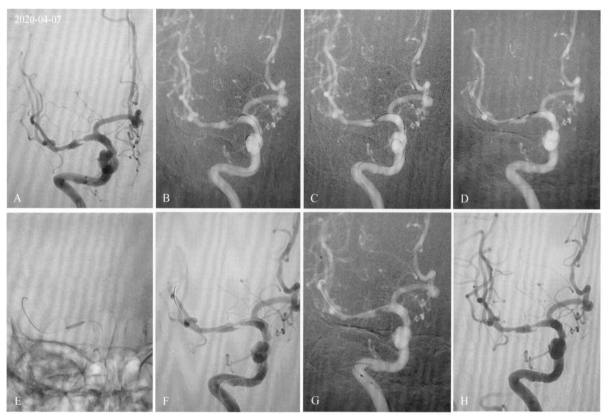

Fig. 5.10.3   The pre-procedural angiogram confirmed severe stenosis in the M1 segment of the right middle cerebral artery (**A**). The Synchro microwire and Echelon-10 microcatheter coaxially advanced through the lesion to the M2 segment of the right middle cerebral artery (**B**). A 2.0 mm×9 mm Gateway balloon was used to dilate the lesion (**C**, **D**), and the Gateway balloon was inflated to its full capacity (**E**). A 2.5 mm×15 mm Neuroform EZ self-expanding stent was employed to cover the lesion (**F**, **G**), it did not fully expand at the narrowest location, resulting in a residual stenosis of approximately 70% (**H**)

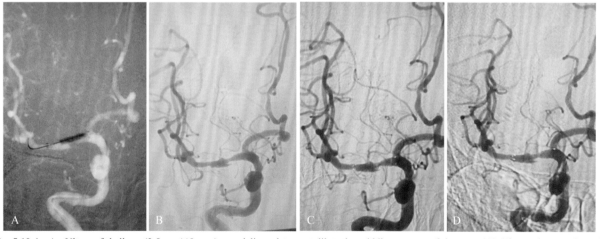

Fig. 5.10.4   An Ultra-soft balloon (2.5 mm×9 mm) was delivered to post-dilate the middle segment of the stent (**A**). The angiogram showed the residual stenosis was about 30% (**B**). There was mural thrombus within the distal and middle segments of the stent (**C**), the thrombus underwent dissolution following the intra-arterial administration of 0.15 mg of tirofiban (**D**)

morphology of stenosis manifested as the focal plaque uplift, concomitant with a filling defect in the distal segment of stenosis. The ulcerative stenosis observed in the M1 segment was attributed to the rupture of the fibrous cap and displacement of the lipid-rich core. It is important to distinguish this ulcerative plaque with its "uplifted plaque morphology" from arterial dissection, which is more commonly seen in the V4 segment of the vertebral artery. Additionally, arterial dissection with a soft structure has the potential to yield more favorable morphological outcomes when undergoing balloon dilatation at a lower pressure or stent implantation. In this particular case, there is an obvious elastic recoil following the balloon dilatation. The occurrence of acute instent thrombosis was also associated with repeated dilations. Choosing a larger-sized balloon with increased dilation pressure during balloon angioplasty could potentially result in a more effective dilation. However, a relatively conservative treatment approach should be considered due to the presence of distal post-stenotic dilation.

(Translated by Rongrong Cui, Revised by Zhikai Hou)

第十一节 烟雾综合征

病例 31 右大脑中动脉近期闭塞

（一）临床病史及影像分析

患者，男性，28 岁，主因"左侧肢体麻木无力 2 周"入院。

既往史：脂蛋白代谢紊乱，吸烟、饮酒。

查体：左上肢肌力 5-级。

头部 MRI：右侧脑室旁新发脑梗死（图 5.11.1 A）。

头部 CTA：右大脑中动脉 M1 段中段重度狭窄（图 5.11.1 B）。

DSA：右大脑中动脉 M1 段中段重度狭窄，右大脑前动脉 A1 段未见显影，考虑缺如或者发育不良（图 5.11.2 A 和 B）；前交通动脉开放，右大脑前动脉经软脑膜动脉向右大脑中动脉供血区域代偿（图 5.11.2 C 和 D）；右大脑后动脉经软脑膜动脉向右大脑中动脉供血区域代偿（图 5.11.3）。

入院后给予双联抗血小板（阿司匹林 100 mg 1 次 / 日＋氯吡格雷 75 mg 1 次 / 日）及阿托伐他汀（20 mg 1 次 / 日）降脂治疗。

（二）诊断

症状性右大脑中动脉 M1 段重度狭窄。

（三）术前讨论

患者因近期左侧肢体无力入院，头颅 MRI 示右大脑半球侧脑室旁新发梗死，血管造影提示责任血管为右大脑中动脉 M1 段，有介入治疗指征。拟先行球囊扩张，再放置自膨式支架。相关风险包括高灌注综合征、急性或亚急性血栓形成、远期支架内再狭窄等。

（四）治疗过程

全麻下将 6F 导引导管放置在右颈内动脉 C1 段，造影示右大脑中动脉 M1 段病变由重度狭窄进展为闭塞，闭塞周围见侧支血管增多；动脉晚期，右大脑中动脉闭塞远端上干缓慢显影（图 5.11.4 A 和 B）。

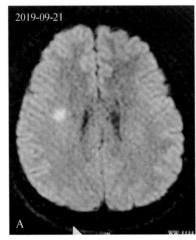
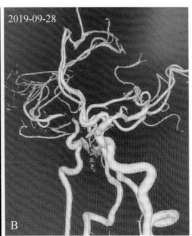

图 5.11.1 **A**. 头部 MRI 示右侧脑室旁新发脑梗死；**B**. 头部 CTA 示右大脑中动脉 M1 段中段重度狭窄

Section 11 Moyamoya Syndrome

Case 31 Recent occlusion of the right middle cerebral artery

1. Clinical presentation and radiological studies

A 28-year-old male patient exhibited a two-week history of left limb weakness and numbness.

The patient had a medical background of lipoprotein metabolism disorder, along with personal habits of smoking cigarettes and consuming alcohol.

The physical examination revealed that the muscle strength in the left upper limb was graded at 5 minus.

The MRI exhibited acute infarctions located in the periventricular area (Fig. 5.11.1 A).

The CT angiography revealed significant stenosis in the middle segment of the M1 segment of the right middle cerebral artery (Fig. 5.11.1 B).

The DSA result revealed significant stenosis in the middle segment of the M1 segment of the right middle cerebral artery, along with the absence or dysplasia of the A1 segment of the right anterior cerebral artery (Fig. 5.11.2 A, B). The anterior communicating artery was patent. The territory of the right middle cerebral artery was compensated by the right anterior cerebral artery and the right posterior cerebral artery via the leptomeningeal artery (Fig. 5.11.2 C, D, and Fig. 5.11.3).

Upon admission, a dual-antiplatelet regimen comprising a daily dosage of 100 mg of Aspirin and 75 mg of Clopidogrel was prescribed, in addition to a daily dosage of 20 mg of Atorvastatin.

2. Diagnosis

Symptomatic severe stenosis of the M1 segment of the right middle cerebral artery.

3. Treatment schedule

Based on the medical history and radiological studies, the patient experienced an acute ischemic stroke within the affected area of the narrowed intracranial artery. The right middle cerebral artery was identified as the responsible artery. Therefore, endovascular therapy was advised. Treatment approach: the stenosis lesion was pre-dilated, followed by the implantation of a self-expanding stent. Potential risks associated with the procedure included hyperperfusion syndrome, acute/subacute in-stent thrombosis, and long-term in-stent restenosis.

4. Treatment

Under general anesthesia, a 6F guiding catheter was placed at the C1 segment of the right internal carotid artery. The angiogram demonstrated the occlusion of the M1 segment of the right middle cerebral artery, which had advanced from significant stenosis. Collateral vessels had established around the occluded area, and the upper division of the right middle cerebral artery could be observed during the late arterial phase (Fig. 5.11.4 A, B).

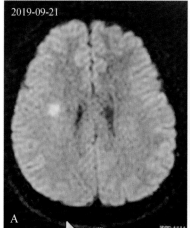
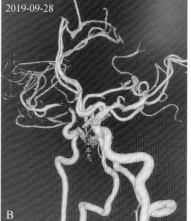

Fig. 5.11.1 MRI exhibited acute infarctions located in the periventricular area (**A**). CT angiography revealed significant stenosis in the middle segment of the M1 segment of the right middle cerebral artery (**B**)

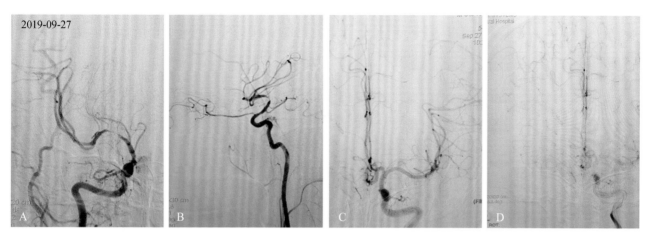

图 5.11.2 DSA 示：**A** 和 **B**. 右大脑中动脉 M1 段中段重度狭窄，右大脑前动脉 A1 段未见显影；**C** 和 **D**. 前交通动脉开放，右大脑前动脉经软脑膜动脉向右大脑中动脉供血区域代偿

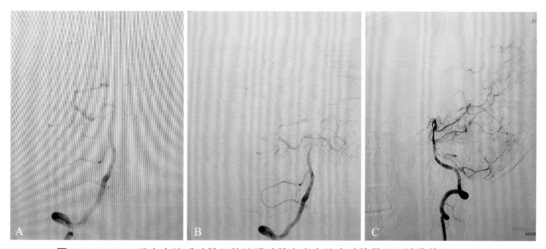

图 5.11.3 DSA 示右大脑后动脉经软脑膜动脉向右大脑中动脉供血区域代偿（**A ～ C**）

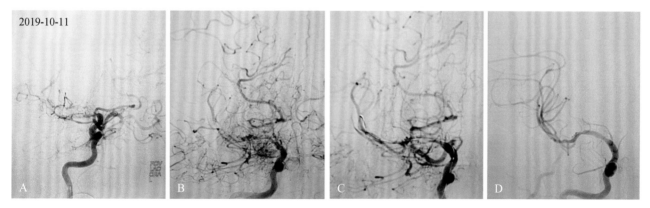

图 5.11.4 血管内介入治疗过程如下：**A** 和 **B**. 术前造影示右大脑中动脉 M1 段闭塞；**C**. 球囊扩张后造影示右大脑中动脉残余狭窄率约 60%，最狭窄处管腔内可见充盈缺损；**D**. 释放支架后造影显示支架贴壁良好，残余狭窄率约 20%

Synchro 微导丝（0.014 in，300 cm）在 Echelon-10 微导管辅助下，越过闭塞段，置于右大脑中动脉 M2 段。经微导管造影证实微导管位于真腔内。其后送入 Gateway 球囊（1.5 mm×15 mm）至狭窄处扩张。扩张后造影，见右大脑中动脉远端分支显影，残余狭窄率约 60%，最狭窄处可见充盈缺

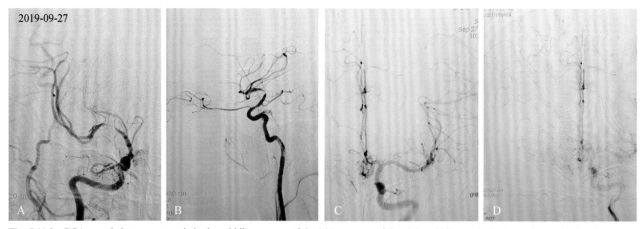

Fig. 5.11.2 DSA revealed severe stenosis in the middle segment of the M1 segment of the right middle cerebral artery, along with the absence or dysplasia of the A1 segment of the right anterior cerebral artery (**A, B**). The anterior communicating artery was patent. The territory of the right middle cerebral artery was compensated by the right anterior cerebral artery via the leptomeningeal artery (**C, D**)

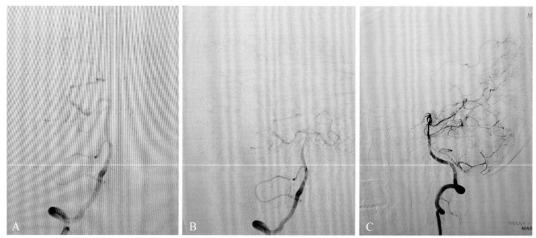

Fig. 5.11.3 DSA revealed the territory of the right middle cerebral artery was compensated by the right posterior cerebral artery via the leptomeningeal artery (**A–C**)

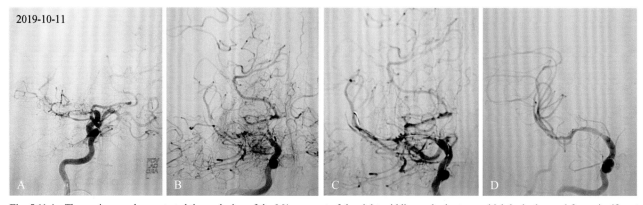

Fig. 5.11.4 The angiogram demonstrated the occlusion of the M1 segment of the right middle cerebral artery, which had advanced from significant stenosis. Collateral vessels had established around the occluded area, and the upper division of the right middle cerebral artery could be observed during the late arterial phase (**A, B**). The post-balloon angiography angiogram showed the residual stenosis was 60%, with a filling defect in the narrowest vessel lumen (**C**). The post-stent implantation angiogram showed excellent stent wall apposition with residual stenosis of about 20% (**D**)

With the assistance of the Echelon-10 microcatheter, the Synchro microwire (0.014 inches, 300 cm) effectively traversed from the lesion segment to the M2 segment of the right middle cerebral artery. The transcatheter angiogram the accurate placement of the microcatheter within the true lumen.

A 1.5 mm×15 mm Gateway balloon was employed to pre-dilate the lesion, and the subsequent angiogram exhibited visualization of the distal branches of the right middle cerebral artery with a residual stenosis of approximately 60%. Furthermore, a filling defect was observed within the

损（图 5.11.4 C）。撤出球囊后放置 Wingspan 自膨式支架（2.5 mm×15 mm）。释放后造影显示支架贴壁良好，前向血流通畅，残余狭窄率约 20%（图 5.11.4 D）。支架释放完毕后观察 10 min，无血栓形成，遂结束手术。

（五）讨论

本例患者前期血管造影提示有症状性右大脑中动脉 M1 段重度狭窄，结合患者有吸烟、脂代谢紊乱等动脉粥样硬化危险因素，考虑动脉粥样硬化性狭窄可能性大。在接受血管内介入治疗时，病变短期内进展，由重度狭窄演变为闭塞性病变。闭塞周围见侧支代偿血管异常增多，呈烟雾样改变。如果无前期血管造影和 CTA 资料，很有可能诊断为烟雾病（Moyamoya disease）。如果患者术前行管壁高分辨率磁共振成像，会有助于与其他非动脉粥样硬化性疾病相鉴别。此外，本例采用 1.5 mm 球囊扩张后，管腔局部见充盈缺损，考虑闭塞处有亚急性血栓可能（也不除外血管夹层），予以自膨式支架贴合后好转。

（黄睿 陈林考 马宁）

narrowest lumen of the vessel (Fig. 5.11.4 C). Following that, a 2.5 mm×15 mm Wingspan self-expanding stent was utilized to cover the lesion. The post-stent implantation angiogram revealed excellent stent wall apposition, with residual stenosis of approximately 20% (Fig. 5.11.4 D). After 10 minutes of observation, there was no thrombus formation in the stent of the middle cerebral artery.

5. Comments

In this particular instance, the prior angiogram exhibited a significant narrowing in the M1 segment of the right middle cerebral artery. The patient's medical history included cigarette smoking, alcohol consumption, and lipoprotein metabolism disorder, the underlying cause of the stenosis was attributed to atherosclerosis. Within a short period, the severe stenosis progressed to an occlusive lesion. The collateral vessels had formed around the occluded region, evidenced by the distinctive "puff-of-smoke" sign. Without the previous angiogram, this presented scenario could have potentially led to the misdiagnosis of Moyamoya disease. High-resolution vessel wall imaging was a useful modality to distinguish intracranial atherosclerotic stenosis from non-atherosclerotic conditions, such as moyamoya disease. During the procedure, a noticeable filling defect was detected at the site of stenosis following balloon angioplasty. This suggested the potential occurrence of thrombus formation or arterial dissection. However, upon the successful implantation of a self-expanding stent, the filling defect vanished.

(Translated by Rongrong Cui, Revised by Zhikai Hou)

第十二节　"蜂巢样"病变

病例 32　基底动脉"蜂巢样"狭窄

（一）临床病史及影像分析

患者，男性，52 岁，主因"反复头晕伴视物旋转 10 个月，加重伴视物成双及行走不稳 5 个月"入院。

当地医院头颅 MRI 示脑桥右侧亚急性梗死（图5.12.1）。CTA 示基底动脉重度狭窄（图 5.12.2）。给予阿司匹林、氯吡格雷抗血小板聚集、阿托伐他汀降脂等治疗，症状仍反复发作。现为进一步行血管内治疗来我院就诊。

既往史：高血压、高脂血症、胃溃疡病史，以及吸烟史。

查体：神经系统查体无阳性定位体征。

入院后头颅 HRMRI：基底动脉起始处管腔内壁环形增厚，斑块形成，内壁粗糙且不规则，斑块呈等 T1 信号，增强扫描提示斑块呈明显均匀强化。诊断考虑为基底动脉起始处管壁斑块形成，表面溃疡形成（图 5.12.3）。

术前 DSA：基底动脉近段狭窄，局部管腔不规则，似有"蜂巢样改变"，管壁不光滑，前向血流减慢（图 5.12.4）。右后交通动脉开放，双侧大脑后动脉、基底动脉尖和基底动脉上段显影（图 5.12.5）。

入院后给予双联抗血小板（西洛他唑 100 mg

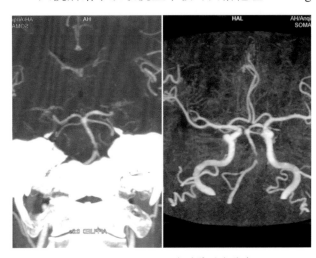

图 5.12.2　CTA 示基底动脉重度狭窄

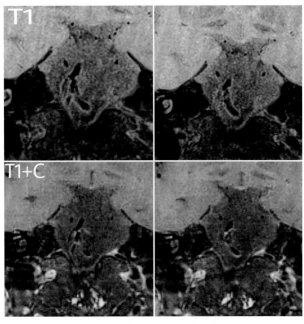

图 5.12.3　HRMRI 示基底动脉起始处管腔内壁环形增厚，斑块形成，内壁粗糙且不规则，斑块呈等 T1 信号，增强扫描提示斑块呈明显均匀强化

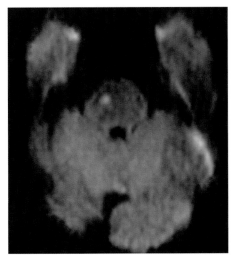

图 5.12.1　头颅 MRI 示脑桥右侧亚急性梗死

Section 12 "Honeycomb" Stenosis

Case 32 "Honeycomb" stenosis of the basilar artery

1. Clinical presentation and radiological studies

A 52-year-old man was admitted to the hospital due to episodes of paroxysmal vertigo for ten months, worsening with double vision and unstable gait for five months.

The MRI findings showed revealed subacute infarctions located on the right side of the pons (Fig. 5.12.1). The CT angiography detected a significant narrowing of the basilar artery (Fig. 5.12.2). Despite receiving intensive medical intervention, the patient's symptoms persisted and recurred.

The patient had a medical history of hypertension, hyperlipidemia, and gastric ulcer. In addition, he had a personal history of cigarette smoking.

Upon admission, the neurological examination of the patient exhibited no abnormalities.

The high-resolution MRI (HRMRI) revealed a concentric thickening of the basilar artery at its origin. The inner wall appeared rough and irregular, while the plaques exhibited an isointense signal on T1 imaging. Furthermore, the enhanced scan demonstrated a significant and uniform enhancement of the plaques. Based on these findings, the diagnosis strongly suggests the presence of plaque formation with the development of ulcerations on the surface of the basilar artery at its origin. (Fig. 5.12.3).

The DSA finding revealed severe stenosis at the proximal basilar artery with an irregular vascular lumen, which exhibited a "honeycomb-like" appearance. (Fig. 5.12.4). The right posterior communicating artery was patent. Furthermore, the bilateral posterior cerebral arteries, basilar artery apex, and upper basilar artery were visualized (Fig. 5.12.5).

Upon admission, he was prescribed a dual antiplatelet regimen consisting of a dosage of 100 mg of the Cilostazol

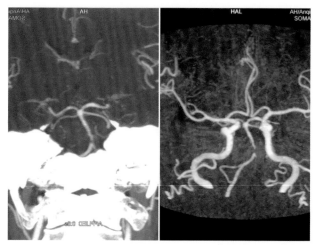

Fig. 5.12.2 CTA detected a significant narrowing of the basilar artery

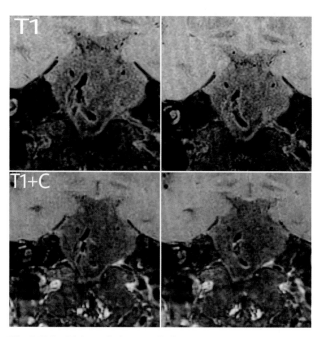

Fig. 5.12.3 High-resolution MRI indicated circumferential thickening of the vessel wall at the origin of the basilar artery, exhibiting iso-signal characteristics on the T1-weighted sequence and strong intra-plaque enhancement on the contrast-enhanced scan

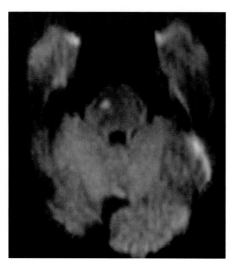

Fig. 5.12.1 The MRI findings showed revealed subacute infarctions located on the right side of the pons

2 次 / 日＋氯吡格雷 75 mg 1 次 / 日）及降脂（阿托伐他汀 20 mg 1 次 / 日）治疗。

（二）诊断

症状性基底动脉重度狭窄。

（三）术前讨论

患者基底动脉症状性狭窄，药物治疗后仍有症

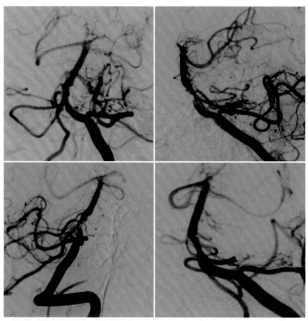

图 5.12.4　DSA 示基底动脉近段狭窄，局部管腔不规则，似有"蜂巢样改变"，管壁不光滑，前向血流减慢

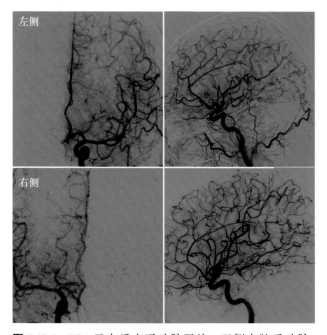

图 5.12.5　DSA 示右后交通动脉开放，双侧大脑后动脉、基底动脉尖和基底动脉上段显影

状反复，具有血管内介入治疗指征。DSA 提示病变局部有充盈缺损，HRMRI 提示基底动脉下段管腔内见斑块掀起，考虑狭窄系不稳定斑块所致。因狭窄病变局部迂曲，通过病变时有一定难度。另外狭窄段毗邻双侧 AICA 及多个细小穿支动脉，治疗风险主要是术后穿支卒中。

（四）治疗过程

全麻下，右股动脉入路，6F 导引导管放至右椎动脉 V2 段远端，Transend 微导丝（0.014 in，300 cm）＋Echelon-10 微导管送至基底动脉狭窄段近端，反复多次尝试不能通过狭窄段（图 5.12.6），遂换用 Traxcess 微导丝（0.014 in，205 cm）越过狭窄段后，重新交换 Transend 微导丝至右大脑后动脉 P2 段，Gateway 球囊（2 mm×9 mm）扩张病变后，放置 Apollo 球囊扩张式支架（2.5 mm×13 mm）至狭窄段，支架释放后贴壁良好，残余狭窄率约15%，前向血流 mTICI 分级 3 级（图 5.12.7）。

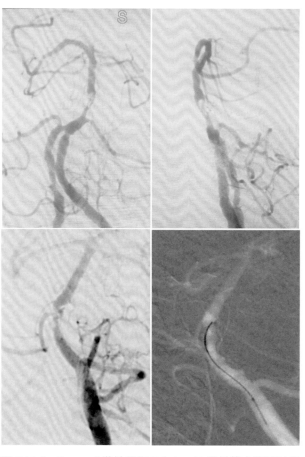

图 5.12.6　Transend 微导丝和 Echelon-10 微导管未能通过基底动脉狭窄段

twice daily and a daily dosage of 75 mg of Clopidogrel, as well as statin therapy with a daily dosage of 20 mg of Atorvastatin.

2. Diagnosis

Symptomatic severe stenosis of the basilar artery.

3. Treatment schedule

Despite receiving intensive medical intervention, the patient's symptoms persisted and recurred. Endovascular treatment was indicated for him. Angiogram showed the

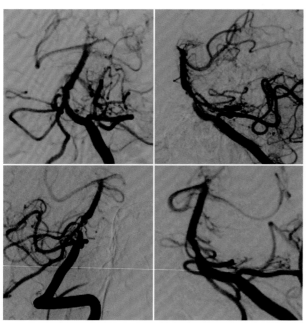

Fig. 5.12.4 The DSA finding revealed severe stenosis at the proximal basilar artery with an irregular vascular lumen, which exhibited a "honeycomb-like" appearance

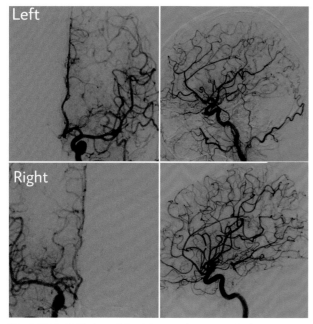

Fig. 5.12.5 DSA showed the right posterior communicating artery was patent. The bilateral posterior cerebral arteries, basilar artery apex, and upper basilar artery were visualized

presence of filling defects situated at the stenotic segment, and vessel wall imaging revealed an uplifted plaque in the lower region of the basilar artery, indicating an unstable plaque as the underlying cause of the stenosis. During the procedure, the tortuosity nature of the stenosis lesion might pose a challenge in navigating through the lesion. Because the stenotic segment was adjacent to the bilateral AICA and multiple perforating arteries, the main potential risk was the occlusion of the perforating arteries.

4. Treatment

Under general anesthesia, a 6F guiding catheter was inserted and positioned at the V2 segment of the right vertebral artery. Despite multiple attempts, the Transend microwire (0.014 in, 300 cm) and Echelon-10 microcatheter failed to traverse through the lesion segment (Fig. 5.12.6). To overcome the challenge, the Traxcess microwire (0.014 in, 205 cm) was utilized to successfully navigate through the lesion. Subsequently, the Transend microwire was reintroduced and advanced to the P2 segment of the right posterior cerebral artery. A Gateway balloon (2 mm×9 mm) was delivered to pre-dilate the lesion. Then an Apollo stent (2.5 mm×13 mm) was used to cover the lesion. A post-stent implantation angiogram showed excellent stent wall apposition, with only a residual stenosis of 15%. The antegrade blood flow in the stented basilar artery was grade 3 (Fig. 5.12.7).

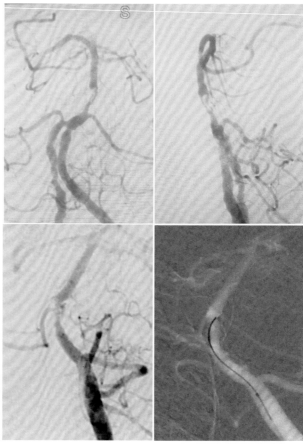

Fig. 5.12.6 Despite multiple attempts, the Transend microwire and Echelon-10 microcatheter failed to traverse through the lesion segment

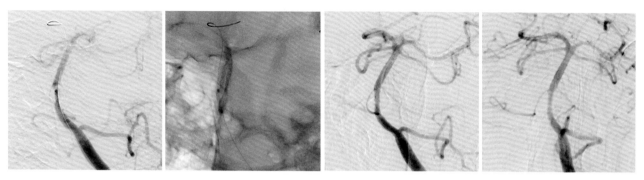

图 5.12.7　支架释放后造影示支架贴壁良好，残余狭窄率约 15%，前向血流 mTICI 分级 3 级

（五）讨论

本例基底动脉"蜂巢样"狭窄形成与重度狭窄病变的斑块内容物脱落有关，形成类似斑块掀起样改变，由于对血流动力学存在影响，产生低灌注缺血症状。本例治疗难点在于使微导丝通过病变，导丝操控时要轻柔，避免大幅度旋转动作，防止形成医源性夹层。具体材料选择上，Traxcess 微导丝通过类似病变的能力似更强一些。

（吴岩峰　胡彦君　刘深龙　宋立刚　马宁）

5.12　手术操作视频
（病例 32）

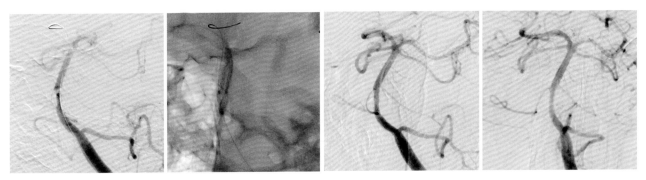

Fig. 5.12.7 A post-stent implantation angiogram showed excellent stent wall apposition, with only residual stenosis of 15%. The antegrade blood flow in the stented basilar artery was grade 3

5. Comments

The development of a honeycomb-like stenosis in the basilar artery in this case was attributed to the dislodgment of the plaque content, resulting in the manifestation of plaque uplift. The ischemic symptoms of hypoperfusion were associated with hemodynamic insufficiency. The challenge of the procedure lies in navigating the microwire through the lesion. During the manipulation of the guidewire, it is important to exercise gentleness and avoid excessive rotational movements to prevent the formation of iatrogenic dissections. In terms of specific device selection, the Traxcess microwire appears to possess a greater ability to navigate through similar lesions.

(Translated by Rongrong Cui, Revised by Zhikai Hou)

5.12   Video of endovascular
therapy (Case 32)

第十三节　狭窄导致穿支动脉灌注不足

病例 33　文丘里效应导致穿支动脉低灌注——左大脑中动脉 M1 段狭窄

（一）临床病史及影像分析

患者，女性，58 岁，主因"发作性右侧肢体无力 1 年余，加重 4 个月"入院。

当地医院行头部 CT 未见异常。头部 MRA 示双侧大脑中动脉 M1 段狭窄（图 5.13.1）。诊断为短暂性脑缺血发作（TIA），给予阿司匹林（100 mg 1 次 / 日）联合氯吡格雷（75 mg 1 次 / 日）双联抗血小板（1 个月后停用氯吡格雷）＋阿托伐他汀（40 mg 1 次 / 日）口服。

4 个月来患者上述症状在活动中反复发作，均持续约 10 min 后自行缓解。每次发病后完善头部 CT 均未见异常，再次给予双联抗血小板治疗。1 个月前（双联抗血小板治疗期间）休息时上述症状再次发作，20 min 后自行缓解，复查头部 CTA 见双侧大脑中动脉 M1 段狭窄，其中左侧 M1 段狭窄与 1 年前 MRA 对比有所加重（图 5.13.2）。头部 CTP 提示双侧大脑半球灌注情况无明显差异。为求进一

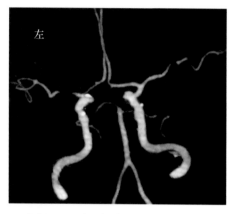

图 5.13.2　头部 CTA 示双侧大脑中动脉 M1 段狭窄，左侧 M1 段狭窄加重

步治疗遂就诊于我院。

既往史：高血压病史 3 年，右手腕粉碎性骨折 1 年。

查体：神经系统查体无阳性体征。

低密度脂蛋白胆固醇（LDL-C）1.51 mmol/L。

血栓弹力图：AA 抑制率 100%，ADP 抑制率 36%。

入院后查大脑中动脉高分辨率 MRI：右大脑中动脉 M1 段分叉部近端前壁、下壁及后壁斑块形成，左大脑中动脉 M1 段起始部斑块形成，左大脑中动脉较右大脑中动脉的管壁强化明显（图 5.13.3）。左大脑中动脉矢状位显示斑块偏下壁，强化也以下壁明显（图 5.13.4）。

DSA 提示双侧大脑中动脉 M1 段轻度狭窄（图 5.13.5）。

入院后给予双联抗血小板（阿司匹林 100 mg 1 次 / 日＋氯吡格雷 75 mg 1 次 / 日）、降脂（阿托伐他汀 20 mg 1 次 / 日）等治疗。

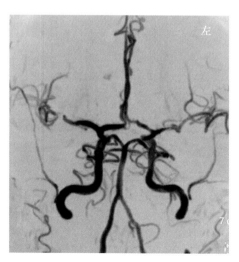

图 5.13.1　头部 MRA 示双侧大脑中动脉 M1 段狭窄

Section 13   ICAS with Perforator Artery Hypoperfusion due to Venturi Effect

Case 33   Perforator artery hypoperfusion due to Venturi effect—Stenosis of the M1 segment of the left middle cerebral artery

1. Clinical presentation and radiological studies

A 58-year-old female patient was admitted to the hospital due to episodes of intermittent weakness in her right-sided limb for over one year, worsening for four months.

The non-contrast CT scan did not reveal any apparent abnormalities. However, the MRA demonstrated stenosis in the M1 segments of both middle cerebral arteries (Fig. 5.13.1). The patient was diagnosed with a transient ischemic attack (TIA). A dual-antiplatelet regimen was prescribed, consisting of a daily dose of 100 mg of Aspirin and a daily dose of 75 mg of Clopidogrel. The Clopidogrel was subsequently discontinued after one month. Additionally, the patient was prescribed statin therapy, with a daily dose of 40 mg of Atorvastatin.

In the past four months, the patient has experienced recurring episodes of the aforementioned ischemic symptoms. Each episode lasted approximately 10 minutes. Despite repeated CT scans showing no notable findings, the dual antiplatelet therapy was reinstated. Unfortunately, even with the administration of dual antiplatelet therapy, the patient suffered a prolonged episode lasting 20 minutes. Subsequent CT angiography indicated severe stenosis in the M1 segment of both middle cerebral arteries. Notably, the stenosis in the left M1 segment had worsened compared to the MRA results from

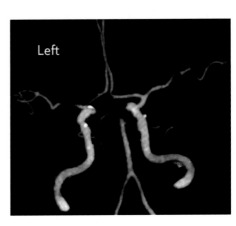

Fig. 5.13.2   CTA showed severe stenosis in the M1 segment of both middle cerebral arteries, and the stenosis in the left M1 segment had worsened than the MRA result from one year ago

one year ago (Fig. 5.13.2). CT perfusion analysis revealed no significant disparity in cerebral hemisphere perfusion between the two sides.

The patient had a three-year history of hypertension. Additionally, she had suffered a comminuted fracture in her right wrist one year ago.

Upon admission, the physical examination indicated the absence of any neurological deficits.

The concentration of LDL-C was measured at 1.51 mmol/L.

The thromboelastography result indicated a 100% inhibition of AA and a 36% inhibition of ADP.

The HRMRI results showed the presence of plaque formation in the proximal anterior, inferior, and posterior walls of the right middle cerebral artery at its bifurcation (M1 segment). Additionally, plaque formation is noted at the beginning of the left middle cerebral artery M1 segment. The arterial wall enhancement is more pronounced in the left middle cerebral artery compared to the right (Figure 5.13.3). The sagittal view of the left middle cerebral artery reveals plaque formation in the inferior wall, with significant enhancement observed in the same region (Figure 5.13.4).

DSA revealed stenosis in the M1 segment of the bilateral middle cerebral arteries (Fig. 5.13.5).

She maintained the administration of a dual-antiplatelet regimen and statin therapy following admission.

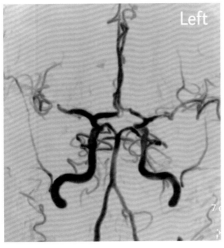

Fig. 5.13.1   The MRA showed stenosis in the M1 segment of the bilateral middle cerebral artery

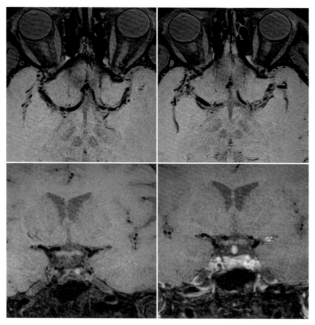

图 5.13.3　高分辨率 MRI 示右大脑中动脉 M1 段分叉部近端前壁、下壁及后壁斑块形成，左大脑中动脉 M1 段起始部斑块形成，左大脑中动脉较右大脑中动脉的管壁强化明显

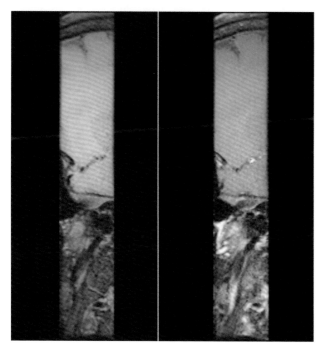

图 5.13.4　高分辨率 MRI 矢状位示左大脑中动脉斑块偏下壁，下壁强化明显

（二）诊断

症状性左大脑中动脉 M1 段狭窄。

（三）术前讨论

该例患者为绝经后女性，有反复发作的右侧肢

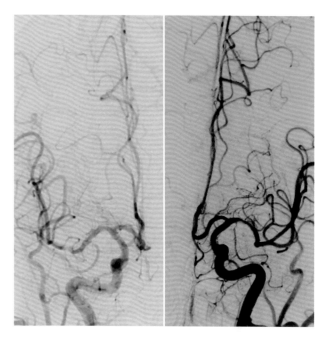

图 5.13.5　DSA 示双侧大脑中动脉 M1 段轻度狭窄

体无力，发作刻板，临床怀疑穿支 TIA，灌注未见明显皮质缺血，结合高分辨率 MRI 所示斑块分布，考虑穿支低灌注系狭窄所致的文丘里效应。双联抗血小板治疗期间仍有发作，提示药物治疗效果不佳。右大脑中动脉 M1 段亦有狭窄，但因无临床症状，故暂不干预。

（四）治疗过程

全麻下，右股动脉置入 6F 鞘，6F 导引导管置于左颈内动脉 C2 段，造影显示左大脑中动脉 M1 段狭窄（图 5.13.6 A）。沿导引导管送入 Transend 微导丝（0.014 in，300 cm）至左大脑中动脉 M2 段，沿微导丝送入 Gateway 球囊（2.0 mm×9 mm），于狭窄处定位准确后扩张（图 5.13.6 B），压力 8 atm，撤出球囊后送入 Wingspan 支架（2.5 mm×15 mm）覆盖狭窄。最后造影显示残余狭窄率约 10%，前向血流 mTICI 分级 3 级（图 5.13.6 C）。

（五）讨论

颅内动脉粥样硬化性狭窄波及穿支动脉开口时可引发穿支动脉闭塞，此外亦有文丘里效应导致穿支动脉低灌注的可能。该效应表现为血流在通过缩小的管腔断面时，流体出现流速增大的现象。而由伯努利定律（Bernoulli's law）可知流速的增大伴

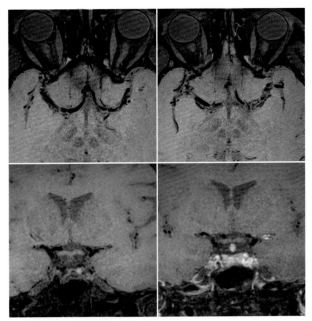

Fig. 5.13.3 The HRMRI results showed the presence of plaque formation in the proximal anterior, inferior, and posterior walls of the right middle cerebral artery at its bifurcation. Additionally, plaque formation is noted at the beginning of the left middle cerebral artery M1 segment. The arterial wall enhancement is more pronounced in the left middle cerebral artery compared to the right

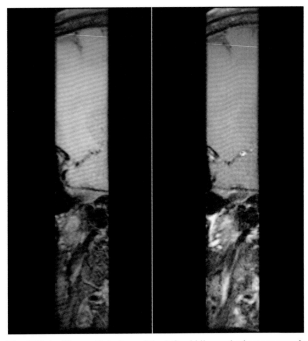

Fig. 5.13.4 The sagittal view of the left middle cerebral artery reveals plaque formation in the inferior wall, with significant enhancement observed in the same region

2. Diagnosis

Symptomatic stenosis of the M1 segment of the left middle cerebral artery.

3. Treatment schedule

The patient in this case was a postmenopausal female who experiences recurrent stereotyped episodes of the right-

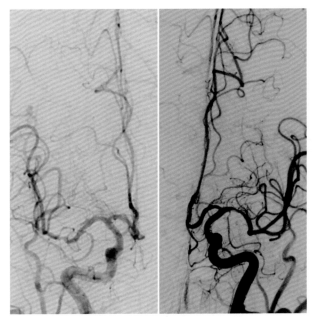

Fig. 5.13.5 DSA showed stenosis in the M1 segment of the bilateral middle cerebral artery

sided limb. These episodes are suspected to be caused by TIAs involving the penetrating arteries. Although the perfusion imaging did not reveal any significant cortical ischemia, a careful analysis of the plaque distribution observed on the high-resolution MRI suggests that the hypoperfusion in the perforating arteries may be attributed to the Venturi effect caused by the stenotic lesion. Despite dual-antiplatelet therapy, episodes continue to occur, suggesting a suboptimal response to medication. Additionally, there is evidence of narrowing in the M1 segment of the right middle cerebral artery; however, the absence of clinical symptoms currently does not warrant intervention.

4. Treatment

Under general anesthesia, a 6F guiding catheter was inserted via the right femoral artery and positioned at the C2 segment of the left internal carotid artery. The angiogram conducted before the procedure showed stenosis in the M1 segment of the left middle cerebral artery (Fig. 5.13.6 A). The Transend microwire (0.014 in, 300 cm) was navigated through the lesion to the M2 segment of the left middle cerebral artery. A 2.0 mm×9 mm Gateway balloon was used to pre-dilate the lesion (Fig. 5.13.6 B). Following that, a 2.5 mm×15 mm Wingspan stent was used to cover the lesion. The post-stent implantation angiogram demonstrated residual stenosis of approximately 10%, while the forward blood flow was assessed as grade 3 (Fig. 5.13.6 C).

5. Comments

The narrowing of intracranial arteries due to atherosclerosis can lead to occlusion of the perforating artery origins. Additionally, there is the possibility of a Venturi effect causing a reduction in perfusion of the perforating artery. This effect is characterized by an increase in fluid velocity as it passes through a narrowed lumen. According to Bernoulli's law, an increase in velocity

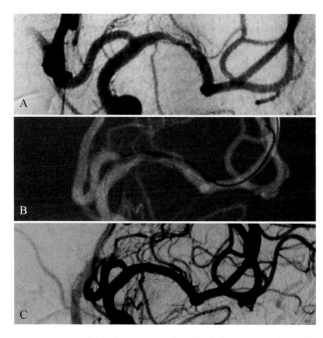

随流体压力的降低，即在狭窄区域有穿支动脉低灌注的可能。理论上对这类型病变进行干预，有望解除穿支动脉低灌注。

（马宁）

5.13　手术操作视频
（病例 33）

图 5.13.6　**A**. 术前造影显示左大脑中动脉 M1 段轻度狭窄；**B**. Gateway 球囊扩张责任病变；**C**. 支架置入后造影显示残余狭窄率约 10%

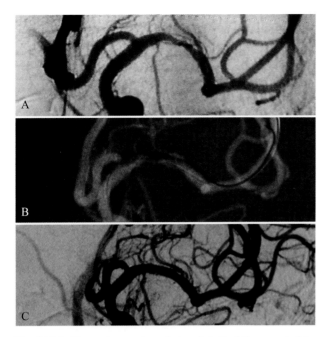

Fig. 5.13.6 The angiogram showed stenosis in the M1 segment of the left middle cerebral artery (**A**). The Gateway balloon was utilized to predilate the lesion (**B**). The post-stent implantation angiogram showed the residual stenosis rate was about 10% (**C**)

is accompanied by a decrease in fluid pressure, indicating the potential for reduced perfusion in the perforating artery of the narrowed region. Theoretically, interventions targeted at this type of lesion hold promise for alleviating the hypoperfusion in the perforating artery.

(Translated by Rongrong Cui, Revised by Zhikai Hou)

5.13   Video of endovascular
therapy (Case 33)

第十四节　球囊通过病变困难

病例 34　基底动脉重度狭窄球囊通过病变困难

（一）临床病史及影像分析

患者，男性，主因"头晕1月余"入院。

既往史：冠心病、高脂血症病史。

查体：神经系统查体无阳性体征。

头部 MRI：无新发梗死灶（图 5.14.1）。

头部 MRA：基底动脉重度狭窄（图 5.14.2）。

DSA：双侧后交通动脉开放（图 5.14.3），双椎动脉 V4 段以后显影浅淡（图 5.14.4）。

入院后给予双联抗血小板（阿司匹林 100 mg 1 次 / 日＋氯吡格雷 75 mg 1 次 / 日）以及强化降脂（阿托伐他汀 40 mg 1 次 / 日）等治疗。

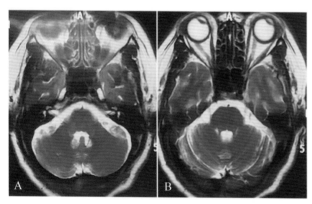

图 5.14.1　头部 MRI 提示无新发梗死灶（**A** 和 **B**）

（二）诊断

症状性基底动脉重度狭窄。

（三）术前讨论

结合患者病史及相关影像学检查，患者后循环缺血症状明确，基底动脉重度狭窄，考虑对基底动脉重度狭窄行血管内介入治疗。相关风险包括医源性夹层、动脉破裂、穿支事件、急性血栓形成、栓子脱落等。

（四）治疗过程

全麻下右股动脉穿刺入路，置入 6F 鞘，将 6F 导引导管送至左椎动脉 V2 段，术前造影明确基底动脉重度狭窄（图 5.14.5 A）。

沿导引导管送入 Synchro 微导丝（0.014 in，300 cm）携 Echelon-10 微导管，反复尝试后微导丝通过狭窄处，但微导管不能通过（图 5.14.5 B），撤出微导丝及微导管，更换支撑力更强的 Asahi Intecc 微导丝，将微导丝送至右大脑后动脉 P1 段（图 5.14.5 C），依次沿微导丝送入 Gateway 球囊（1.5 mm×15 mm）和 Emerge 球囊（1.2 mm×15 mm），均未能通过狭窄段，撤出微导丝造影显示

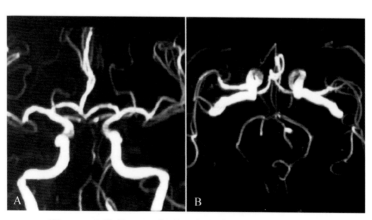

图 5.14.2　头部 MRA 提示基底动脉重度狭窄（**A** 和 **B**）

Section 14   Difficulty in Crossing the Lesion with a Balloon

Case 34   Difficulty in crossing the lesion with a balloon— Severe stenosis of basilar artery

1. Clinical presentation and radiological studies

A male patient was admitted to the hospital because of persistent dizziness lasting over one month.

The patient had a history of coronary heart disease and hyperlipidemia.

Upon admission, his neurological status was found to be intact.

The MRI revealed no indications of acute cerebral infarction (Fig. 5.14.1).

The MRA revealed severe stenosis of the basilar artery (Fig. 5.14.2).

The digital subtraction angiography (DSA) revealed the bilateral posterior communicating arteries were patent (Fig. 5.14.3), and the visualization of the V4 segments of the bilateral vertebral arteries was poor (Fig. 5.14.4).

Upon admission, a prescription was given consisting of

a dual-antiplatelet regimen comprising a daily intake of 100 mg Aspirin and 75 mg Clopidogrel, alongside a statin therapy consisting of a daily dose of 40 mg Atorvastatin.

2. Diagnosis

Symptomatic severe stenosis of the basilar artery.

3. Treatment schedule

Upon assessment of the patient's clinical presentation and radiological findings, it was determined that the patient experienced repeated episodes of dizziness, with severe basilar artery stenosis identified as the underlying cause. Consequently, endovascular therapy was advised. Potential risks included iatrogenic dissection, arterial rupture, perforating artery occlusion, acute in-stent thrombosis, and dislodgement of emboli.

4. Treatment

Under general anesthesia, a 6F guiding catheter was inserted via the right femoral artery and placed at the V2 segment of the left vertebral artery. The angiogram revealed severe stenosis of the basilar artery (Fig. 5.14.5 A).

After multiple attempts, the Synchro microwire (0.014 in, 300 cm) successfully navigated across the lesion. However, the Echelon-10 microcatheter was unsuccessful in crossing the lesion (Fig. 5.14.5 B). The Synchro microwire was subsequently substituted with the Asahi Intecc microwire, which had superior support capabilities. The Asahi Intecc microwire was carefully advanced to the P1 segment of the right posterior cerebral artery (Fig. 5.14.5 C). However, neither the Gateway balloon (1.5 mm×15 mm) nor the Emerge balloon (1.2 mm×15 mm)

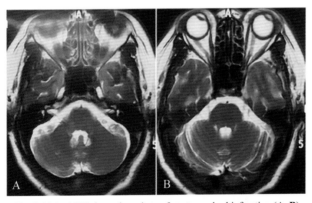

Fig. 5.14.1   MRI showed no signs of acute cerebral infarction (**A, B**)

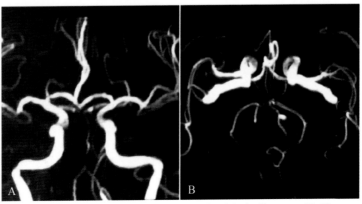

Fig. 5.14.2   MRA revealed severe stenosis of the basilar artery (**A, B**)

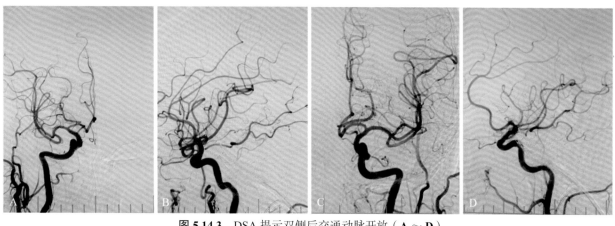

图 5.14.3　DSA 提示双侧后交通动脉开放（**A ～ D**）

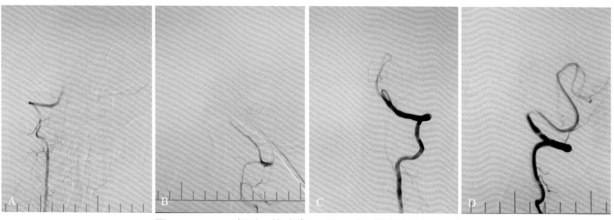

图 5.14.4　DSA 提示双椎动脉 V4 段以后显影浅淡（**A ～ D**）

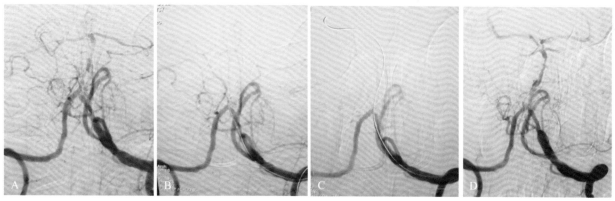

图 5.14.5　血管内介入治疗过程如下：**A**.术前造影；**B**.微导管未能通过狭窄处；**C**. Asahi Intecc 微导丝送至右大脑后动脉 P1 段；**D**.球囊未能通过狭窄段，撤出微导丝后造影显示前向血流明显改善

前向血流较前明显改善（图 5.14.5 D）。观察 10 min 后造影，血流通畅，无急性血栓形成，撤出导管，结束手术。

（五）讨论

本例患者基底动脉重度狭窄，微导丝顺利通过，微导管和球囊不能通过狭窄段，强行通过会导致血管破裂。结束手术时发现前向血流较前明显改善，可能与微导丝在狭窄段的机械作用有关，治疗结果满意。

（阎龙　马宁）

5.14　手术操作视频
（病例 **34**）

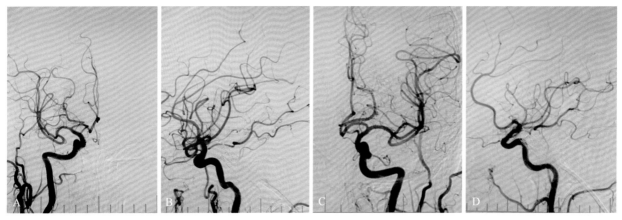

Fig. 5.14.3   DSA showed the bilateral posterior communicating arteries were patent (**A**–**D**)

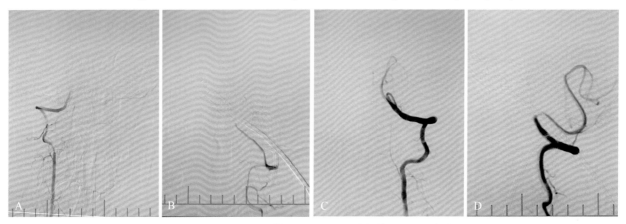

Fig. 5.14.4   DSA showed the visualization of the V4 segments of the bilateral vertebral arteries was poor (**A**–**D**)

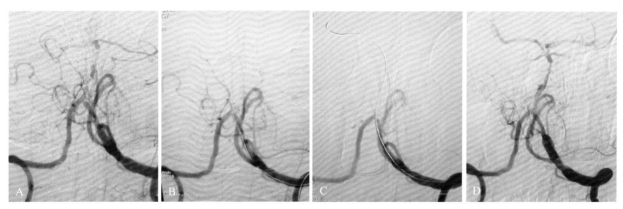

Fig. 5.14.5   (**A**) The angiogram before the procedure. (**B**) The microcatheter failed to navigate the lesion. (**C**) The Asahi Intecc microwire was advanced into the P1 segment of the right posterior cerebral artery. (**D**) Upon withdrawal of the microwire, an improvement in antegrade blood flow was observed in the angiogram

achieved successful passage through the narrowed segment. Upon withdrawal of the microwire, an improvement in antegrade blood flow was observed in the angiogram (Fig. 5.14.5 D). Following a 10-minute observation period, the angiogram exhibited no signs of acute thrombosis.

5. Comments

In this case, the patient exhibited severe stenosis of the basal artery. The microwire successfully traversed through, however, both the microcatheter and balloon were unable to pass through the narrowed segment. Forcing passage could result in vessel rupture. It was noted that there was a marked improvement in antegrade blood flow after the procedure, potentially attributed to the mechanical effect of the microwire in the stenotic segment. The treatment outcome was deemed satisfactory.

(Translated by Rongrong Cui, Revised by Zhikai Hou)

5.14   Video of endovascular therapy (Case 34)

第十五节 钙化病变

病例 35 左椎动脉 V4 段粥样硬化性钙化性狭窄

（一）临床病史及影像分析

患者，男性，主因"头晕半年"入院。

既往史：高血压病史，吸烟。

查体：神经系统查体无阳性体征。

头部 MRI：双侧小脑半球多发急性梗死灶（图 5.15.1）。

头部 MRA：左椎动脉 V4 段重度狭窄（图 5.15.2）。

头部 CTP：脑干、双侧小脑半球低灌注（图 5.15.3）。

高分辨率 MRI：左椎动脉 V4 段重度狭窄，管壁可见钙化（图 5.15.4）。

DSA：左后交通动脉开放（图 5.15.5 A ~ D），后循环造影显示左椎动脉 V4 段串联狭窄（图 5.15.5 E 和 F）。

入院后给予双联抗血小板（阿司匹林 100 mg 1 次 / 日＋氯吡格雷 75 mg 1 次 / 日）以及强化降脂（阿托伐他汀 40 mg 1 次 / 日）等治疗。

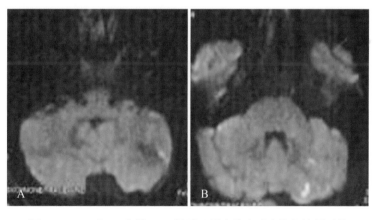

图 5.15.1 **A** 和 **B**. 头部 MRI 提示双侧小脑半球多发急性梗死灶

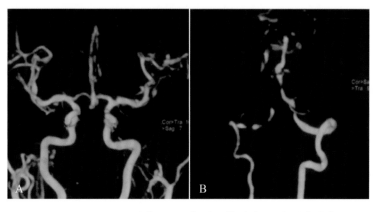

图 5.15.2 **A** 和 **B**. 头部 MRA 提示左椎动脉 V4 段重度狭窄

Section 15　Calcific Stenosis

Case 35　Severe calcific stenosis of the V4 segment of the left vertebral artery

1. Clinical presentation and radiological studies

A male patient was admitted to the hospital due to persistent dizziness for half a year.

The patient had a history of hypertension and cigarette smoking.

Upon admission, his neurological status was found to be intact.

The MRI showed multiple acute infarctions in the bilateral cerebellar hemispheres (Fig. 5.15.1).

The MRA revealed severe stenosis at the V4 segment of the left vertebral artery (Fig. 5.15.2).

The CT perfusion revealed hypoperfusion in the brainstem and bilateral cerebellar hemispheres (Fig. 5.15.3).

The high-resolution MRI indicated significant stenosis at the V4 segment of the left vertebral artery, accompanied by intra-plaque calcification (Fig. 5.15.4).

DSA examination demonstrated the left posterior communicating artery to be patent (Fig. 5.15.5 A–D), while revealing tandem stenosis at the V4 segment of the left vertebral artery (Fig. 5.15.5 E, F).

Upon admission, a prescription was given consisting of a dual-antiplatelet regimen comprising a daily intake of 100 mg Aspirin and 75 mg Clopidogrel, alongside a statin therapy consisting of a daily dose of 40 mg Atorvastatin.

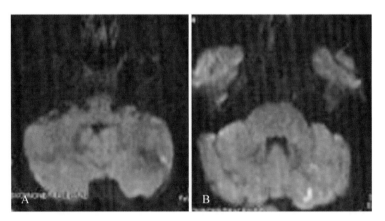

Fig. 5.15.1　The MRI showed multiple acute infarcts in the bilateral cerebellar hemispheres (**A**, **B**)

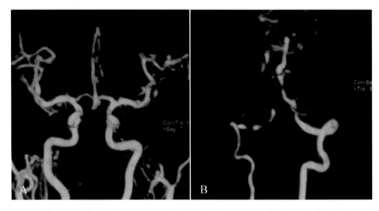

Fig. 5.15.2　The MRA showed severe stenosis at the V4 segment of the left vertebral artery (**A**, **B**)

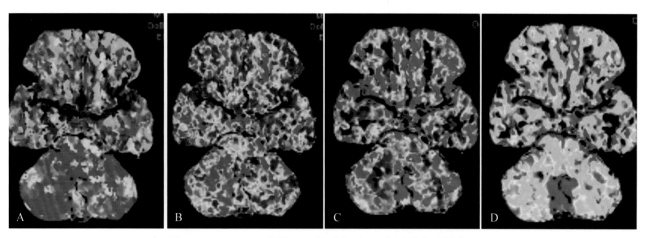

图 **5.15.3**　**A ～ D**. 头部 CTP 提示脑干、双侧小脑半球低灌注

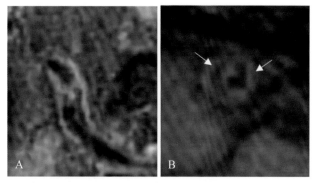

图 **5.15.4**　**A** 和 **B**. 高分辨率 MRI 提示左椎动脉 V4 段重度狭窄，管壁可见钙化（箭头示）

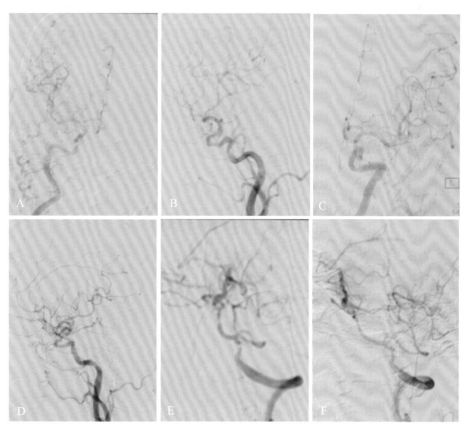

图 **5.15.5**　DSA 示：**A ～ D**. 左后交通动脉开放；**E** 和 **F**. 左椎动脉 V4 段串联狭窄

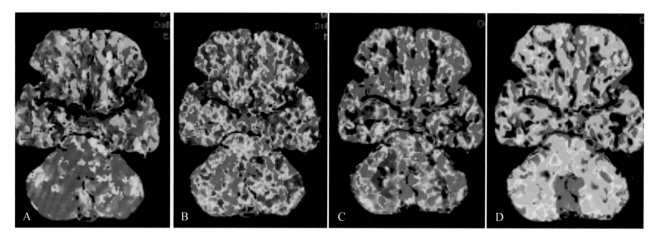

Fig. 5.15.3   The CT perfusion showed hypoperfusion in the brainstem and bilateral cerebellar hemispheres (**A**–**D**)

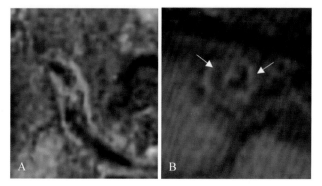

Fig. 5.15.4   The high-resolution MRI indicated significant stenosis at the V4 segment of the left vertebral artery, accompanied by intra-plaque calcification (arrow) (**A**, **B**)

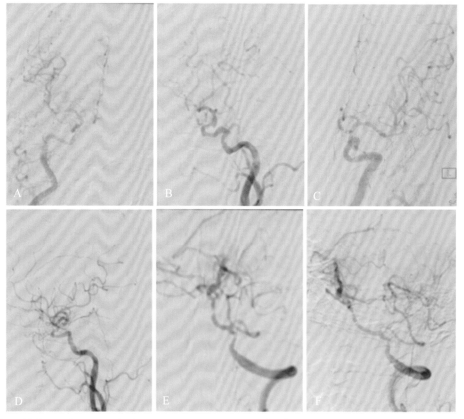

Fig. 5.15.5   DSA showed left posterior communicating artery was patent (**A**–**D**), and tandem stenoses at the V4 segment of the left vertebral artery (**E**, **F**)

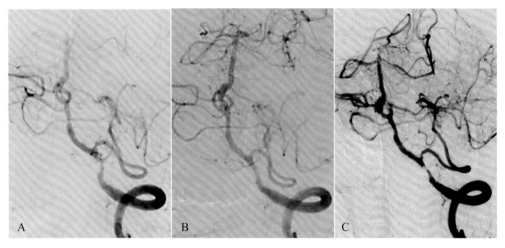

图5.15.6 血管内介入治疗过程如下：**A**.术前造影；**B**.释放支架后残余狭窄率约35%；**C**.术后2年复查DSA提示近端狭窄处再狭窄

（二）诊断

症状性左椎动脉V4段重度狭窄。

（三）术前讨论

结合患者病史及相关影像学检查，患者后循环缺血症状反复发作，小脑半球新发梗死，左椎动脉V4段重度狭窄，考虑行左椎动脉重度狭窄血管内介入治疗。相关风险包括医源性夹层、动脉破裂、穿支事件、急性血栓形成、栓子脱落等。

（四）治疗过程

全麻下右股动脉穿刺入路，置入6F鞘，将6F导引导管送至左椎动脉V2段，造影明确左椎动脉串联狭窄（图5.15.6 A），沿导引导管送入Transend微导丝携Echelon-10微导管，将微导丝送至左大脑后动脉P1段，撤出Echelon-10微导管，沿微导丝送入Gateway球囊（2.0 mm×9.0 mm），由远及近依次扩张两处狭窄，远端狭窄处扩张效果满意，近端狭窄处残余狭窄率约60%，撤出球囊，沿微导丝送入Select Plus微导管，撤出微导丝，沿微导管送入Enterprise支架（4.5 mm×9.0 mm）并释放，造影显示前向血流良好，残余狭窄率约35%（图5.15.6 B）。观察10 min后造影，血流通畅，无急性血栓形成，撤出导管，结束手术。

2年后复查见近端狭窄处再狭窄（图5.15.6 C）。

（五）讨论

本例患者椎动脉串联狭窄，球囊扩张后近端病变残余狭窄较重，遂给予支架置入术。术后2年复查，支架内再狭窄，可能与钙化病变有关。

（阎龙 马宁）

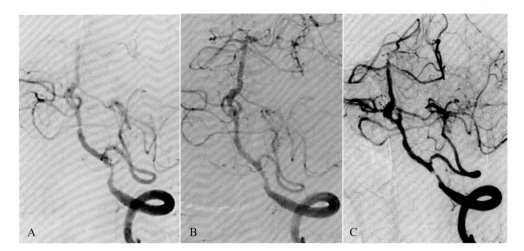

Fig. 5.15.6   (**A**) The angiogram before the procedure. (**B**) The angiogram conducted after the stent implantation revealed a residual stenosis of 35%. (**C**) The 2-year follow-up angiogram indicated the occurrence of in-stent restenosis in the proximal stenosis segment

2. Diagnosis

Symptomatic severe stenosis of the V4 segment of the left vertebral artery.

3. Treatment schedule

The patient had recurrent episodes of dizziness. The radiological findings showed multiple new infarctions in both cerebellar hemispheres. Furthermore, significant stenosis was identified at the V4 segment of the left vertebral artery, which was considered the responsible vessel. In light of these findings, endovascular therapy was proposed as a recommended course of action. Potential risks associated with the procedure included iatrogenic dissection, arterial rupture, perforating artery occlusion, acute in-stent thrombosis, and dislodgement of emboli.

4. Treatment

Under general anesthesia, the right femoral artery was punctured as the entry point. A 6F guiding catheter was inserted and positioned at the V2 segment of the left vertebral artery. The angiogram confirmed the presence of tandem stenosis at the V4 segment of the left vertebral artery (Fig. 5.15.6 A). A Transend microwire and an Echelon-10 microcatheter coaxially navigated through the lesion to the P1 segment of the left posterior cerebral artery. Following that, a Gateway balloon (2.0 mm×9.0 mm) was employed to perform sequential dilation of the tandem stenosis starting from the distal region and moving towards the proximal region. Subsequent angiography after the balloon dilation procedure indicated a minor degree of residual stenosis at the distal stenosis site, while the proximal stenosis revealed an approximate 60% residual stenosis. Upon withdrawing the balloon, a Select Plus microcatheter was smoothly guided along the previously placed microwire. Subsequently, an Enterprise stent (4.5 mm×9.0 mm) was navigated through the Select Plus microcatheter, precisely positioning it to fully cover the lesion. The angiogram conducted after the stent implantation revealed a residual stenosis of 35% and a notable enhancement in antegrade blood flow (Fig. 5.15.6 B). Following a monitoring period of 10 minutes, a subsequent angiogram confirmed the patency of the stent in the V4 segment of the left vertebral artery, with no indications of acute in-stent thrombosis.

Two years later, The follow-up angiogram revealed the occurrence of in-stent restenosis in the proximal stenosis segment. (Fig. 5.15.6 C).

5. Comments

In this case, the patient exhibited tandem stenoses in the left vertebral artery. Significant residual stenosis remained in the proximal lesion after balloon dilation. Consequently, stent placement was performed. The 2-year follow-up angiogram indicated the occurrence of in-stent restenosis, which was likely associated with the existence of calcified lesions in the plaque.

(Translated by Rongrong Cui, Revised by Zhikai Hou)

第六章

手术相关不良事件的处理

第一节　术中血管痉挛

病例 36　右大脑中动脉重度狭窄血管内治疗术中发生血管痉挛

（一）临床病史及影像分析

患者，男性，45 岁，主因"左侧肢体无力伴言语不清 15 个月"入院。

当地医院头颅 MRI 示右侧脑室旁及右颞叶多发陈旧性缺血灶（图 6.1.1）。头颅 MRA 示右大脑中动

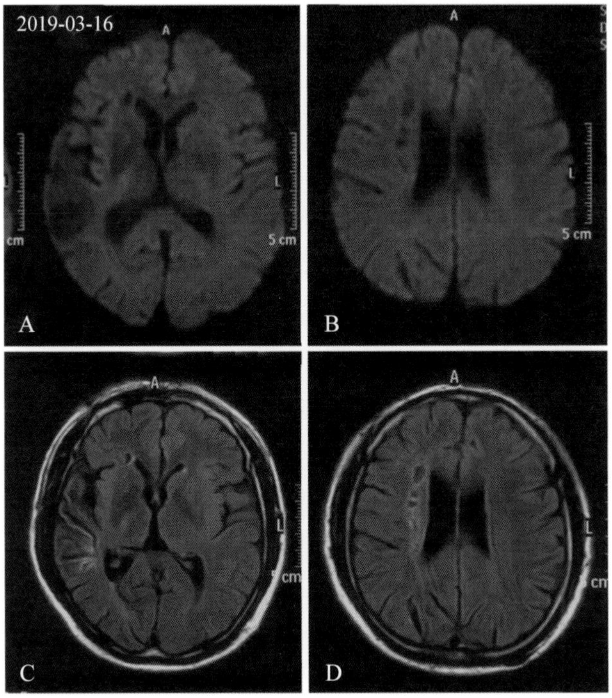

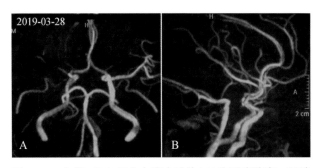

图 6.1.1　头颅 MRI 示右侧脑室旁及右颞叶多发陈旧性缺血灶

脉 M1 段重度狭窄，远端分支显影不良（图 6.1.2）。

头部 CTA 示右大脑中动脉重度狭窄（图 6.1.3 A 和 B），CTP 示相关供血区域低灌注（图 6.1.3 C ～ F）。

予以双联抗血小板等内科药物治疗后，患者病情仍有反复，为行血管内介入治疗而收入我院。

既往史：糖尿病病史。

查体：构音障碍，左上肢肌力 4 级，余体征阴性。

入院后 DSA：右大脑中动脉 M1 段近分叉处长段重度狭窄，可见少许同侧大脑后动脉经软脑膜动脉向大脑中动脉供血区域代偿，同侧大脑前动脉代偿不明显（图 6.1.4）。

HRMRI：右大脑中动脉 M1 段中远段见偏心性斑块，有中度强化（图 6.1.5）。

图 6.1.2　头颅 MRA 示右大脑中动脉 M1 段重度狭窄，远端分支显影不良

Chapter 6

Procedure-Related Adverse Events

Section 1   Periprocedural Vasospasm

Case 36   Vasospasm during endovascular treatment of a severe stenosis of the right middle cerebral artery

1. Clinical presentation and radiological studies

A 45-year-old male patient was admitted to the hospital due to left-sided limb weakness and dysarthria for fifteen months.

The MRI findings revealed the presence of multiple old infarctions in the right periventricular area and right temporal lobe (Fig. 6.1.1). The MRA results showed severe stenosis in the M1 segment of the right middle cerebral artery, accompanied by suboptimal visualization of its distal branches (Fig. 6.1.2).

The CT angiography revealed severe stenosis in the M1 segment of the right middle cerebral artery (Fig. 6.1.3 A, B), and CT perfusion showed hypoperfusion in the territory of the right middle cerebral artery (Fig. 6.1.3 C–F).

Despite aggressive medical treatment, the patient continues to experience recurrent symptoms.

He had a medical history of diabetes mellitus.

Physical examination showed dysarthria and 4/5 muscle strength in the left upper limb.

DSA revealed severe and long-segment stenosis in the M1 segment of the right middle cerebral artery, with limited compensation observed from the ipsilateral posterior cerebral artery through the leptomeningeal arteries to the supply region of the middle cerebral artery. However, compensatory blood flow from the ipsilateral anterior cerebral artery was not readily apparent (Fig. 6.1.4).

The High-resolution MRI revealed eccentric plaques in the middle segments of the M1 segment of the right middle cerebral artery, with moderate intra-plaque enhancement (Fig. 6.1.5).

Fig. 6.1.1   The MRI findings revealed the presence of multiple old infarctions in the right periventricular area and right temporal lobe

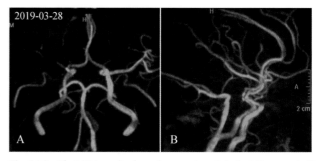

Fig. 6.1.2   The MRA results showed severe stenosis in the M1 segment of the right middle cerebral artery, accompanied by suboptimal visualization of its distal branches

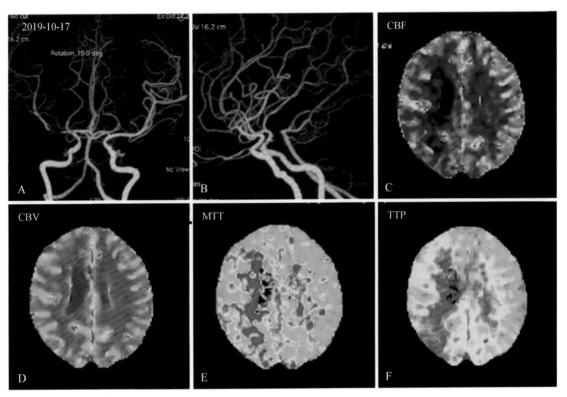

图 6.1.3 **A** 和 **B**. 头部 CTA 示右大脑中动脉重度狭窄；**C ~ F**. CTP 示右大脑中动脉供血区域低灌注

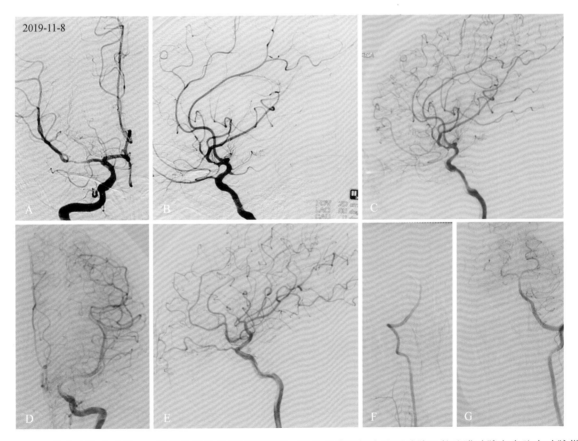

图 6.1.4 DSA 示右大脑中动脉 M1 段近分叉处长段重度狭窄，可见少许同侧大脑后动脉经软脑膜动脉向大脑中动脉供血区域代偿，同侧大脑前动脉代偿不明显

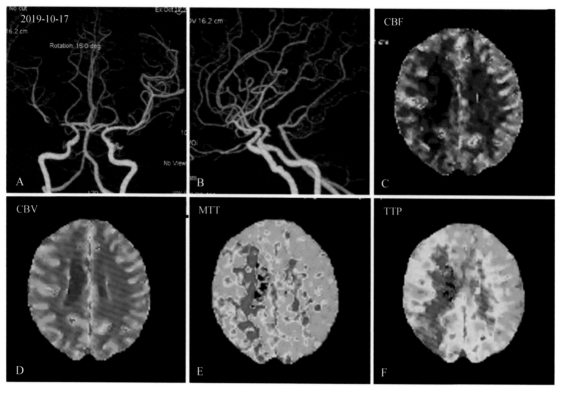

Fig. 6.1.3 The CTA revealed severe stenosis in the M1 segment of the right middle cerebral artery (**A, B**). The CTP showed hypoperfusion in the right middle cerebral artery territory (**C–F**)

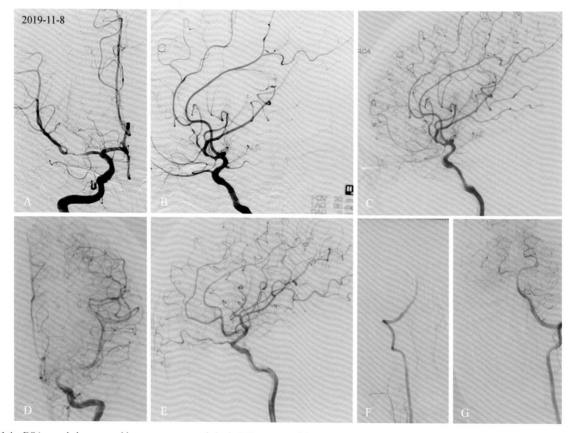

Fig. 6.1.4 DSA revealed severe and long-segment stenosis in the M1 segment of the right middle cerebral artery, with limited compensation observed from the ipsilateral posterior cerebral artery through the leptomeningeal arteries to the supply region of the middle cerebral artery. However, compensatory blood flow from the ipsilateral anterior cerebral artery was not readily apparent

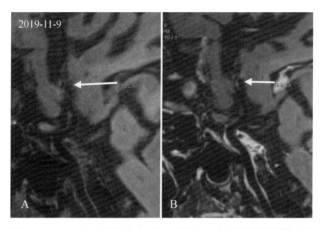

图 6.1.5　HRMRI 显示右大脑中动脉 M1 段中远段见偏心性斑块，有中度强化

目前予以双联抗血小板（阿司匹林 100 mg 1 次 / 日＋氯吡格雷 75 mg 1 次 / 日）、降脂（阿托伐他汀 20 mg 1 次 / 日）治疗。

（二）诊断

症状性右大脑中动脉 M1 段重度狭窄。

（三）术前讨论

患者症状为左侧肢体无力伴言语不清，影像学检查提示右侧内分水岭区脑梗死，右大脑中动脉 M1 段重度狭窄，考虑右大脑中动脉为责任病变。因相关供血区域低灌注且药物治疗效果欠佳，拟行血管内介入治疗。微导丝结合微导管先通过狭窄病变，其后行球囊预扩张和置入自膨式支架。相关风险包括急性或亚急性血栓形成、动脉夹层等。

（四）治疗过程

全麻下右股动脉入路，将 6F 导引导管头端置于右颈内动脉 C1 段远端，造影显示右大脑中动脉 M1 段中远段重度狭窄（图 6.1.6 A）。

Synchro 微导丝（0.014 in，300 cm）顺利通过狭窄段至右大脑中动脉下干 M3 段（图 6.1.6 B），送入 Gateway 球囊（1.5 mm×15 mm）至狭窄段，缓慢扩张（图 6.1.6 C 和 D）。其后造影示狭窄程度明显改善，残余狭窄率约 40%（图 6.1.6 E）。撤出球囊，送入并释放 Wingspan 自膨式支架（2.5 mm×

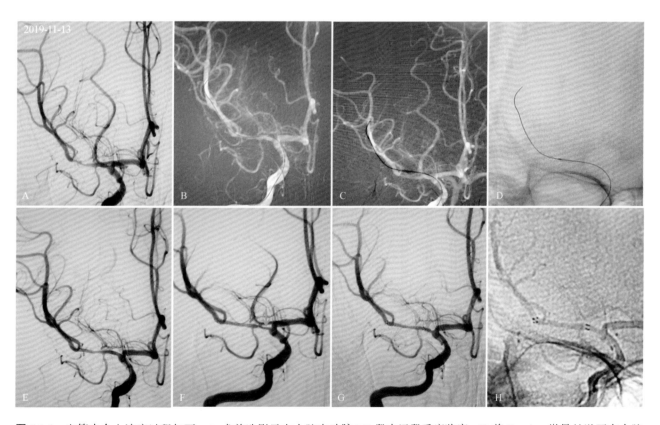

图 6.1.6　血管内介入治疗过程如下：**A**. 术前造影示右大脑中动脉 M1 段中远段重度狭窄；**B**. 将 Synchro 微导丝送至右大脑中动脉下干 M3 段；**C** 和 **D**. Gateway 球囊扩张狭窄病变；**E**. 球囊扩张后造影示残余狭窄率约 40%；**F**. 置入支架后造影示支架近端管腔变细，考虑有血管痉挛可能（箭头）；**G** 和 **H**. 给予尼莫地平后血管痉挛缓解（箭头）

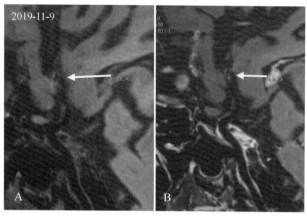

Fig. 6.1.5 HRMRI revealed eccentric plaques in the middle segments of the M1 segment of the right middle cerebral artery, with moderate intraplaque enhancement

Following admission, the patient was prescribed a daily regimen of 100 mg of Aspirin and 75 mg of Clopidogrel, as well as statin therapy with a daily dose of 20 mg of Atorvastatin.

2. Diagnosis

Symptomatic severe stenosis in the M1 segment of the right middle cerebral artery.

3. Treatment schedule

The patient presented with left-sided hemiplegia and dysarthria, and imaging results revealed ischemic lesions in the internal border-zone, as well as severe stenosis in the M1 segment of the right middle cerebral artery. The stenosis in the right middle cerebral artery was identified as the primary culprit lesion. Considering the presence of hypoperfusion in the affected vascular territory and the limited effectiveness of medical treatment, endovascular therapy has been scheduled. The treatment plan involves initial pre-dilation of the stenotic lesion, followed by the placement of a self-expanding stent. Potential risks associated with this procedure include acute/subacute in-stent thrombosis and arterial dissection.

4. Treatment

Under general anesthesia, the right femoral artery was punctured as the access, a 6F guide catheter was then positioned at the C1 segment of the right internal carotid artery. The angiogram revealed severe stenosis in the middledistal portions of the M1 segment of the right middle cerebral artery (Fig. 6.1.6 A).

A Synchro microwire (0.014 in, 300 cm) was navigated through the lesion to reach the M3 segment of the right middle cerebral artery (Fig. 6.1.6 B). A 1.5 mm×15 mm Gateway balloon was used to pre-dilate the lesion (Fig. 6.1.6 C, D). The subsequent angiogram showed a residual stenosis of approximately 40% (Fig. 6.1.6 E). Following that, a 2.5 mm×15 mm Wingspan stent was employed to fully cover the

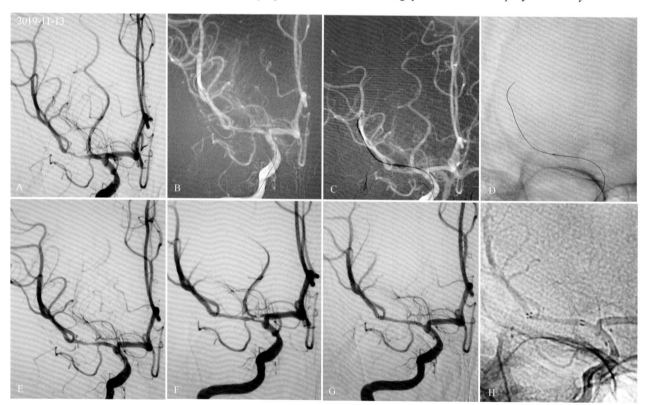

Fig. 6.1.6 (**A**) Preprocedural angiogram revealed severe stenosis in the middle-distal segment of the M1 segment of the right middle cerebral artery. (**B**) A Synchro microwire successfully passed through the lesion to reach the M3 segment of the lower division. (**C, D**) A Gateway balloon was used to pre-dilated the lesion. (**E**) The angiogram after the balloon dilatation showed a residual stenosis of 40%. (**F**) The angiogram after the stent implantation showed a constriction in the vessel lumen proximal to the stent, indicating the possibility of vasospasm (arrow). (**G, H**) After administration of nimodipine, a follow-up angiogram revealed the alleviation of the vasospasm (arrow)

15 mm)，造影显示原病变狭窄率进一步改善，支架近端见管腔变细，此时考虑有血管痉挛可能（图6.1.6 F）。予以尼莫地平4 ml/h静脉泵入，观察10 min后造影显示血管痉挛缓解，前向血流mTICI分级3级，（图6.1.6 G和H），遂结束手术。

术后第2日复查头颅CTA及CTP：支架内血流通畅，右大脑中动脉供血区域低灌注状况较术前明显改善（图6.1.7）。

窄毗邻分叉，但未波及上、下干开口，将平顺及直径较粗的下干作为微导丝着陆区，以减少跨越分叉扩张病变时对穿支血管的损伤。支架置入后支架近心端管腔变细，考虑血管痉挛所致，予以静脉泵入尼莫地平后，影像学改变迅速好转。此外，本例豆纹动脉以内侧组为著，其开口与狭窄近端有一定的解剖距离，血管内介入治疗术后发生穿支卒中并发症的风险相对较小。

（五）讨论

本例右大脑中动脉M1段中远段重度狭窄，狭

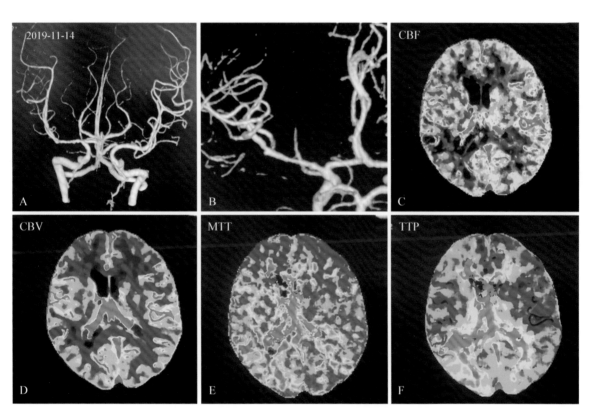

图6.1.7　术后复查头部CTA示支架内血流通畅，CTP示右大脑中动脉供血区域低灌注状况较术前明显改善

6.1　手术操作视频
（**病例36**）

（孙勇　何子骏　孙立倩　马宁）

lesion. Subsequent angiography revealed an improvement in the degree of stenosis. Nevertheless, a constriction was detected in the vessel lumen proximal to the stent, suggesting the possibility of vasospasm (Fig. 6.1.6 F). Intravenous administration of Nimodipine at a rate of 4 ml/h was initiated. After 10 minutes, a follow-up angiogram revealed the alleviation of the vasospasm. The antegrade blood flow was rated as grade 3 in the modified Thrombolysis In Cerebral Infarction (mTICI) scale (Fig. 6.1.6 G, H).

The postprocedural CTA revealed a patent stent in the right middle cerebral artery. Additionally, the CTP scans exhibited a significant improvement in hypoperfusion within the region supplied by the right middle cerebral artery (Fig. 6.1.7).

5. Comments

In this particular case, the patient presented with a severe stenosis of the M1 segment of the right middle cerebral artery. The stenosis lesion was adjacent to the M1 bifurcation but did not affect the origins of the upper and lower divisions. To reduce the damage to the perforator vessels during the angioplasty, the straight and widecaliber lower division was chosen as the landing site for the microwire. Upon review of the angiogram following the implantation of the stent, a constriction in the vessel lumen was observed proximal to the stent, indicating potential vasospasm. The administration of nimodipine successfully alleviated this vasospasm. There was a significant anatomical distance between the origin of the lenticulostriate artery and the proximal end of the stenosis, reducing the risk of perforating artery occlusion after the procedure.

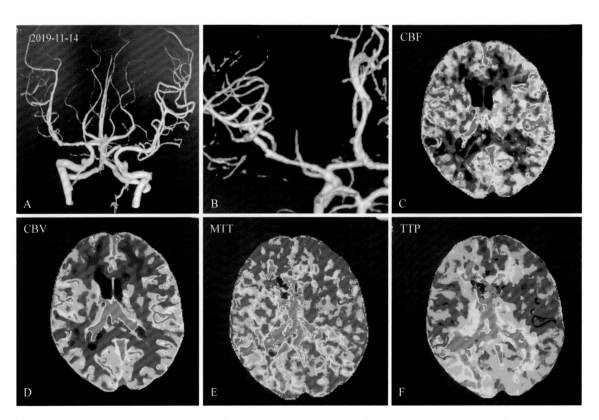

Fig. 6.1.7 Postprocedural CTA revealed the right middle cerebral artery was patent, and the CTP indicated the hypoperfusion in the right middle cerebral artery territory was significantly improved

6.1 Video of endovascular therapy (Case 36)

(Translated by Rongrong Cui, Revised by Zhikai Hou)

第二节 术中夹层形成

病例 37 基底动脉闭塞血管内治疗术中发生血管夹层

（一）临床病史及影像分析

患者，女性，69 岁，主因"头晕 9 个月，加重伴行走不稳 4 个月"入院。

当地医院影像学检查提示后循环梗死（资料丢失）。DSA 提示双侧前循环无明显异常（图 6.2.1）。右椎动脉优势，基底动脉中段中度狭窄，左椎动脉 V4 段闭塞（图 6.2.2）。予以双联抗血小板聚集以及他汀类药物调脂治疗。

4 个月前患者症状加重。当地医院头颅 MRI 提示脑干急性梗死灶（图 6.2.3）。为行血管内介入治疗收入我院。

既往史：高血压、糖尿病病史。

查体：左侧肢体肌力 4 级。

入院后头部 CTA 示基底动脉闭塞（图 6.2.4），CTP 示后循环供血区域低灌注（图 6.2.5）。

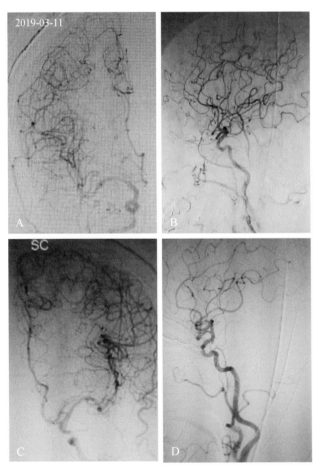

图 6.2.1 DSA 提示双侧前循环无明显异常

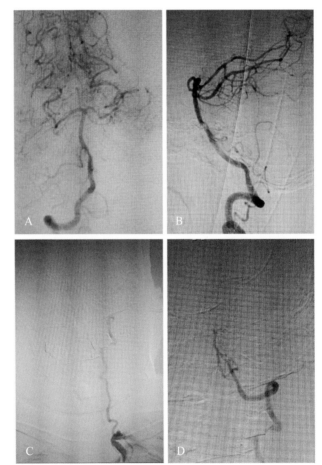

图 6.2.2 DSA 提示右椎动脉优势，基底动脉中段中度狭窄，左椎动脉 V4 段闭塞

Section 2 Periprocedural Dissection

Case 37 Arterial dissection during endovascular treatment of a basilar artery occlusion

1. Clinical presentation and radiological studies

A 69-year-old female patient was admitted to the hospital due to dizziness for nine months, accompanied by gait instability for four months.

Imaging examinations conducted at a local hospital revealed the presence of acute infarction within the posterior circulation (with data loss). The digital subtraction angiography (DSA) results exhibited no notable abnormalities within the anterior circulation (Fig. 6.2.1). The right vertebral artery displayed dominance, while moderate stenosis was identified in the middle section of the basilar artery. Additionally,

occlusion was detected in the V4 segment of the left vertebral artery. (Fig. 6.2.2). The patient was prescribed dual-antiplatelet therapy and statin treatment.

Four months ago, the patient's symptoms were exacerbated. The follow-up MRI results indicated focal acute brainstem infarction (Fig. 6.2.3).

Her medical history included hypertension and diabetes.

The physical examination indicated that the muscle strength in the left limbs was graded at 4.

The CT angiography (CTA) revealed the presence of basilar artery occlusion (Fig. 6.2.4). While the CT perfusion revealed hypoperfusion in the posterior circulation territory (Fig. 6.2.5).

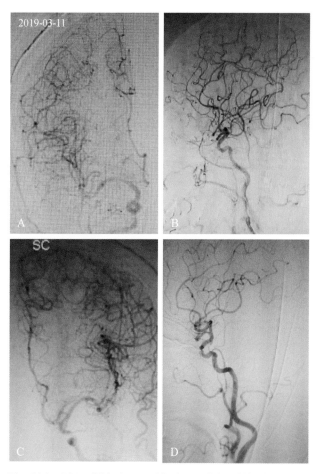

Fig. 6.2.1 DSA exhibited no notable abnormalities within the anterior circulation

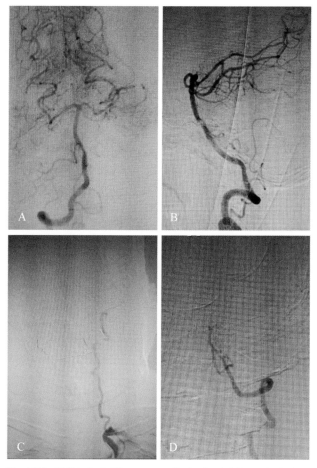

Fig. 6.2.2 DSA indicated the presence of a dominant right vertebral artery, accompanied by a moderate stenosis in the middle segment of the basilar artery. Furthermore, occlusion was identified in the V4 segment of the left vertebral artery

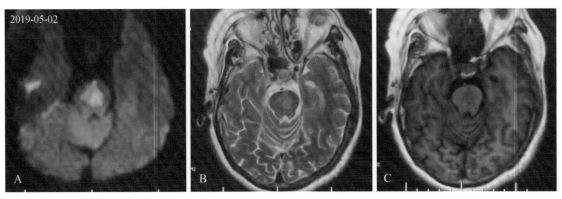

图 6.2.3 头颅 MRI 示脑干急性梗死灶

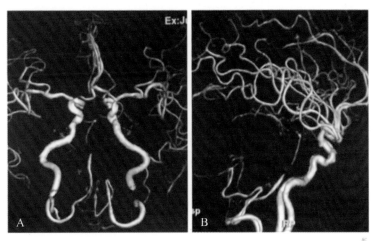

图 6.2.4 头颅 CTA 示基底动脉闭塞

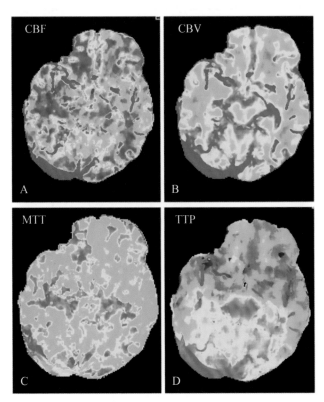

图 6.2.5 头颅 CTP 示后循环供血区域低灌注

高分辨率 MRI：基底动脉中段管壁增厚且未见管腔，考虑闭塞（图 6.2.6）。

目前予以双联抗血小板（阿司匹林 100 mg 1 次 / 日＋氯吡格雷 75 mg 1 次 / 日）、降脂（阿托伐他汀 20 mg 1 次 / 日）治疗。

（二）诊断

症状性基底动脉闭塞。

（三）术前讨论

患者后循环供血区域复发性脑梗死，影像学检查提示 5 个月内基底动脉由中度狭窄进展为闭塞。基底动脉闭塞后患者依然存在头晕症状，考虑基底动脉供血区域存在低灌注，拟行血管内介入治疗。患者闭塞时间相对较长，存在开通治疗不成功的可能。血管造影提示基底动脉闭塞段存在一定角度，通过闭塞病变有引发医源性夹层的风险，此外还有穿支卒中、急性或亚急性支架内血栓形成、术后高灌注等其他风险。

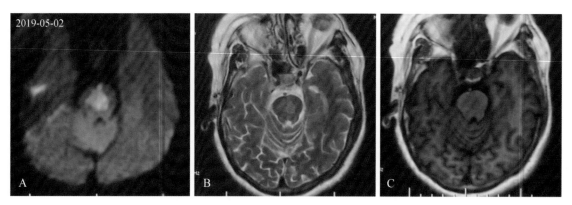

Fig. 6.2.3   The MRI revealed acute brainstem infarction

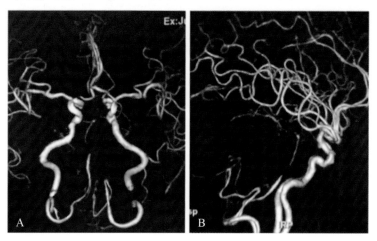

Fig. 6.2.4   The CTA revealed the presence of the basilar artery occlusion

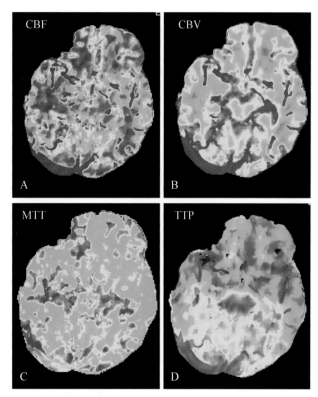

Fig. 6.2.5   The CTP showed hypoperfusion in the posterior circulation territory

The high-resolution MRI (HRMRI) indicated a thickened vessel wall and complete occlusion of the middle portion of the basilar artery (Fig. 6.2.6).

She had been prescribed a regimen of dual antiplatelet therapy, consisting of daily doses of Aspirin (100 mg) and Clopidogrel (75 mg), as well as statin therapy with Atorvastatin (20 mg).

2. Diagnosis

Symptomatic occlusion of the basilar artery.

3. Treatment schedule

The patient presented with recurrent ischemic stroke in the posterior circulation. Over five months, moderate stenosis of the basilar artery progressed to complete occlusion. Following the occlusion of the basilar artery, the patient experienced symptoms of dizziness, likely attributed to hypoperfusion within the basilar artery territory. Endovascular intervention was recommended. However, the extended duration of occlusion (5 months), posed a potential risk of unsuccessful recanalization. The angiogram revealed an angulated segment at the site of basilar artery occlusion, which poses a potential risk of iatrogenic dissection. Other associated risks include perforator stroke, acute/subacute in-stent thrombosis, and hyperperfusion syndrome.

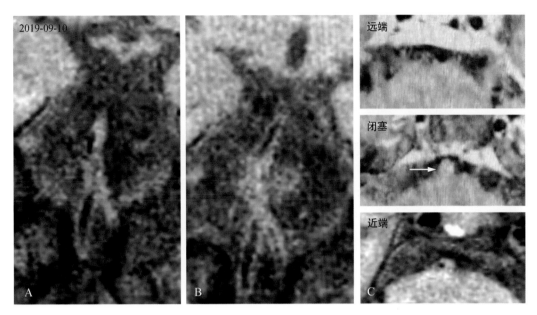

图 6.2.6　高分辨率 MRI 示基底动脉中段管壁增厚且未见管腔，考虑闭塞

（四）治疗过程

全麻下右股动脉入路，将 6F 导引导管头端置于左椎动脉 V1 段造影显示，左椎动脉发出 PICA 以远有少许顺向血流，基底动脉未见显影，小脑上动脉由 PICA 经小脑软脑膜动脉代偿显影（图 6.2.7 A）。右椎动脉优势，右椎动脉 V1 和 V2 段迂曲，右 PICA 起源于右椎动脉颅外段，基底动脉中下段闭塞，闭塞远端代偿血供主要来自右 PICA 和 AICA 间的侧支代偿（图 6.2.7 B ～ D）。

Echelon 微导管与 Synchro 微导丝（0.014 in，300 cm）同轴，经多次尝试微导丝通过闭塞段，但微导管始终不能越过闭塞段，遂撤出微导管（图 6.2.8 A 和 B）。经微导丝送入 Gateway 球囊（1.5 mm×15 mm），对位后两次扩张闭塞段（图 6.2.8 C 和 D）。造影可见狭窄明显改善，但原闭塞远端形成夹层，尤以侧位明显（图 6.2.9 A 和 B）。送入 Select Plus 微导管至基底动脉远段，置入无头型 Enterprise 支架（4.5 mm×28 mm）完全覆盖闭塞段及闭塞远端夹层。支架术后造影显示支架覆盖夹层，狭窄程度进一步改善，观察 10 min 无改变后结束手术（图 6.2.9 C 和 D）。

术后立即复查头部 CT 未见出血。

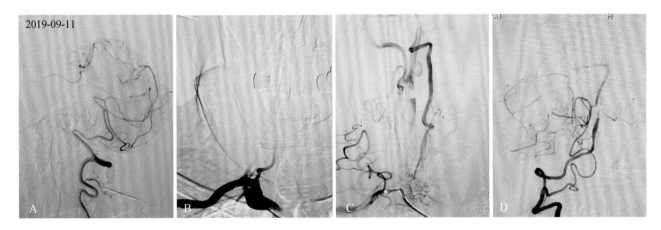

图 6.2.7　术前造影如下：**A**. 左椎动脉发出 PICA 以远有少许顺向血流，基底动脉未见显影，小脑上动脉由 PICA 经小脑软脑膜动脉代偿显影；**B ～ D**. 右椎动脉优势，右椎动脉 V1 和 V2 段迂曲，右 PICA 系右椎动脉颅外段起源，基底动脉中下段闭塞，闭塞远端代偿血供主要来自右 PICA 和 AICA 间的侧支代偿

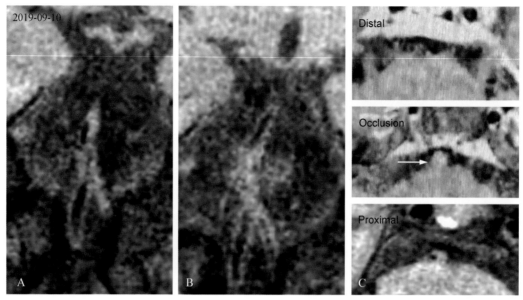

Fig. 6.2.6 HRMRI indicated a thickened vessel wall and complete occlusion of the middle portion of the basilar artery

4. Treatment

Under general anesthesia, the right femoral artery was inserted as the access, and a 6F guiding catheter was positioned at the V1 segment of the left vertebral artery. The angiogram showed limited visualization distal to the origin of the left posterior inferior cerebellar artery (PICA), and the basilar artery was not visualized. Furthermore, the superior cerebellar artery was visualized through collateral blood supply from the pial arteries originating from the PICA (Fig. 6.2.7 A). The right vertebral artery was dominant, with tortuous V1 and V2 segments. The right PICA originated from the extracranial segment of the right vertebral artery. The middle-to-lower segment of the basilar artery was occluded, while the distal segment beyond the occlusion was visualized due to the compensatory blood flow from the branches of the right PICA and the AICA (Fig. 6.2.7 B–D).

After multiple attempts, the Synchro microwire (0.014 in, 300 cm) successfully traversed the occluded segment. However, the Echelon microcatheter failed to traverse the occlusion and was subsequently withdrawn (Fig. 6.2.8 A, B). The lesion was pre-dilated twice using a 1.5 mm×15 mm Gateway balloon (Fig. 6.2.8 C, D). The angiogram revealed an improvement in the extent of stenosis, however, with the presence of an iatrogenic dissection distal to the occlusion, which displayed notable prominence, particularly in the lateral view (Fig. 6.2.9 A, B). Subsequently, a headless Enterprise stent (4.5 mm×28 mm) was used to cover both the occluded segment and the iatrogenic dissection. A post-stent implantation angiogram demonstrated the successful coverage of the arterial dissection, accompanied by a notable improvement in the degree of stenosis (Fig. 6.2.9 C, D).

Postprocedural CT scans showed no evidence of intracranial hemorrhage.

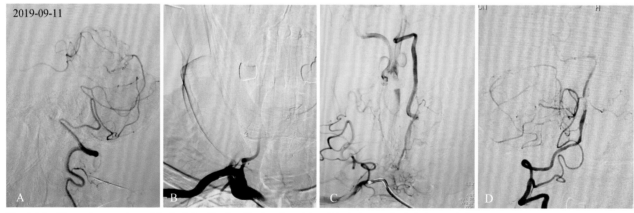

Fig. 6.2.7 The angiogram showed limited visualization distal to the origin of the left posterior inferior cerebellar artery (PICA), and the basilar artery was not visualized. Furthermore, the superior cerebellar artery was visualized through collateral blood supply from the pial arteries originating from the PICA (**A**). The right vertebral artery was dominant, with tortuous V1 and V2 segments. The right PICA originated from the extracranial segment of the right vertebral artery. The middle-to-lower segment of the basilar artery was occluded, while the distal segment beyond the occlusion was visualized due to the compensatory blood flow from the branches of the right PICA and the AICA (**B–D**)

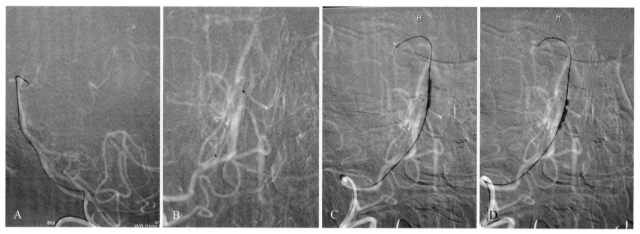

图 6.2.8 血管内介入治疗过程如下：**A** 和 **B**. 微导丝通过闭塞段，微导管始终不能越过闭塞段，撤出微导管；**C** 和 **D**. Gateway 球囊两次扩张闭塞段

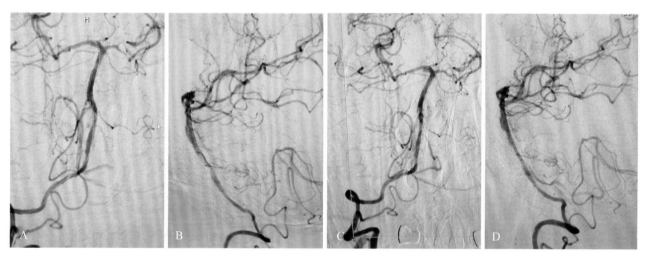

图 6.2.9 **A** 和 **B**. 球囊扩张后造影显示狭窄改善，但闭塞远端形成夹层，尤以侧位明显；**C** 和 **D**. 置入支架后狭窄进一步改善，夹层稳定

（五）讨论

本例基底动脉闭塞，干预治疗过程中出现医源性夹层，考虑与微导丝通过病变时损伤血管或与球囊扩张相关。结合闭塞段及闭塞远端夹层长度，个体化选择了长度 28 mm 的无头型 Enterprise 支架。术中微导丝与微导管同轴，但微导管不能越过病变，遂保留微导丝后送入 1.5 mm 小球囊，因其头端硬度大，较微导管更容易穿越闭塞病变，但相关血管损伤的风险也会相应增高。

（连瑜 王坤 张义森

孙立倩 马宁）

6.2 手术操作视频
（病例 **37**）

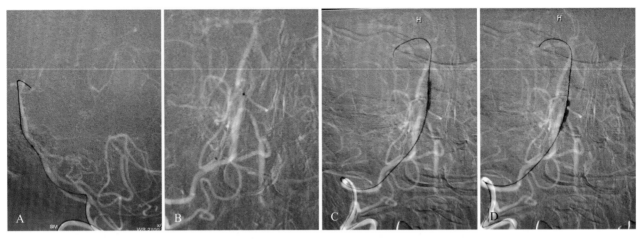

Fig. 6.2.8 The Synchro microwire successfully traversed the occluded segment. The Echelon microcatheter failed to traverse the occlusion and was withdrawn (**A**, **B**). The Gateway balloon was utilized to pre-dilate the lesion twice (**C**, **D**)

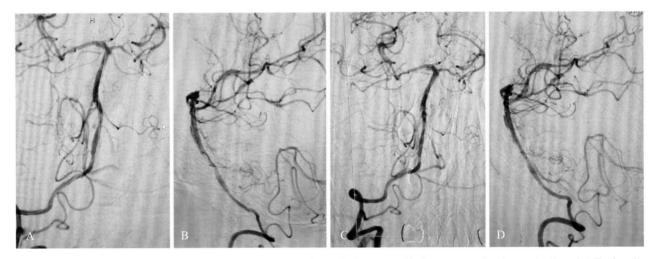

Fig. 6.2.9 The angiogram revealed an improvement in the extent of stenosis, however, with the presence of an iatrogenic dissection distal to the occlusion, which displayed notable prominence, particularly in the lateral view (**A**, **B**). A post-stent implantation angiogram demonstrated the successful coverage of the arterial dissection, accompanied by a notable improvement in the degree of stenosis (**C**, **D**)

5. Comments

In this particular case, a patient was diagnosed with occlusion of the basilar artery. The occurrence of iatrogenic dissection during the procedure can be attributed to vascular injury caused by the microwire's navigation through the lesion or the balloon dilation. Taking into account the length of the occluded segment and the presence of the arterial dissection distal to the occlusion, a specifically selected 28 mm Enterprise stent was employed to provide coverage for the affected area. During the procedure, the microwire and microcatheter were coaxially aligned, although the microcatheter was unable to pass through the lesion. Therefore, the microwire was retained and a 1.5 mm small balloon was introduced instead. The increased rigidity at the tip of the balloon facilitated easier traversal through the occluded lesion compared to the microcatheter, albeit raising the corresponding risk of vascular injury.

(Translated by Rongrong Cui, Revised by Zhikai Hou)

6.2 Video of endovascular therapy (Case 37)

病例 38　左大脑中动脉 M1 段闭塞血管内治疗术中发生血管夹层

（一）临床病史及影像分析

患者，男性，主因"右侧肢体活动不利 2 月余"入院。

既往史：饮酒 30 年，吸烟 10 年，高血压及冠心病病史 1 年。

查体：伸舌右偏，右下肢肌力 4 级。

头部 MRI：左侧基底节区梗死灶（图 6.2.10 A 和 B）。

头部 MRA：左大脑中动脉 M1 段闭塞（图 6.2.10 C 和 D）。

DSA：右大脑前动脉 A1 段发育不良，右胚胎型大脑后动脉（图 6.2.11 A 和 B），左大脑中动脉 M1 段闭塞，同侧大脑前动脉通过软脑膜动脉向左大脑中动脉供血区域代偿供血（图 6.2.11 C 和 D），左大脑后动脉也通过软脑膜动脉向左大脑中动脉供血区域代偿（图 6.2.12）。

高分辨率 MRI：左大脑中动脉管腔消失，全程高信号（图 6.2.13）。

病后一直接受双联抗血小板（阿司匹林 100 mg 1 次 / 日，氯吡格雷 75 mg 1 次 / 日）和他汀类药物（阿托伐他汀 20 mg 1 次 / 日）调脂治疗。

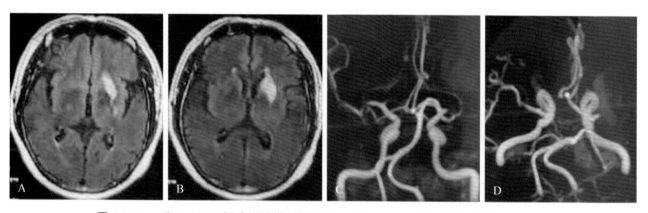

图 6.2.10　**A** 和 **B**. MRI 示左侧基底节区梗死灶；**C** 和 **D**. MRA 示左大脑中动脉 M1 段闭塞

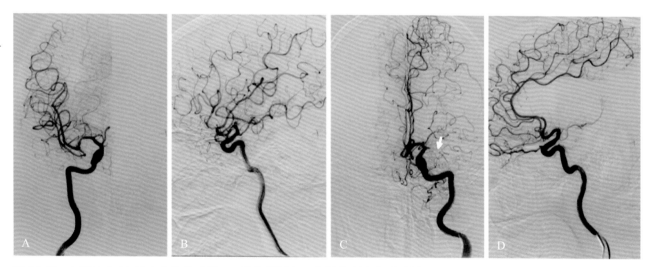

图 6.2.11　**A** 和 **B**. DSA 示右大脑前动脉 A1 段发育不良，右胚胎型大脑后动脉；**C** 和 **D**. DSA 示左大脑中动脉 M1 段闭塞（箭头），同侧大脑前动脉通过软脑膜动脉向左大脑中动脉供血区域代偿供血

Case 38   Arterial dissection during endovascular treatment of a left middle cerebral artery occlusion

1. Clinical presentation and radiological studies

A male patient was admitted to the hospital due to right-sided limb paralysis for over two months.

The patient had a three-decade alcohol consumption record, a decade of smoking cigarettes, as well as a one-year history of both hypertension and coronary heart disease.

The physical examination revealed a rightward deviation during tongue extension, as well as grade 4 muscle strength in the right lower limb.

The MRI results revealed acute infarctions in the left basal ganglia (Fig. 6.2.10 A, B).

The MRA results indicated the occlusion of the M1 segment of the left middle cerebral artery (Fig. 6.2.10 C, D).

The DSA indicated a hypoplastic A1 segment of the right anterior cerebral artery, and a posterior cerebral artery of fetal type on the right side (Fig. 6.2.11 A, B). The M1 segment of the left middle cerebral artery was occluded. The territory of the left middle cerebral artery was compensated through the pial arteries originating from both the ipsilateral anterior cerebral artery (Fig. 6.2.11 C, D) and the ipsilateral posterior cerebral artery (Fig. 6.2.12).

The high-resolution MRI revealed the presence of high signal intensity throughout the entire lumen of the left middle cerebral artery (Fig. 6.2.13).

Following the onset of symptoms, the patient has been prescribed a dual-antiplatelet regimen consisting of a daily administration of 100 mg of Aspirin and 75 mg of Clopidogrel, in addition to statin therapy involving a daily dosage of 20 mg of Atorvastatin.

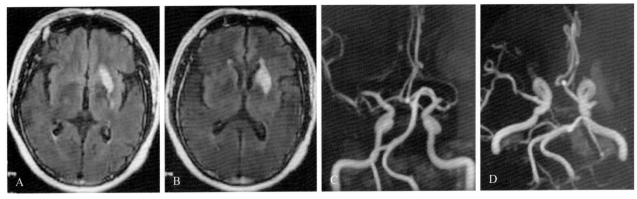

Fig. 6.2.10   MRI showed acute infarction in the left basal ganglia (**A, B**). MRA showed occlusion of the M1 segment of the left middle cerebral artery (**C, D**)

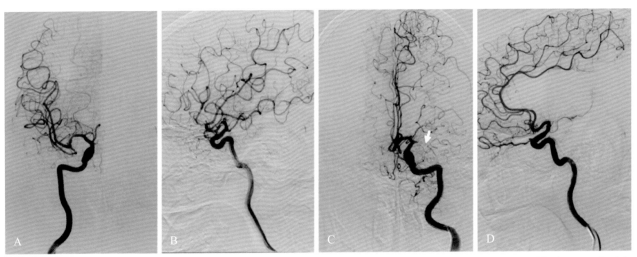

Fig. 6.2.11   The DSA indicated a hypoplastic A1 segment of the right anterior cerebral artery, and a posterior cerebral artery of fetal type on the right side (**A, B**). The M1 segment of the left middle cerebral artery was occluded. The territory of the left middle cerebral artery was compensated through the pial arteries originating from the ipsilateral anterior cerebral artery (**C, D**)

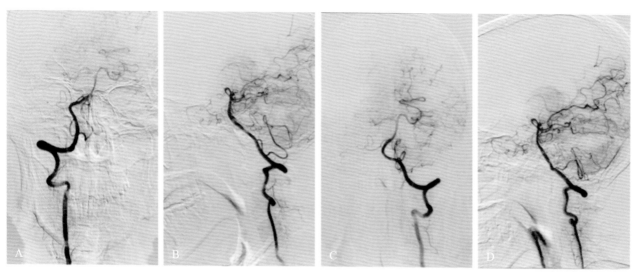

图 6.2.12　DSA 示左大脑后动脉通过软脑膜动脉向左大脑中动脉供血区域代偿（ **A ～ D** ）

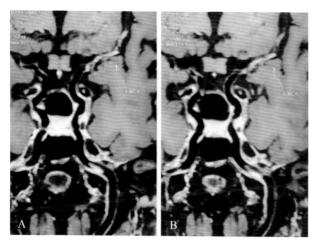

图 6.2.13　高分辨率 MRI 示左大脑中动脉管腔消失，全程高信号（ **A 和 B** ）

（二）诊断

症状性左大脑中动脉 M1 段闭塞。

（三）术前讨论

结合患者病史及相关影像学检查，考虑左大脑中动脉 M1 段为本次发病的责任血管，拟行血管内介入治疗。相关风险包括开通治疗失败、医源性夹层、动脉破裂、穿支损伤、急性血栓形成、术后高灌注等。

（四）治疗过程及随访

全麻下右股动脉穿刺入路，置入 6F 鞘，将 6F 导引导管送至左颈内动脉 C2 段，血管造影显示左大脑中动脉 M1 段闭塞（图 6.2.14 A）。

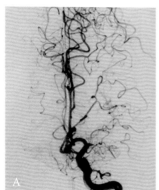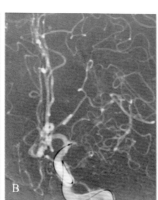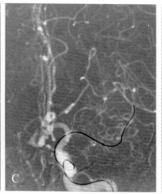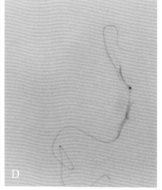

图 6.2.14　**A**. 术前造影；**B**. 微导丝携微导管尝试通过闭塞段；**C**. 微导丝通过闭塞段至 M2 段；**D**. 经微导管造影证实微导管位于真腔

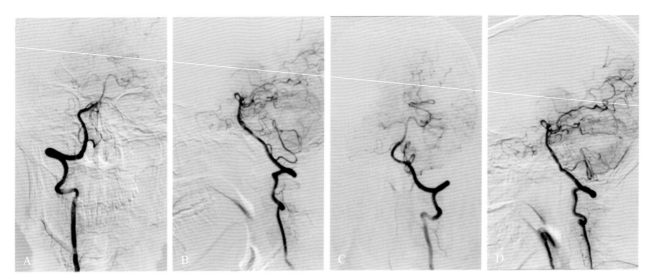

Fig. 6.2.12   The territory of the left middle cerebral artery was compensated through the pial arteries originating from the ipsilateral posterior cerebral artery (**A–D**)

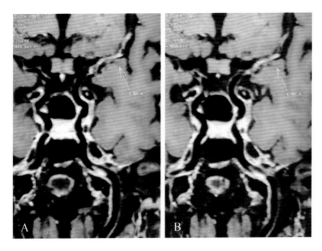

Fig. 6.2.13   HRMRI revealed the presence of high signal intensity throughout the entire lumen of the left middle cerebral artery (**A, B**)

2. Diagnosis

Symptomatic occlusion in the M1 segment of the left middle cerebral artery.

3. Treatment schedule

Considering the patient's clinical presentation and imaging results, the M1 segment of the left middle cerebral artery was identified as the responsible vessel in the occurrence of the ischemic stroke. Endovascular intervention was proposed as a recommended course of action. Potential procedural risks included recanalization failure, iatrogenic dissection, arterial rupture, perforating artery occlusion, acute in-stent thrombosis, and hyperperfusion syndrome.

4. Treatment and follow-up

Under general anesthesia, a 6F guiding catheter was positioned at the C2 segment of the left internal carotid artery. The angiogram indicated the occlusion of the M1 segment of the left middle cerebral artery (Fig. 6.2.14 A).

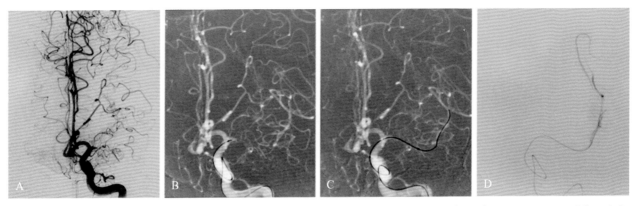

Fig. 6.2.14   (**A**) The angiogram before the procedure. (**B, C**) The Synchro microwire and an Echelon-10 microcatheter were maneuvered through the occlusive region, reaching the M2 segment of the left middle cerebral artery. (**D**) The angiogram confirmed that the microcatheter was in the true lumen

Synchro 微导丝（0.014 in，300 cm）携 Echelon-10 微导管尝试通过闭塞段（图 6.2.14 B）至 M2 段（图 6.2.14 C），撤出微导丝，经微导管手推造影证实位于真腔（图 6.2.14 D）。沿微导管送入微导丝后撤出微导管，沿微导丝送入 Maverick 球囊（1.5 mm×15 mm），由远及近扩张 3 次（图 6.2.15 A ～ C），撤出球囊，造影显示残留狭窄率约 50%，M1 段远端形成夹层（图 6.2.15 D），动脉内给予 0.15 mg 替罗非班。观察 10 min 后再次造影，血流通畅，无血栓形成，结束手术。

28 天后复查 DSA：左大脑中动脉 M1 段管腔轻度狭窄，远端夹层修复，前向血流 3 级（图 6.2.16）。其与术前、术后即刻的造影对比见图 6.2.16。

（五）讨论

本例处理左大脑中动脉闭塞，闭塞段较长，术中微导丝经尝试顺利通过闭塞段，球囊扩张有夹层形成，但考虑夹层位于 M1-M2 段交界区，放置自膨式支架存在进一步血管损伤的风险，且动脉内给予替罗非班后，经观察夹层未有进展且未影响血流，遂未予以支架置入。28 天后复查显示夹层修复，管腔残留轻度狭窄。

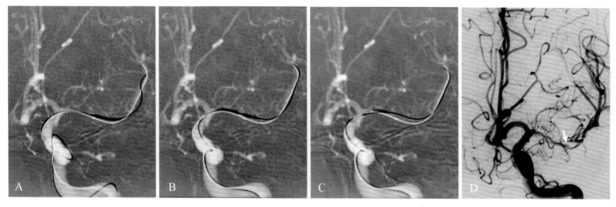

图 6.2.15　**A ～ C**. Maverick 球囊由远及近扩张 3 次；**D**. 球囊扩张后造影显示 M1 段远端夹层形成（箭头）

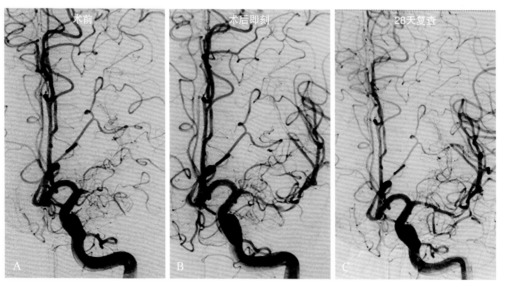

图 6.2.16　**A**. 术前造影；**B**. 术后即刻造影；**C**. 术后 28 天复查造影

（孙勇　刘亚辉　张增权　马宁）

The Synchro microwire (0.014 in, 300 cm) and an Echelon-10 microcatheter were maneuvered through the occlusive region, reaching the M2 segment of the left middle cerebral artery (Fig. 6.2.14 B, C). Microcatheter angiography validated the accurate positioning of the microcatheter within the true lumen (Fig. 6.2.14 D). The occlusive segment underwent three sequential dilations utilizing a Maverick balloon (1.5 mm × 15 mm), progressing from the distal to the proximal direction (Fig. 6.2.15 A–C). The angiogram exhibited a 50% residual stenosis, along with an arterial dissection occurring at the distal segment of the M1 segment (Fig. 6.2.15 D). A dosage of 0.15 mg of tirofiban was administered through the guiding catheter. Following a 10-minute monitoring interval, the angiogram exhibited no signs of acute thrombus formation.

The subsequent angiogram performed after 28 days showed mild stenosis in the M1 segment of the left middle cerebral artery with a grade 3 of antegrade blood flow. The arterial dissection at the distal segment of the left middle cerebral artery was healed (Fig. 6.12.16). The 28-day follow-up angiogram images were compared with the pre-procedure and immediate post-procedure angiograms, as illustrated in Fig. 6.2.16.

5. Comments

The presented case involved a patient presenting with occlusion of the left middle cerebral artery. Despite the considerable length of the occlusion segment, the microwire successfully navigated through the occlusion after several attempts. However, a dissection in the arterial wall occurred at the junction of the M1-M2 segments during balloon dilatation, potentially posing a risk of further vascular injury during the placement of a selfexpanding stent. Following the intraarterial administration of tirofiban, the arterial dissection remained stable without compromising blood flow. A subsequent angiogram conducted 28 days later revealed healing of the dissection and a mild residual stenosis of the arterial lumen.

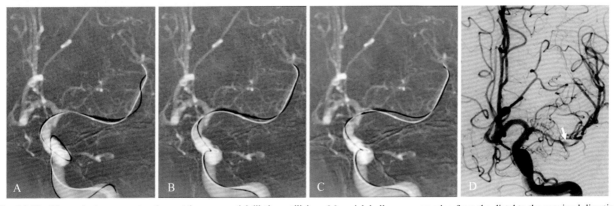

Fig. 6.2.15   The occlusive segment underwent three sequential dilations utilizing a Maverick balloon, progressing from the distal to the proximal direction (**A**–**C**). The angiogram exhibited a 50% residual stenosis, along with an arterial dissection occurring at the distal segment of the M1 segment (arrow) (**D**)

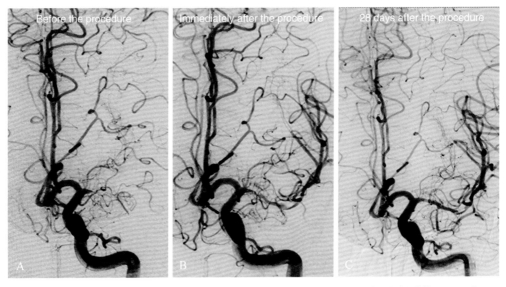

Fig. 6.2.16   (**A**) The pre-procedure angiogram (**B**) The post-procedure angiogram. (**C**) The 28-day follow-up angiogram

(Translated by Rongrong Cui, Revised by Zhikai Hou)

第三节　术中血栓形成

病例 39　右大脑中动脉 M1 段闭塞血管内治疗术中血栓形成

（一）临床病史及影像分析

患者，女性，62 岁，主因"言语不利及左侧肢体无力 2 月余"入院。

既往史：高血压病史。

查体：轻度构音障碍，左侧中枢性面瘫，左侧肢体肌力 4 级。

头部 MRI：右侧脑室旁、半卵圆中心区急性梗死灶（图 6.3.1 A～C）。

头部 MRA：右大脑中动脉未见显影（图 6.3.1 D）。

DSA：右大脑中动脉闭塞，同侧大脑前动脉及胚胎型大脑后动脉经软脑膜动脉向右大脑中动脉代偿（图 6.3.2 A），左颈内动脉系统未见异常（图 6.3.2 B），左大脑后动脉管壁不光滑（图 6.3.2 C 和 D）。

头部 CTA 示右大脑中动脉 M1 段闭塞（图 6.3.3 A），

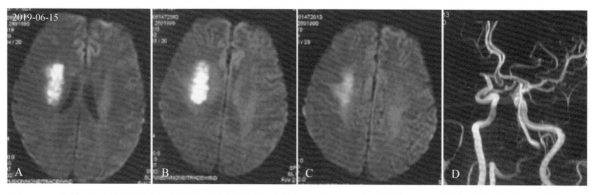

图 6.3.1　头部 MRI 示右侧脑室旁、半卵圆中心区急性梗死灶（**A～C**）。头部 MRA 示右大脑中动脉未见显影（**D**）

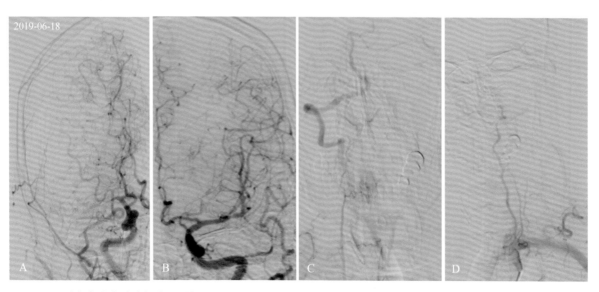

图 6.3.2　DSA 示右大脑中动脉闭塞，同侧大脑前动脉及胚胎型大脑后动脉经软脑膜动脉向右大脑中动脉代偿（**A**），左颈内动脉系统未见异常（**B**），左大脑后动脉管壁不光滑（**C 和 D**）

Section 3   Periprocedural Thrombosis

Case 39   Thrombus formation during endovascular treatment of a right middle cerebral artery occlusion

1. Clinical presentation and radiological studies

A 62-year-old female patient was admitted to the hospital due to dysarthria and left-sided weakness for more than two months.

She had a medical history of hypertension.

The physical examination showed dysarthria, left-sided central facial paralysis, and grade 4 muscle strength in the left limbs.

The MRI results revealed acute infarctions in the right periventricular area and centrum semiovale regions (Fig. 6.3.1 A–C).

The MRA results showed occlusion of the right middle cerebral artery (Fig. 6.3.1 D).

The digital subtraction angiography (DSA) revealed occlusion of the right middle cerebral artery, which was compensated by blood flow from the ipsilateral anterior cerebral artery and fetal-type posterior cerebral artery through the leptomeningeal arteries (Fig. 6.3.2 A). The left internal carotid artery displayed no abnormalities (Fig. 6.3.2 B). The left posterior cerebral artery exhibited irregularity in the vascular wall (Fig. 6.3.2 C, D).

The CT angiography (CTA) revealed the occlusion in the M1

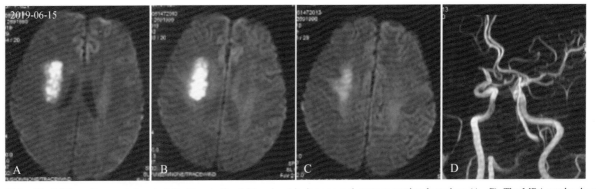

Fig. 6.3.1   The MRI results revealed acute infarctions in the right periventricular area and centrum semiovale regions (A–C). The MRA results showed occlusion of the right middle cerebral artery (D)

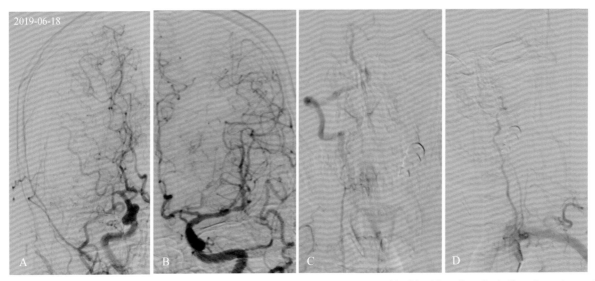

Fig. 6.3.2   DSA revealed occlusion of the right middle cerebral artery, which was compensated by blood flow from the ipsilateral anterior cerebral artery and fetal-type posterior cerebral artery through the leptomeningeal arteries (A). The left internal carotid artery displayed no abnormalities (B). The left posterior cerebral artery exhibited irregularity in the vascular wall (C, D)

CT 灌注示右大脑中动脉供血区域低灌注（图 6.3.3 B）。

高分辨率 MRI：右大脑中动脉闭塞，闭塞段内血栓形成，闭塞远端血管通畅，管腔较对侧纤细（图 6.3.4）。

入院后给予双联抗血小板（阿司匹林 100 mg 1 次 / 日＋氯吡格雷 75 mg 1 次 / 日）以及降脂（瑞舒伐汀 10 mg 1 次 / 日）等治疗。

（二）诊断

症状性右大脑中动脉 M1 段闭塞。

（三）术前讨论

患者 2 个月前出现局灶性神经功能缺损症状，影像学检查显示右大脑中动脉分布区脑梗死，右大

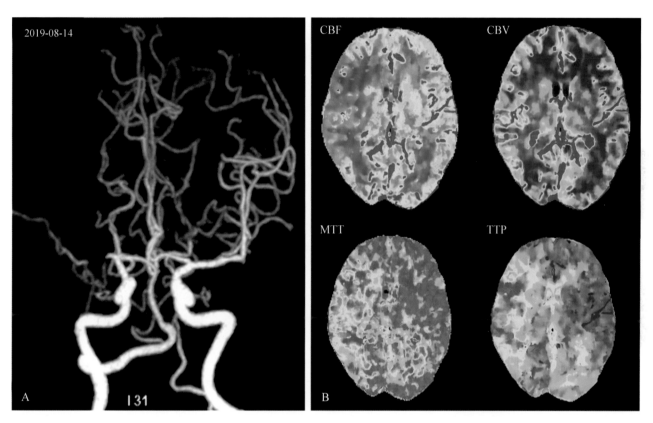

图 6.3.3　CTA 示右大脑中动脉 M1 段闭塞（A），CTP 示右大脑中动脉供血区域低灌注（B）

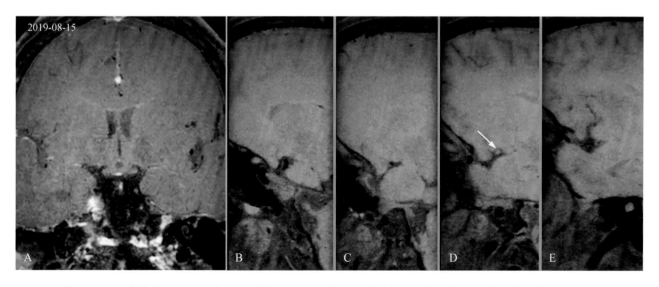

图 6.3.4　高分辨率 MRI 示右大脑中动脉闭塞，闭塞段内血栓形成，闭塞远端血管通畅，管腔较对侧纤细

segment of the right middle cerebral artery (Fig. 6.3.3 A). The CT perfusion indicated hypoperfusion in the territory supplied by the occluded right middle cerebral artery. (Fig. 6.3.3 B).

The high-resolution MRI unveiled the occlusion of the right middle cerebral artery, accompanied by the thrombus formation within the occluded segment. However, the distal segment beyond the occluded segment remained patent. (Fig. 6.3.4).

Upon admission, the patient was initiated on a dual-antiplatelet regimen comprising a daily dose of 100 mg of aspirin and a daily dose of 75 mg of Clopidogrel, in addition to statin therapy with a daily dose of 10 mg of Rosuvastatin.

2. Diagnosis

Symptomatic occlusion in the M1 segment of the right middle cerebral artery.

3. Treatment schedule

Two months prior, the patient exhibited focal neurological deficits. The imaging results indicated acute infarction within the territory of the right middle cerebral artery, which was attributed to the occlusion of the afore-mentioned artery. CT perfusion further confirmed a hypoperfused state within the

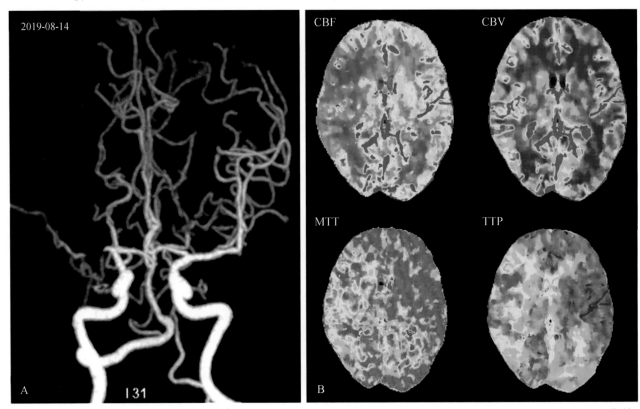

Fig. 6.3.3 The CTA revealed the occlusion in the M1 segment of the right middle cerebral artery (**A**). CTP showed hypoperfusion in the territory supplied by the occluded right middle cerebral artery (**B**)

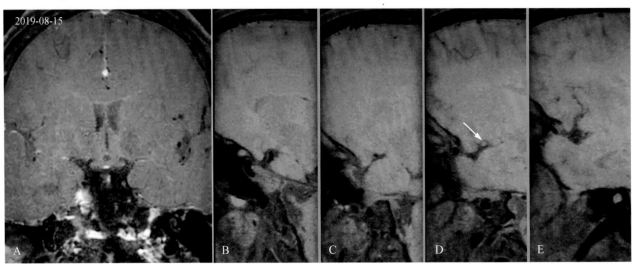

Fig. 6.3.4 HRMRI the occlusion of the right middle cerebral artery, accompanied by the thrombus formation within the occluded segment. However, the distal segment beyond the occluded segment remained patent

脑中动脉闭塞，且 CTP 显示责任动脉供血区域存在低灌注，有血管内介入治疗指征。拟微导管结合微导丝越过病变，稍小球囊预扩张，其后放置自膨式支架。相关风险包括开通失败、医源性夹层、穿支卒中、急性或亚急性血栓形成、高灌注综合征等。

（四）治疗过程

全麻下右股动脉入路，将 6F 导引导管头端置于右颈内动脉 C1 段远端。造影显示右大脑中动脉 M1 段闭塞（图 6.3.5 A 和 B）。

路径图下将 Pilot 50 微导丝（0.014 in，150 cm）结合 Echelon-10 微导管越过闭塞段后，跟进微导管较为困难，遂更换为 Synchro 微导丝（0.014 in，300 cm）并输送至 M2 段以增强支撑力（图 6.3.5 C）。微导管到位后行微导管造影证实微导管位于真腔内（图 6.3.5 D）。经微导丝送入 Gateway 球囊（1.5 mm×15 mm）至闭塞段，准确定位后球囊逐渐加压至 6 atm，可见球囊完全张开（图 6.3.6 A），

抽瘪并后撤球囊，造影示闭塞段较前明显改善，残余狭窄率约为 60%（图 6.3.6 B）。送入 XT-27 微导管，经其送入 Neuroform EZ 支架（2.5 mm×15 mm）并释放，复查造影提示支架贴壁可，残余狭窄率约为 40%。支架放置后观察期间，支架内见充盈缺损，考虑血栓形成（图 6.3.6 C）。将 Synchro 微导丝携 Echelon-10 微导管送至支架近端，给予替罗非班微导管内推注及同时静脉泵入。10 min 后观察支架内充盈缺损消失，前向血流正常，遂结束治疗（图 6.3.6 D）。

术后复查 CTA ＋ CTP：右大脑中动脉管腔通畅，相关区域血流灌注较术前明显改善（图 6.3.7）。

患者术后无明显神经功能缺损症状。

（五）讨论

本例右大脑中动脉 M1 段闭塞，影像学检查结果提示闭塞主要累及大脑中动脉 M1 段中远段，

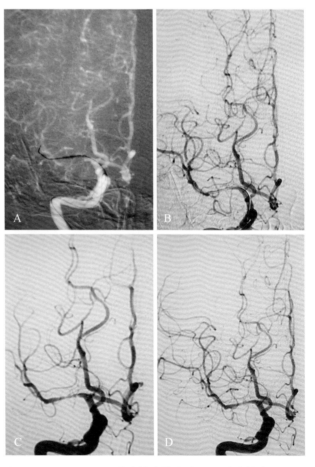

图 6.3.6 **A**. Gateway 球囊扩张狭窄段；**B**. 球囊扩张后造影示残余狭窄率约为 60%；**C**. 支架置入后造影示支架内充盈缺损，考虑血栓形成；**D**. 给予替罗非班后充盈缺损消失，前向血流正常

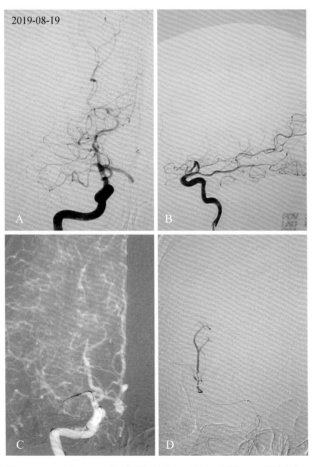

图 6.3.5 **A** 和 **B**. 术前造影示右大脑中动脉 M1 段闭塞；**C**. Synchro 微导丝被输送至 M2 段；**D**. 微导管造影证实微导管位于真腔内

corresponding territory. Endovascular intervention was deemed necessary for this patient. A microcatheter, in conjunction with a microwire, was employed to navigate through the occlusive lesion. Subsequently, the lesion was predilated utilizing a small-sized balloon, followed by the placement of a self-expanding stent. Potential risks included unsuccessful recanalization, iatrogenic dissection, occlusion of perforating arteries, acute/subacute in-stent thrombosis, and hyperperfusion syndrome.

4. Treatment

Under general anesthesia, a 6F guiding catheter was advanced at the distal C1 segment of the right internal carotid artery. The angiogram confirmed the occlusion in the M1 segment of the right middle cerebral artery (Fig. 6.3.5 A, B).

Under the roadmap, the Echelon-10 microcatheter, in conjunction with the Pilot 50 microwire (0.014 in, 150 cm), was navigated through the occlusion segment. However, the advancement of the microcatheter presented challenges. Therefore, the Pilot 50 microwire was substituted with the Synchro microwire (0.014 in, 300 cm) and was advanced to the M2 segment to provide enhanced support force (Fig.6.3.5 6.3.5 D). A Gateway balloon (1.5 mm×15 mm) was inflated at a pressure of 6 atm (Fig. 6.3.6 A). An angiogram conducted after balloon dilation revealed a residual stenosis of approximately

60%. (Fig. 6.3.6 B). Subsequently, a 2.5 mm×15 mm Neuroform EZ self-expanding stent was released using the XT-27 microcatheter to cover the lesion. The angiogram showed excellent stent wall apposition, with a residual stenosis of 40%. Throughout the observation period, a filling defect within the stent became evident, implying the thrombus formation within the stent. (Fig. 6.3.6 C). The Echelon-10 microcatheter was positioned close to the stent. Intra-arterial administration of tirofiban was carried out, followed by intravenous administration of tirofiban. After ten minutes, the previously observed filling defect vanished, with an antegrade blood flow grade of 3 (Fig. 6.3.6 D).

Postprocedural CTA revealed the stent in the right middle cerebral artery was patent (Fig. 6.3.7 A). The CTP showed an improvement in the hypoperfusion of the right cerebral hemisphere (Fig. 6.3.7 B).

The patient displayed no evident focal neurological deficit.

5. Comments

This case involved an individual with occlusion of the right middle cerebral artery. Upon evaluation of the imaging findings, the occlusive lesion primarily affected the middleto-distal portion of the M1 segment of the right middle cerebral

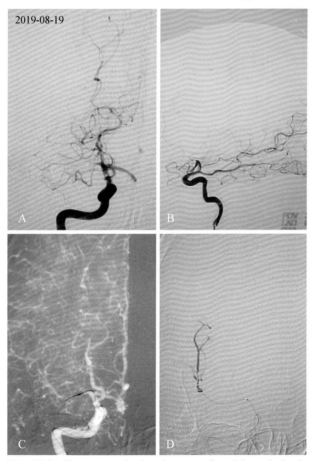

Fig. 6.3.5 The pre-procedural angiogram confirmed the occlusion in the M1 segment of the right middle cerebral artery (**A**, **B**). The Synchro microwire was delivered to the M2 segment (**C**). The transcatheter angiogram confirmed that the microcatheter was in the true lumen (**D**)

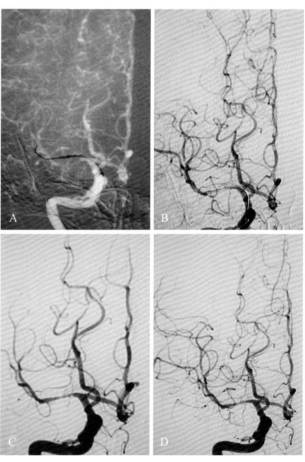

Fig. 6.3.6 A Gateway balloon was utilized to pre-dilated the lesion (**A**). Post-balloon dilation angiogram revealed a residual stenosis of approximately 60% (**B**). A filling defect within the stent became evident, implying the thrombus formation within the stent (**C**). The final angiogram showed the filling defect vanished, with an antegrade blood flow grade of 3 (**D**)

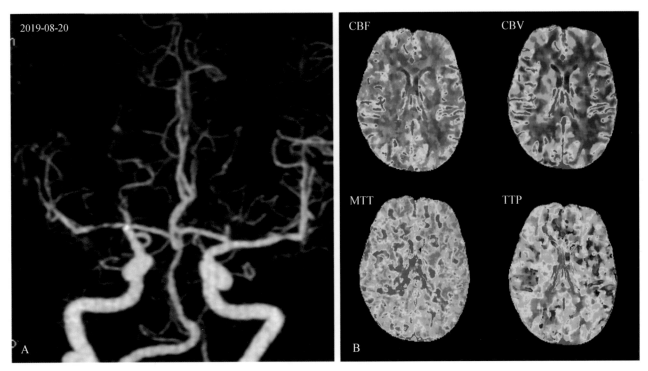

图 6.3.7 术后 CTA 示右大脑中动脉管腔通畅（**A**），CTP 示右大脑中动脉供血区域低灌注较术前明显改善（**B**）

闭塞远端有正常血管床，但管腔直径较为纤细。此外，因右大脑中动脉供血区域低灌注明显，我们选用最小直径球囊扩张以期减少高灌注发生的概率。本例显示少量替罗非班动脉内局部灌注及同期静脉泵入，有助于崩解支架置入后形成的急性血栓。

6.3 手术操作视频
（病例 39）

（杨连琦 王坤 张义森 马宁）

病例 40 左颈内动脉 C7 段闭塞血管内治疗术中血栓形成

（一）临床病史及影像分析

患者，男性，主因"右侧肢体活动不利 4 周"入院。

既往史：饮酒史 40 年，吸烟史 40 年，高血压病史 10 年。

查体：右侧中枢性面瘫，右侧肢体肌力 4 级。

头部 MRI：左侧侧脑室旁及放射冠区新发梗死灶（图 6.3.8 A 和 B）。

头颈部 CTA：左颈内动脉颅内段闭塞（图 6.3.8 C 和 D）。

DSA：右颈动脉系统无明显血管狭窄，前交通动脉未开放（图 6.3.9 A 和 B）。左颈内动脉 C7 段闭塞（图 6.3.9 C 和 D）。后循环系统无明显血管狭窄，左大脑后动脉通过软脑膜支向左侧前循环区域代偿供血（图 6.3.10）。

高分辨率 MRI：左颈内动脉 C7 段及左大脑中动脉 M1 段近端管腔闭塞，M1 段远端可见流空的血管床（图 6.3.11）。

发病后一直接受双联抗血小板（阿司匹林 100 mg 1 次/日、氯吡格雷 75 mg 1 次/日）以及

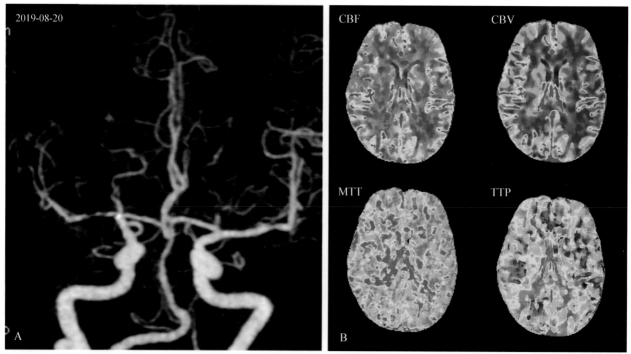

Fig. 6.3.7 Postprocedural CTA showed the stent in the right middle cerebral artery was patent (**A**). The CTP showed an improvement in the hypoperfusion of the right cerebral hemisphere (**B**)

artery. However, the vascular bed beyond the occlusion site remained unobstructed. CT perfusion scans revealed notable hypoperfusion in the area supplied by the right middle cerebral artery. To reduce the risk of hyperperfusion syndrome, we employed a small-size diameter balloon for pre-dilation. Furthermore, the patient experienced acute thrombus formation within the stent during the procedure.

The in-stent thrombus was successfully dissolved following the administration of a small dose of tirofiban via arterial infusion, which was then followed by a sequential intravenous infusion.

(Translated by Rongrong Cui, Revised by Zhikai Hou)

6.3 Video of endovascular therapy (Case 39)

Case 40　Thrombus formation during endovascular treatment of a left internal carotid artery occlusion

1. Clinical presentation and radiological studies

A male patient was admitted to the hospital due to right-sided limb weakness for four weeks.

He possessed a medical history including 40 years of alcohol consumption, 40 years of smoking, and 10 years of hypertension.

Upon physical examination, it was observed that the patient displayed right-sided central facial paralysis, alongside a muscle strength grade of 4 in the right limbs.

The MRI findings revealed the presence of acute infarctions in the periventricular area and corona radiata on the left side (Fig. 6.3.8 A, B).

The CT angiography revealed occlusion in the intracranial segment of the left internal carotid artery (Fig. 6.3.8 C, D).

The DSA findings revealed no significant stenosis in the right carotid artery system. The anterior communicating artery was found to be non-patent (Fig. 6.3.9 A, B). Moreover, there was occlusion observed in the C7 segment of the left internal carotid artery (Fig. 6.3.9 C, D). As for the posterior circulation system, no significant stenosis was identified. The left posterior cerebral artery served as compensation for the left anterior circulation through pial branches (Fig. 6.3.10).

The HRMRI revealed a complete occlusion in both the C7 segment of the left internal carotid artery and the proximal M1 segment of the left middle cerebral artery. Furthermore, a patent vascular bed beyond the distal M1 segment of the left middle cerebral artery was represented as a "flow void" (Fig. 6.3.11).

At the onset of symptoms, the patient had been receiving a

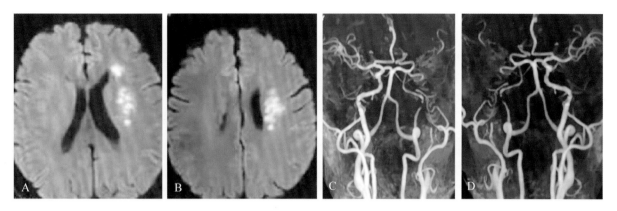

图 6.3.8　**A** 和 **B**. 头颅磁共振 DWI 序列示左侧侧脑室旁及放射冠区新发梗死灶；**C** 和 **D**. 头颈部 CTA 示左颈内动脉颅内段闭塞

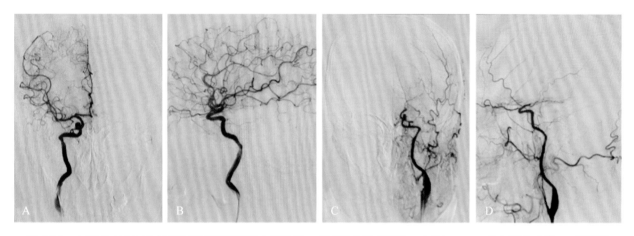

图 6.3.9　**A** 和 **B**. DSA 示右颈动脉系统无明显血管狭窄，前交通动脉未开放；**C** 和 **D**. DSA 示左颈内动脉 C7 段闭塞

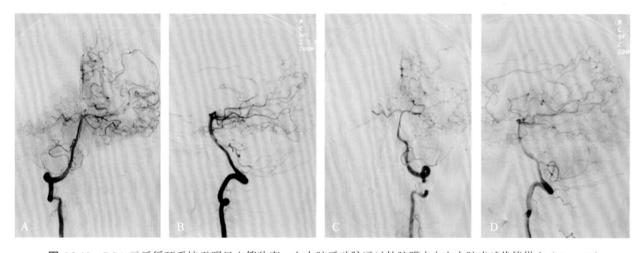

图 6.3.10　DSA 示后循环系统无明显血管狭窄，左大脑后动脉通过软脑膜支向左大脑半球代偿供血（**A ～ D**）

他汀类药物（阿托伐他汀 20 mg 1 次 / 日）调脂等治疗。

（二）诊断

症状性左颈内动脉 C7 段闭塞。

（三）术前讨论

结合患者病史及相关影像学检查，考虑左颈内动脉 C7 段闭塞为本次发病的责任病变，拟行血管内介入治疗。相关风险包括开通不成功、医源性夹

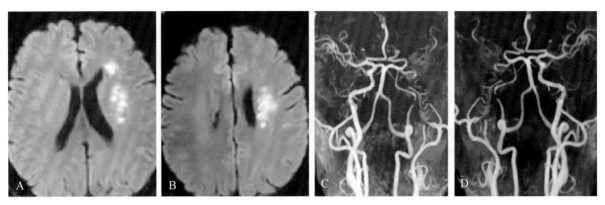

Fig. 6.3.8 The MRI showed acute infarctions in the left periventricular area and corona radiata (**A, B**). The CTA results showed occlusion of the intracranial segment of the left internal carotid artery (**C, D**)

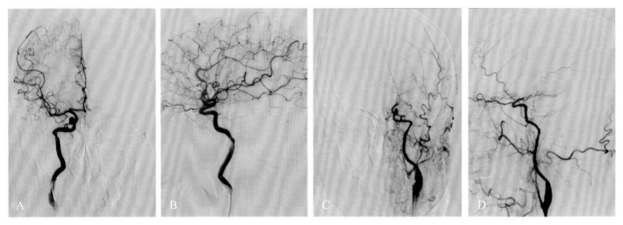

Fig. 6.3.9 The DSA findings revealed no significant stenosis in the right carotid artery system. The anterior communicating artery was found to be non-patent (**A, B**). There was occlusion observed in the C7 segment of the left internal carotid artery (**C, D**)

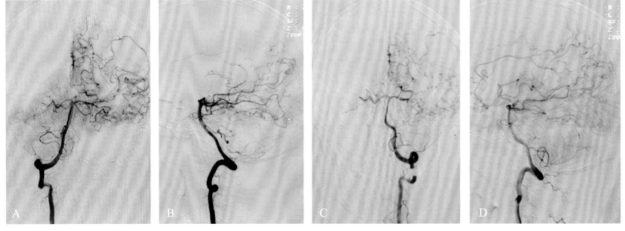

Fig. 6.3.10 DSA showed no significant stenosis identified in the posterior system. The left posterior cerebral artery served as compensation for the left anterior circulation through pial branches (**A–D**)

combination therapy consisting of dual antiplatelet agents (daily intake of 100 mg Aspirin and 75 mg Clopidogrel) along with statin therapy (daily intake of 20 mg Atorvastatin).

2. Diagnosis

Symptomatic occlusion in the C7 segment of the left internal carotid artery.

3. Treatment schedule

Based on the patient's medical history and relevant imaging examinations, the left internal carotid artery occlusion in the C7 segment was considered to be the responsible lesion for the current onset. Endovascular intervention was proposed as a treatment option. Relevant risks associated with this

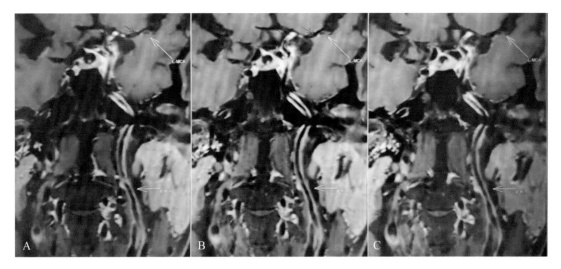

图 6.3.11　高分辨率 MRI 示左颈内动脉 C7 段及左大脑中动脉 M1 段近端管腔闭塞，M1 段远端可见流空的血管床（箭头）（**A ~ C**）

层、动脉破裂、急性血栓形成等。

（四）治疗过程

全麻下右股动脉穿刺入路，置入 6F 鞘，将 6F 导引导管送至左颈内动脉 C2 段，造影显示左颈内动脉 C7 段闭塞，并可见静脉早显（图 6.3.12 A）。

Synchro 微导丝（0.014 in，300 cm）在 Echelon-10 微导管辅助下到达闭塞处，多次尝试后顺利通过闭塞段（图 6.3.12 B），沿 Synchro 微导丝将 Echelon-10 微导管送至左大脑中动脉 M2 段，撤出微导丝，经微导管手推造影显示微导管位于真腔（图 6.3.12 C），通过交换技术撤出微导管，再次送入 Synchro 微导丝。沿微导丝送入 Maverick 球囊（1.5 mm×15 mm）准确到达闭塞处，加压充盈球囊扩张血管，回撤球囊，造影显示 M1 段近端仍残留重度狭窄（图 6.3.12 D）。再次送入球囊扩张（图 6.3.13 A），路径图显示形态满意（图 6.3.13 B），撤出球囊，沿微导丝送入 XT-27 微导管，微导管到位后送入 Neuroform EZ 支架（2.5 mm×15 mm），准确释放（图 6.3.13 C），即刻造影提示支架完全覆盖病变，支架内血流通畅，残余狭窄率约 20%，远端血管显影良好（图 6.3.13 D）。

观察 10 min 后造影，颈内动脉末端显影较前浅淡，支架内局部可见充盈缺损（图 6.3.14 A），考虑血栓形成，动脉内给予替罗非班 4 ml。20 min 后再次造影，支架近端仍有少量充盈缺损（图 6.3.14 B），路径图下送入微导丝，在支架内按摩（图 6.3.14 C），

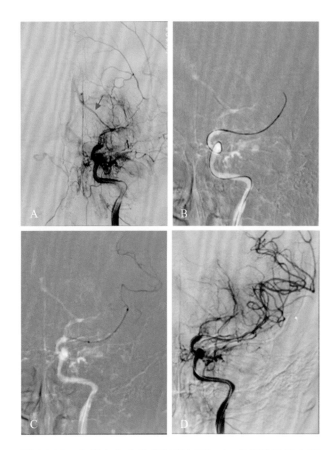

图 6.3.12　血管内介入治疗过程如下：**A**. 术前造影示左颈内动脉 C7 段闭塞，并可见静脉早显（箭头示）；**B**. Synchro 微导丝通过闭塞段到达 M2 段；**C**. 造影证实微导管位于真腔；**D**. 第一次球囊扩张并造影

造影显示局部充盈缺损消失，血流通畅，病变有一定程度的弹性回缩，残余狭窄率约 35%（图 6.3.14 D）。观察 10 min 后无改变，结束治疗。

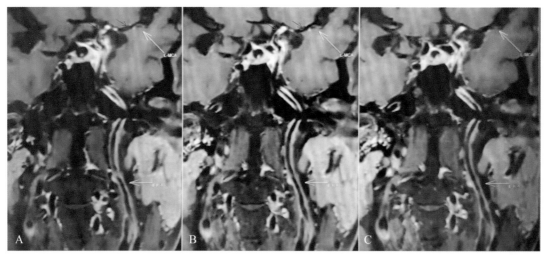

Fig. 6.3.11   HRMRI revealed a complete occlusion in both the C7 segment of the left internal carotid artery and the proximal M1 segment of the left middle cerebral artery. Furthermore, a patent vascular bed beyond the distal M1 segment of the left middle cerebral artery was represented as a "flow void" (arrow)

procedure include unsuccessful recanalization, iatrogenic dissection, arterial rupture, and acute thrombus formation.

4. Treatment

Under general anesthesia, a 6F guiding catheter was advanced to the C2 segment of the left internal carotid artery. The angiogram verified the presence of occlusion in the C7 segment of the left internal carotid artery. Additionally, the veins were observed to exhibit early visualization during the procedure (Fig. 6.3.12 A).

After multiple attempts, a Synchro microwire (0.014 inches, 300 cm), with the assistance of the Echelon-10 microcatheter, was successfully maneuvered through the occlusion segment, reaching the M2 segment of the left middle cerebral artery (Fig. 6.3.12 B). The Echelon-10 microcatheter was positioned in the M2 segment along the microwire. The microcatheter angiogram confirmed the accurate placement of the microcatheter within the true lumen (Fig. 6.3.12 C). A Maverick balloon (1.5 mm × 15 mm) was delivered to pre-dilate the occlusion. However, The following angiogram showed severe residual stenosis in the proximal M1 segment (Fig. 6.3.12 D). Subsequently, a repeated balloon dilation was carried out (Fig. 6.3.13 A). The roadmap showed an efficient dilation outcome (Fig. 6.3.13 B). Following that, a Neuroform EZ self-expanding stent (2.5 mm × 15 mm) was accurately deployed using the XT-27 microcatheter to fully cover the lesion (Fig. 6.3.13 C). The post-stent implantation angiogram displayed an approximate residual stenosis of 20% (Fig. 6.3.13 D).

After a 10-minute observation period, an angiogram revealed the presence of a filling defect within the stent, suggesting the thrombus formation (Fig. 6.3.14 A). An intra-arterial injection of tirofiban at a dosage of 4 ml was administered. However, even after 20 minutes, a filling defect persisted in the proximal site of the stent (Fig. 6.3.14 B). Under the roadmap, the microcatheter was maneuvered

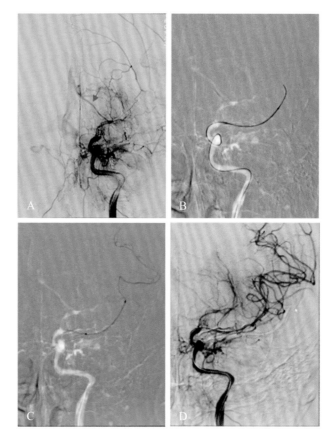

Fig. 6.3.12   (**A**) Preprocedural angiogram showed the occlusion of the C7 segment of the left internal carotid artery (arrow). (**B**) A Synchro microwire maneuvered through the occlusion segment to the M2 segment. (**C**) The angiogram confirmed that the microcatheter was in the true lumen. (**D**) The angiogram after the first balloon dilation

towards the stent for gentle massage (Fig. 6.3.14 C). The angiogram showed the the disappearance of filling defect, leaving behind a residual stenosis of approximately 35% (Fig. 6.3.14 D). Following a 10-minute interval, a conclusive angiogram confirmed the successful patency of the stent in the left C7, devoid of any indications of thrombus formation.

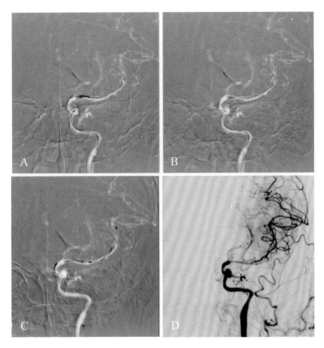

图 6.3.13　**A**.再次球囊扩张；**B**.球囊扩张后造影；**C**.Neuroform EZ 支架释放；**D**.支架释放后造影

（五）讨论

本例术中出现支架内血栓，动脉内给予替罗非班结合支架内微导丝按摩是有效的处理办法。本例支架置入的即刻效果良好，但是短期内即有轻度的弹性回缩，可能与选用的支架有关。

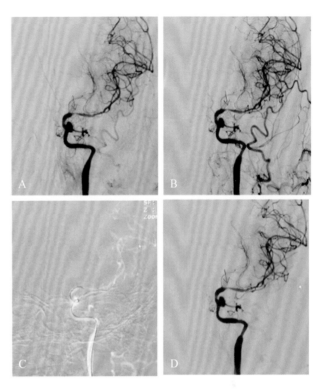

图 6.3.14　**A**.支架内局部可见充盈缺损（箭头）；**B**.动脉内给予替罗非班后支架近端仍有少量充盈缺损（箭头）；**C**.送入微导丝，在支架内按摩；**D**.术后造影示局部充盈缺损消失，病变有一定程度的弹性回缩，残余狭窄率约 35%（箭头）

（刘亚辉　孙勇　李鑫　张增权）

病例 41　左椎基底动脉交界区重度狭窄血管内治疗术中血栓形成

（一）临床病史及影像分析

患者，女性，59 岁，主因"发作性眩晕伴右侧肢体无力 1 年余"入院。

8 个月前行 DSA 检查示左椎基底动脉交界区重度狭窄，给予内科药物治疗后症状缓解。6 个月前患者再次出现发作性眩晕，严重时伴右侧肢体麻木无力，低血压时可诱发上述症状。

既往史：高血压和 2 型糖尿病病史。

查体：神经系统查体阴性。

入院后复查 DSA：左椎动脉优势，左椎基底动脉交界区重度狭窄（图 6.3.15 A 和 B）；右椎动脉

V3 ～ V4 段闭塞（图 6.3.15 C）。前循环向后循环未见明显代偿（图 6.3.16）。

头部 MRI：动脉自旋标记（ASL）序列提示右枕叶及右侧小脑半球低灌注（图 6.3.17）。

CYP2C19 基因型：中间代谢型。

入院后给予双联抗血小板（阿司匹林 100 mg 1 次 / 日＋替格瑞洛 90 mg 2 次 / 日）、降脂（阿托伐他汀 20 mg 1 次 / 日）等治疗。

（二）诊断

左椎基底动脉交界区症状性重度狭窄。

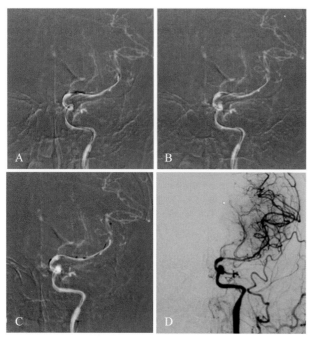

Fig. 6.3.13   (**A**) The second balloon dilatation. (**B**) The angiogram after the second balloon dilatation. (**C**) The Neuroform EZ stent was used to cover the lesion. (**D**) The angiogram after stent implantation

5. Comments

Upon the implantation of the stent, the patient experienced the development of acute in-stent thrombosis. The combination of intra-arterial tirofiban administration with the microwire massage within the stent was an effective treatment to resolve the thrombus. It is worth noting that the immediate elastic recoil of the stent may be attributed to the specific stent type that was selected.

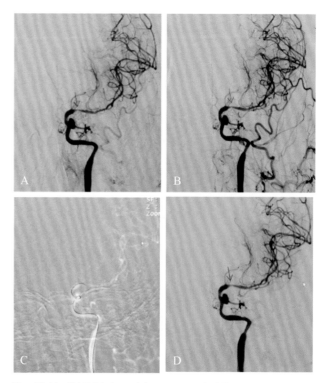

Fig. 6.3.14   (**A**) DSA showed the presence of a filling defect in the stent (arrow). (**B**) There was still a filling defect in the proximal site of the stent after intra- arterial administration of tirofiban (arrow). (**C**) The microwire was delivered to massage mildly in the stent. (**D**) The angiogram showed the the disappearance of filling defect, leaving behind a residual stenosis of approximately 35% (arrow)

(Translated by Rongrong Cui, Revised by Zhikai Hou)

Case 41   Thrombus formation during endovascular treatment of a severe vertebro-basilar junction stenosis

1. Clinical presentation and radiological studies

A 59-year-old woman was admitted to the hospital due to episodes of paroxysmal vertigo and right-sided limb weakness for over one year.

The DSA examination conducted eight months ago revealed the presence of severe stenosis at the junction of the left vertebro-basilar artery. The symptoms were alleviated with medical treatment. However, before 6 months, the patients experienced paroxysmal vertigo episodes along with numbness and weakness in the right limb, particularly under conditions of hypotension.

The patient had a medical history of hypertension and type 2 diabetes mellitus.

Upon admission, her neurological condition remained intact.

The follow-up DSA findings indicated that the left vertebral artery was the dominant vessel, and a significant stenosis was observed at the junction of the left vertebro-basilar artery (Fig.

6.3.15 A, B). Additionally, the V3–V4 segments of the right vertebral artery were found to be completely occluded (Fig. 6.3.15 C). Moreover, there was inadequate compensation from the anterior circulation to the posterior circulation (Fig. 6.3.16).

The arterial spin labeling (ASL) sequence showed hypoperfusion in the right occipital lobe and right cerebellar hemisphere (Fig. 6.3.17).

The CYP2C19 genotype corresponded to an intermediate metabolizer phenotype.

Upon admission, the patient had been prescribed a dual-antiplatelet regimen comprising a daily dose of 100 mg of Aspirin and twice-daily doses of 90 mg of Ticagrelor, in addition to statin therapy with a daily dose of 20 mg of Atorvastatin.

2. Diagnosis

Symptomatic severe stenosis of the left vertebro-basilar junction.

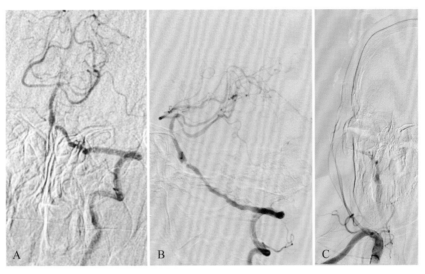

图 6.3.15　DSA 示左椎动脉优势，左椎基底动脉交界区重度狭窄（**A** 和 **B**）；右椎动脉 V3 ～ V4 段闭塞（**C**）

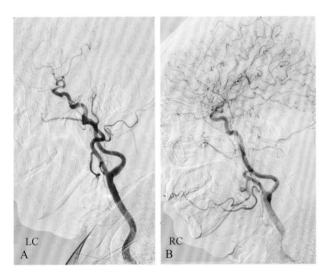

图 6.3.16　DSA 未见明显前循环向后循环代偿

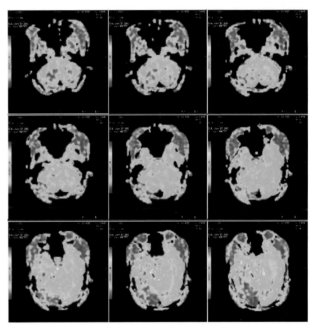

图 6.3.17　头部 MR 动脉自旋标记（ASL）序列提示右枕叶及右侧小脑半球低灌注

（三）术前讨论

结合患者病史及相关影像学检查，患者反复发作眩晕伴右侧肢体无力，血压下降时加重，平卧位休息时缓解，考虑左椎动脉为后循环唯一供血血管及责任血管，可通过介入治疗改善狭窄远端血流低灌注状态。相关风险包括急性血栓形成、医源性夹层、动脉破裂、穿支事件等。

（四）治疗过程

全麻下右股动脉穿刺入路，路径图见左椎动脉开口处轻度狭窄，血管迂曲（图 6.3.18 A）。泥鳅导丝同轴 5F 多功能导管（125 cm）将 6F 导引导管（Cordis Envoy）送至左椎动脉 V2 段远端，造影显示左椎动脉 V3 段以远未见显影且对比剂滞留（图 6.3.18 B）。将 Synchro 微导丝（0.014 in，200 cm）与 Echelon-10 微导管同轴通过闭塞段至左侧大脑后动脉（图 6.3.18 C）。

更换为 Synchro 微导丝（0.014 in，300 cm）同时交换撤出微导管，沿微导丝送入 Sinomed 球囊（1.5 mm×10 mm）至狭窄段，准确定位后缓慢扩张病变，路径图显示左侧大脑后动脉及右侧小脑上

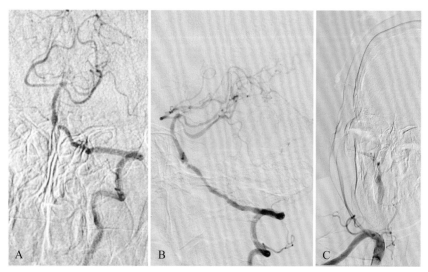

Fig. 6.3.15   DSA findings indicated that the left vertebral artery was the dominant vessel and a significant stenosis was observed at the junction of the left vertebro-basilar artery (**A**, **B**), the V3–V4 segments of the right vertebral artery were found to be completely occluded (**C**)

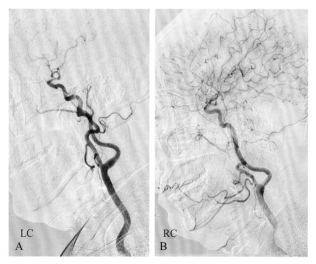

Fig. 6.3.16   There was inadequate compensation from the anterior circulation to the posterior circulation

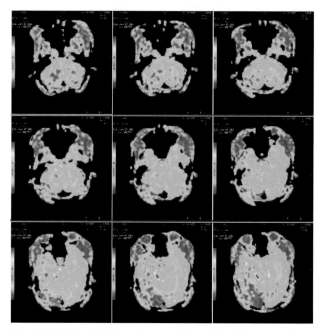

Fig. 6.3.17   The ASL showed hypoperfusion in the right occipital lobe and right cerebellar hemisphere

3. Treatment schedule

Based on the patient's medical history and relevant imaging examinations, the patient presented with recurrent vertigo episodes and weakness in the right limbs, particularly in the presence of hypotension. The left vertebral artery, being the sole supplied artery of the posterior circulation, was identified as the responsible artery. Endovascular intervention was suggested to enhance hypoperfusion in the posterior region. Potential procedural risks included acute in-stent thrombosis, iatrogenic dissection, arterial rupture, and occlusion of the perforating artery.

4. Treatment

Under general anesthesia, vascular access was established via the right femoral artery. The roadmap angiogram showed mild stenosis at the origin of the left vertebral artery, along with a tortuous access (Fig. 6.3.18 A). Using a loach Guidewire and a 5F multifunctional catheter (125 cm), and a 6F guiding catheter (Cordis Envoy) were navigated to the distal V2 segment of the left vertebral artery. The angiogram showed the V3 segment of the left vertebral artery was not visualized, with the contrast agent retention (Fig. 6.3.18 B). A Synchro microwire (0.014 in, 200 cm) in conjunction with an Echelon-10 microcatheter coaxially maneuvered through the occluded segment to reach the left posterior cerebral artery (Fig. 6.3.18 C).

A Synchro microwire (0.014 in, 300 cm) was employed as a replacement, and a Sinomed balloon (1.5 mm × 10 mm) along the microwire was positioned at the stenotic segment to predilate the lesion. The roadmap showed the left posterior cerebral artery and right superior cerebellar artery were not visualized (Fig. 6.3.19 A). A dosage of 3ml of tirofiban

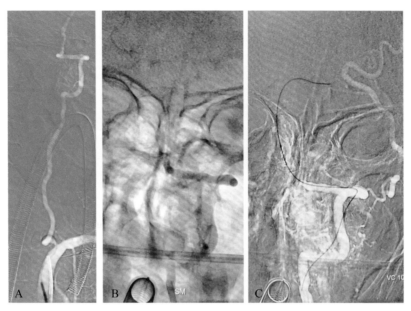

图 6.3.18　路径图显示左椎动脉开口处轻度狭窄，血管迂曲（**A**）；导引导管到位后造影显示左椎动脉 V3 段以远未见显影且对比剂滞留（**B**）；Synchro 微导丝与 Echelon-10 微导管通过闭塞段至左侧大脑后动脉（**C**）

动脉显影欠佳（图 6.3.19 A）。经 6F 导引导管给予替罗非班 3 ml（150 μg），同时以 4 ml/h（200 μg/h）持续静脉泵入，复查造影仍未显影（图 6.3.19 B）。

撤出球囊，沿微导丝送入 Echelon-10 微导管置于左侧大脑后动脉 P2 段（图 6.3.20 A），造影证实位于真腔（图 6.3.20 B），交换技术更换为 Rebar-18 微导管（图 6.3.20 C）。置入取栓支架 Trevo XP（4 mm×20 mm）行支架取栓（图 6.3.21 A 和 B），

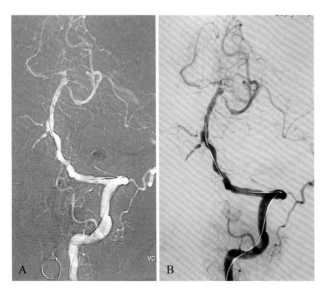

图 6.3.19　球囊扩张后路径图显示左侧大脑后动脉及右侧小脑上动脉显影欠佳（**A**），给予替罗非班后仍未显影（**B**）

同时配合 6F 导引导管抽吸，可见取出条状红色血栓（图 6.3.21 C）。

取栓后复查造影提示基底动脉尖端、左侧大脑后动脉及右侧小脑上动脉血流恢复（图 6.3.22 A）。Transend EX 微导丝（205 cm）带 Apollo 球囊扩张式支架（2.5 mm×13 mm）至狭窄段，到位后释放支架（图 6.3.22 B），复查造影提示支架位置满意、贴壁良好，残余狭窄率约 20%，双侧大脑后动脉及小脑上动脉显影（图 6.3.22 C）。观察 10 min 后，造影见基底动脉主干及分支血流通畅，前向血流 3 级（图 6.3.22 D），结束治疗。

（五）讨论

本例病变为后循环单椎动脉供血，且狭窄程度极重，6F 导引导管到位过程中血流阻断，可能是通过迂曲病变时引发动脉-动脉栓塞，导致左椎动脉 V3 段以远不显影，在球囊扩张病变后血管再通，但造影提示左大脑后动脉及右小脑上动脉不显影，考虑基底动脉尖急性血栓形成。支架取栓后恢复 mTICI 3 级血流。因原狭窄病变在球囊扩张后残余狭窄率较高，在远端血管再通后置入直径较短的球囊扩张式支架。术后患者头晕症状较前改善，远期疗效待随访。

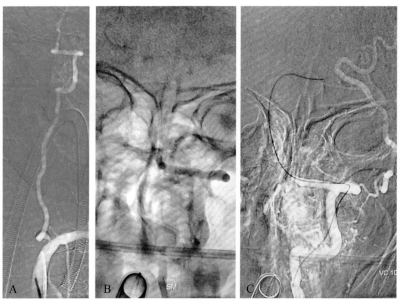

Fig. 6.3.18   The roadmap angiogram showed mild stenosis at the origin of the left vertebral artery, along with a tortuous access (**A**). The angiogram showed the V3 segment of the left vertebral artery was not visualized, with the contrast agent retention (**B**). A Synchro microwire (0.014 in, 200 cm) in conjunction with an Echelon-10 microcatheter coaxially maneuvered through the occluded segment to reach the left posterior cerebral artery (**C**)

was administered through a 6F guiding catheter, while the simultaneous intravenous infusion of tirofiban at a rate of 4 ml/h. However, the subsequent angiogram indicated the target arteries remained not visualized (Fig. 6.3.19 B).

The Echelon-10 microcatheter was advanced to the P2 segment of the left posterior cerebral artery (Fig. 6.3.20 A). The catheter angiogram confirmed the accurate position of the catheter in the true lumen (Fig. 6.3.20 B). Utilizing the exchange approach, a Rebar-18 microcatheter was employed (Figure 6.3.20 C) to successfully release a Trevo XP stent (4 mm×20 mm) for the efficient retrieval of the clot. (Fig. 6.3.21 A, B). In combination with the catheter aspiration with a 6F guiding catheter, a substantial length of red thrombus was effectively retrieved (Fig. 6.3.21 C).

Following the retrieval of the clot, the angiogram revealed

a successful restoration of blood flow in the distal segment of the basilar artery, as well as the left posterior cerebral artery and the right superior cerebellar artery (Fig. 6.3.22 A). A 2.5 mm× 13 mm Apollo balloon-mounted stent was advanced to the stenotic segment and sequentially implanted after its accurate in place (Fig. 6.3.22 B). The post-stent implantation angiogram showed excellent stent wall apposition, with residual stenosis of 20%. Additionally, both the bilateral posterior cerebral arteries and superior cerebellar arteries were visualized (Fig. 6.3.22 C). Following an observation period of 10 minutes, the angiogram displayed unobstructed blood flow within the main trunk as well as the branches of the basilar artery, with a grade 3 of antegrade blood flow (Fig. 6.3.22 D).

5. Comments

This case involved a patient who exhibited a severe stenosis at the left vertebro-basilar junction, serving as the sole source of blood supply to the posterior circulation. During the procedure, the antegrade blood flow was obstructed upon the proper position of the guide catheter. The occlusion of the V3 segment of the left vertebral artery may be attributed to the plaque embolism during the catheter's passage through the tortuous lesion. Following the balloon angioplasty, the occlusion lesion was successfully recanalized. Nonetheless, the angiogram revealed the absence of visualization in the left posterior cerebral artery and right superior cerebellar artery, implying the acute thrombus formation at the distal end of the basilar artery. After the mechanical thrombectomy, the antegrade flow of blood was restored to a grade 3 in mTICI. Due to significant residual stenosis in situ following the balloon dilation, a balloon-mounted stent was inserted after the recanalization of the distal branch. The patient's symptoms of dizziness an alleviation after the procedure. The long-term efficacy of the treatment need to be further followed-up.

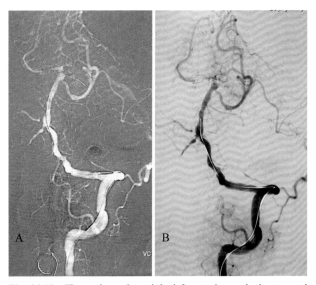

Fig. 6.3.19   The roadmap showed the left posterior cerebral artery and the right superior cerebellar artery were not visualized (**A**), the subsequent angiogram indicated the target arteries remained not visualized (**B**)

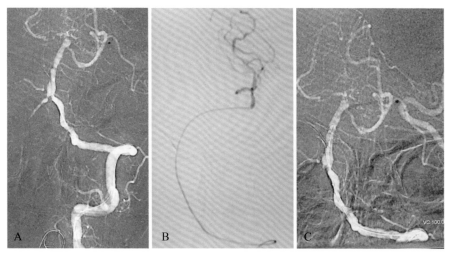

图 6.3.20　将 Echelon-10 微导管置于左侧大脑后动脉 P2 段（**A**），造影证实微导管位于真腔（**B**），交换技术更换为 Rebar-18 微导管（**C**）

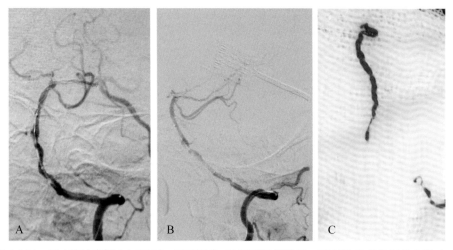

图 6.3.21　置入取栓支架（**A** 和 **B**），同时配合 6F 导引导管抽吸，可见取出条状红色血栓（**C**）

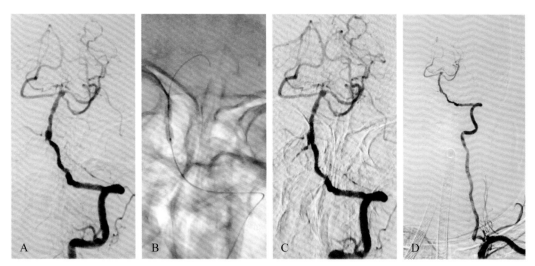

图 6.3.22　取栓后复查造影提示基底动脉尖端、左侧大脑后动脉及右侧小脑上动脉血流恢复（**A**）。释放 Apollo 球囊扩张式支架（**B**），复查造影提示支架贴壁良好，残余狭窄率约 20%，双侧大脑后动脉及小脑上动脉显影（**C**）。观察 10 min 后，造影显示基底动脉主干及分支血流通畅（**D**）

（马宁）

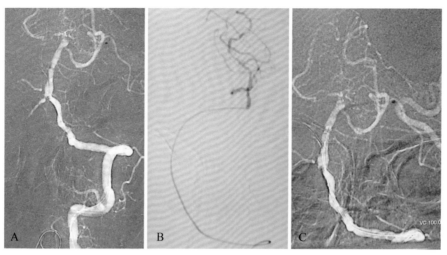

Fig. 6.3.20 The Echelon-10 microcatheter was advanced to the P2 segment of the left posterior cerebral artery (**A**) The catheter angiogram confirmed the accurate position of the catheter in the true lumen (**B**). Utilizing the exchange approach, a Rebar-18 microcatheter was employed (**C**)

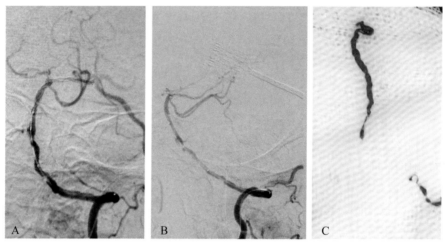

Fig. 6.3.21 The Trevo XP stent was released (**A, B**). A substantial length of red thrombus was effectively retrieved (**C**)

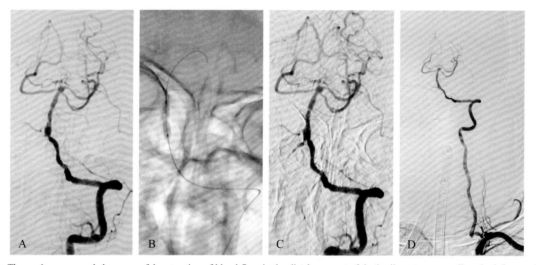

Fig. 6.3.22 The angiogram revealed a successful restoration of blood flow in the distal segment of the basilar artery, as well as the left posterior cerebral artery and the right superior cerebellar artery (**A**). A Apollo balloon-mounted stent was advanced to the stenotic segment and sequentially implanted after its accurate in place (**B**). The post-stent implantation angiogram showed excellent stent wall apposition, with residual stenosis of 20%, Additionally, both the bilateral posterior cerebral arteries and superior cerebellar arteries were visualized (**C**). The angiogram displayed unobstructed blood flow within the main trunk as well as the branches of the basilar artery (**D**)

(Translated by Rongrong Cui, Revised by Zhikai Hou)

第四节 术中血管破裂

病例 42 右大脑中动脉 M1 段串联狭窄血管内治疗术中血管破裂

（一）临床病史及影像分析

患者，女性，69 岁，主因"头晕 17 个月，加重 2 个月"入院。

17 个月前于当地医院检查，头部 MRI 未见急性梗死灶（图 6.4.1），头部 MRA 示右大脑中动脉重度狭窄（图 6.4.2）。头部 CTA 示右大脑中动脉 M1 段串联重度狭窄（图 6.4.3）。头部 CTP 示右大脑中动脉供血区域低灌注（图 6.4.4）。

全脑血管造影（DSA）提示右大脑中动脉 M1 段串联重度狭窄（图 6.4.5 A 和 B），左颈动脉系统通过软脑膜支向对侧代偿（图 6.4.5 C 和 D）。后循环系统未见明显异常（图 6.4.6）。

发病后口服阿司匹林（100 mg 1 次 / 日）、氯吡格雷（75 mg 1 次 / 日）以及瑞舒伐他汀（10 mg 1 次 / 日）治疗。2 个月前患者自觉头晕症状较前加重。外院头部 CTA 提示右大脑中动脉串联重度狭窄，狭窄程度较前有所加重（图 6.4.7）。患者为求进一步治疗收入我院。

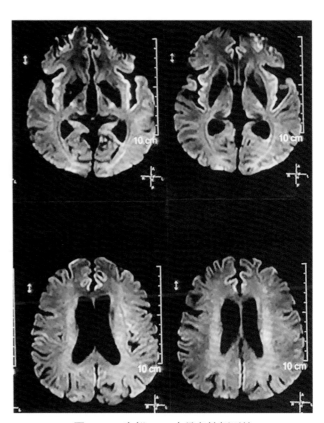

图 6.4.1 头部 MRI 未见急性梗死灶

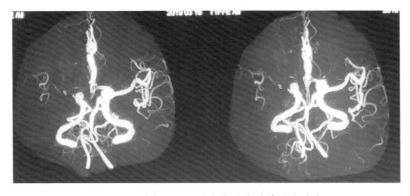

图 6.4.2 头部 MRA 示右大脑中动脉重度狭窄

Section 4   Periprocedural Vascular Rupture

Case 42   Arterial rupture during endovascular treatment of tandem stenosis of the right middle cerebral artery M1 segment

1. Clinical presentation and radiological studies

A 69-year-old woman was admitted to the hospital because of dizziness for 17 months, with the symptoms worsening over the past two months.

The MRI findings from seventeen months prior indicated the absence of any indications of acute infarction (Fig. 6.4.1). The MRA results revealed the presence of severe stenosis in the right middle cerebral artery (Fig. 6.4.2). Furthermore, the CT angiography (CTA) demonstrated tandem severe stenosis in the M1 segment of the right middle cerebral artery (Fig. 6.4.3). The CT perfusion scan exhibited notable hypoperfusion within the territory of the right middle cerebral artery (Fig. 6.4.4).

The angiogram findings revealed the presence of tandem severe stenosis within the M1 segment of the right middle cerebral artery (Fig. 6.4.5 A, B), while the compensatory flow was observed from the left carotid artery through the pial arteries (Fig. 6.4.5 C, D). Additionally, the vertebro-basilar artery system displayed no significant abnormalities (Fig. 6.4.6).

Upon the onset of symptoms, the patient was prescribed a daily regimen of 100 mg of Aspirin and 75 mg of Clopidogrel, as well as statin therapy with a daily dose of 10 mg of Rosuvastatin. However, two months ago, there was a notable exacerbation of dizziness symptoms. Subsequent CTA examination revealed a worsening of the stenosis in the right middle cerebral artery (Fig. 6.4.7).

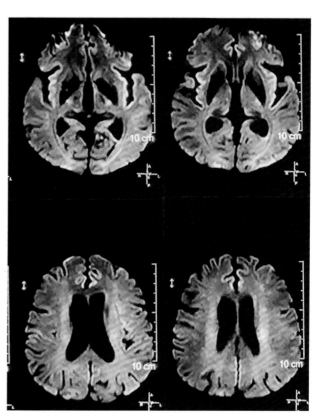

Fig. 6.4.1   The MRI showed the absence of any indications of acute infarction

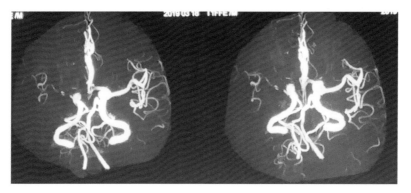

Fig. 6.4.2   The MRA results revealed the presence of severe stenosis in the right middle cerebral artery

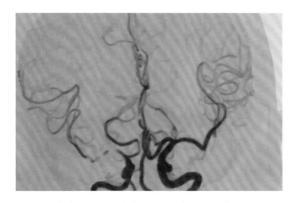

图 6.4.3　头部 CTA 示右大脑中动脉 M1 段串联重度狭窄

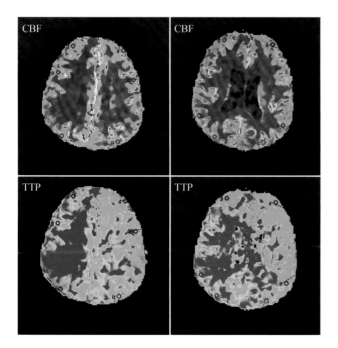

图 6.4.4　头部 CTP 示右大脑中动脉供血区域低灌注

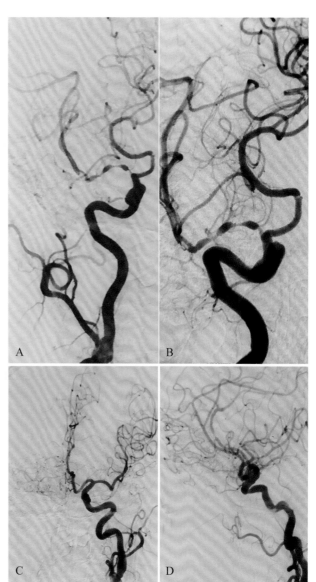

图 6.4.5　DSA 示右大脑中动脉 M1 段串联重度狭窄（**A** 和 **B**），左颈动脉系统通过软脑膜支向对侧代偿（**C** 和 **D**）

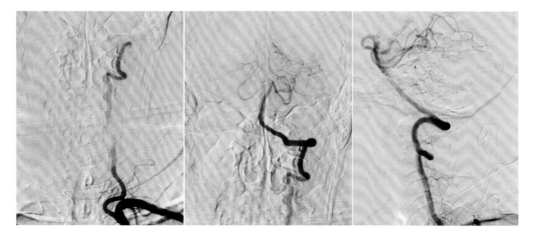

图 6.4.6　DSA 示后循环系统未见明显异常

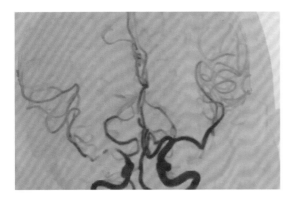

Fig. 6.4.3 The CT angiography demonstrated tandem severe stenosis in the M1 segment of the right middle cerebral artery

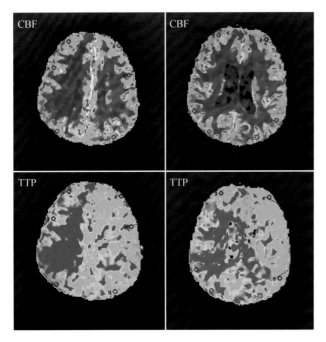

Fig. 6.4.4 The CT perfusion scan exhibited notable hypoperfusion within the territory of the right middle cerebral artery

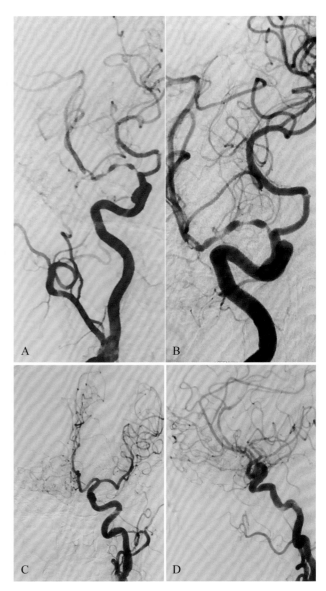

Fig. 6.4.5 DSA showed the presence of tandem severe stenosis within the M1 segment of the right middle cerebral artery (**A**, **B**), while the compensatory flow was observed from the left carotid artery through the pial arteries (**C**, **D**)

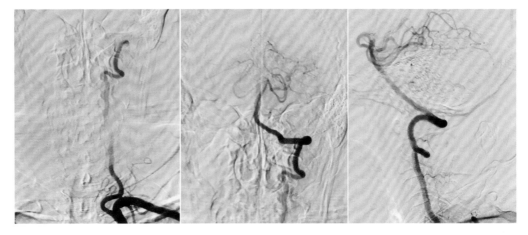

Fig. 6.4.6 The vertebro-basilar artery system displayed no significant abnormalities

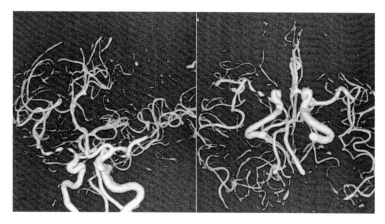

图 6.4.7 2 个月前头部 CTA 提示右大脑中动脉串联重度狭窄，且狭窄程度较前加重

既往史：高血压、糖尿病及脑梗死病史。

查体：神经系统查体无阳性体征。

入院后复查 DSA：右大脑中动脉 M1 段串联重度狭窄（图 6.4.8）。

高分辨率 MRI：右大脑中动脉 M1 段管壁增厚，管腔串联重度狭窄（图 6.4.9）。

入院后给予双联抗血小板（阿司匹林 100 mg 1 次 / 日＋氯吡格雷 75 mg 1 次 / 日）及降脂（瑞舒伐他汀 10 mg 1 次 / 日）治疗。

（二）诊断

症状性右大脑中动脉 M1 段串联重度狭窄。

（三）术前讨论

结合患者病史及相关影像学检查，考虑右大脑中动脉 M1 段串联狭窄为责任病变，且药物治疗效果欠佳，拟行右大脑中动脉血管内治疗。相关风险包括栓子脱落、医源性夹层、动脉破裂、穿支事件、急性血栓形成等。

（四）治疗过程及随访

全麻下右股动脉穿刺入路，置入 8F 鞘，将 8F 导引导管送至右颈内动脉 C2 段，6F Navien 导管送至右颈内动脉海绵窦段（C4 段），造影明确右大脑中动脉 M1 段串联重度狭窄（图 6.4.10）。

在路径图下将 Synchro 微导丝（0.014 in，200 cm）小心通过狭窄段至右大脑中动脉 M2 段，沿微导丝将 Sino 球囊（1.5 mm×10 mm）送至病变处，由远及近依次扩张（图 6.4.11），撤出球囊，造影见狭窄程度较前改善，对比剂未见滞留（图 6.4.12 A）。

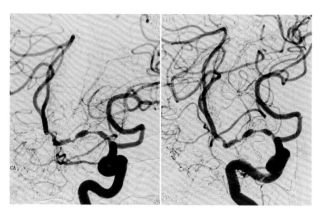

图 6.4.8 入院后复查 DSA 示右大脑中动脉 M1 段串联重度狭窄

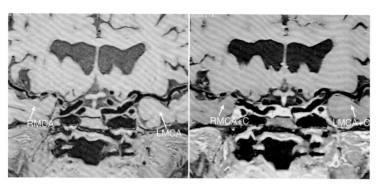

图 6.4.9 高分辨率 MRI 示右大脑中动脉 M1 段管腔串联重度狭窄

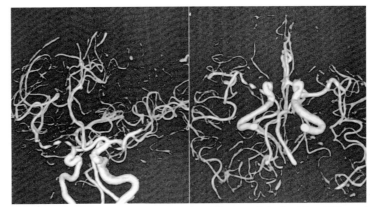

Fig. 6.4.7   Two months ago, CTA revealed a worsening of the stenosis in the right middle cerebral artery

She had a medical history of hypertension, diabetes mellitus, and cerebral infarction.

Upon admission, the physical examination revealed an intact neurological function.

The repeated DSA results indicated the presence of severe tandem stenosis within the M1 segment of the right middle cerebral artery (Fig. 6.4.8).

The high-resolution MRI revealed a thickening of the vessel wall along the entire course of the right middle cerebral artery, leading to the occurrence of tandem severe stenosis in the M1 segment (Fig. 6.4.9).

She maintained a consistent intake of a dual antiplatelet regimen and statin therapy.

2. Diagnosis

Symptomatic tandem severe stenosis in the M1 segment

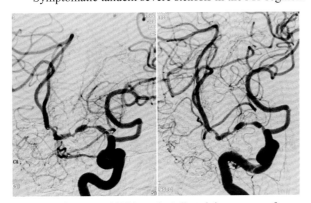

Fig. 6.4.8   The repeated DSA results indicated the presence of severe tandem stenosis within the M1 segment of the right middle cerebral artery

of the right middle cerebral artery.

3. Treatment schedule

Based on the patient's clinical presentation and relevant imaging studies, the M1 segment of the right middle cerebral artery was identified as the responsible artery, displaying unresponsiveness to aggressive medical intervention. Consequently, endovascular therapy was suggested as the recommended course of action. potential risks associated with the procedure included the dislodgement of emboli, iatrogenic dissection, arterial rupture, the occlusion of the perforating arteries, and acute in-stent thrombosis.

4. Treatment and follow-up

Under general anesthesia, an 8F guiding catheter was positioned at the C2 segment of the right internal carotid artery. And a 6F Navien catheter was advanced to the cavernous segment of the right internal carotid artery. The angiogram confirmed tandem severe stenoses in the M1 segment of the right middle cerebral artery (Fig. 6.4.10).

Under the roadmap, a Synchro microwire (0.014 in, 200 cm) carefully maneuvered through the stenotic segment to reach the M2 segment of the right middle cerebral artery. A 1.5 mm × 10 mm Sino balloon was employed to perform a distal-to-proximal dilation of the lesion (Fig. 6.4.11). The subsequent angiogram revealed an improvement in the degree of stenosis, with no residual contrast agent observed (Fig. 6.4.12 A). Intra-arterial administration of tirofiban was performed. The subsequent angiogram, taken 10 minutes later, indicated

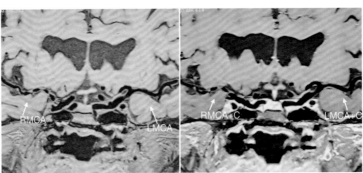

Fig. 6.4.9   The HRMRI revealed a thickening of the vessel wall along the entire course of the right middle cerebral artery, leading to the occurrence of tandem severe stenosis in the M1 segment

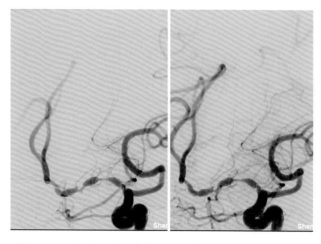

图 6.4.10　术前造影示右大脑中动脉 M1 段串联重度狭窄

动脉内给予替罗非班，观察 10 min，造影提示血管通畅，M1 段末端局部高信号影，考虑医源性夹层形成，对比剂未见滞留（图 6.4.12 B）。

沿导引导管送入 Transend 微导丝（0.014 in，300 cm）携 Echelon-10 微导管小心通过病变处至右大脑中动脉 M2 段，造影见血管破裂形成（图 6.4.13）。顺微导丝将 Sino 球囊（2.0 mm×10 mm）送至右大脑中动脉 M1 段末端，加压扩张（图 6.4.14 A 和 B），复查造影未见对比剂渗出（图 6.4.14 C）。10 min 后回撤球囊，复查造影提示血管通畅，远端血管显影差（图 6.4.14 D）。行 Dyna-CT 可见蛛网膜下腔出血（图 6.4.15）。

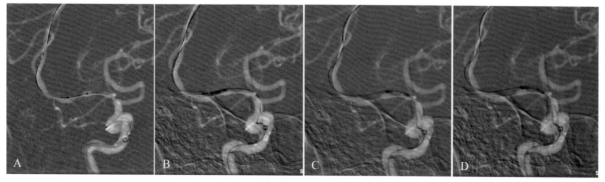

图 6.4.11　Sino 球囊由远及近依次扩张病变

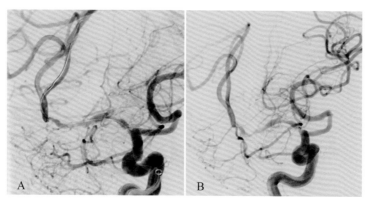

图 6.4.12　**A**. 球囊扩张后造影显示狭窄程度较前改善，无对比剂滞留；**B**. 观察 10 min 后造影提示右大脑中动脉 M1 段末端局部高信号影，考虑医源性夹层形成

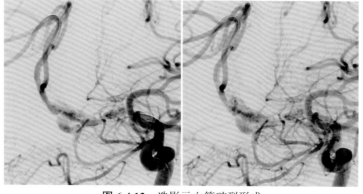

图 6.4.13　造影示血管破裂形成

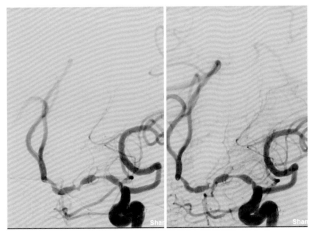

Fig. 6.4.10 The angiogram confirmed tandem severe stenoses in the M1 segment of the right middle cerebral artery

a patent blood vessel with a focal hyperintensity observed at the distal end of the M1 segment, implying the development of an iatrogenic dissection, without any contrast agent retention (Fig. 6.4.12 B).

The Transend microwire (0.014 in, 300 cm), in combination with an Echelon-10 microcatheter, coaxially advanced through the lesion to the M2 segment. The angiogram revealed arterial rupture (Fig. 6.4.13). A 2.0 mm × 10 mm Sino balloon was advanced to the distal end of the right M1 segment for pressurized dilation (Fig. 6.4.14 A, B). The Subsequent angiogram showed there was no contrast agent exudation (Fig. 6.4.14 C). Following 10 minutes, the balloon was gradually withdrawn. The subsequent angiogram revealed an unobstructed vessel, albeit with limited visualization of the distal branches. (Fig. 6.4.14 D). Dyna-CT imaging displayed the presence of subarachnoid hemorrhage. (Fig. 6.4.15).

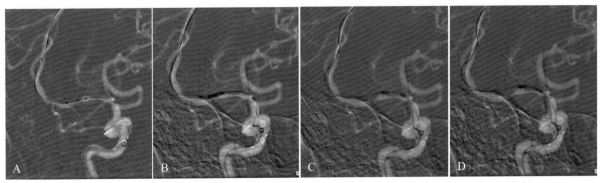

Fig. 6.4.11 A 1.5 mm × 10 mm Sino balloon was employed to perform a distal-to-proximal dilation of the lesion

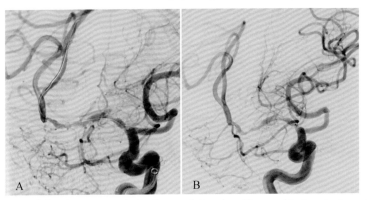

Fig. 6.4.12 (**A**). The angiogram revealed an improvement in the degree of stenosis, with no residual contrast agent observed (**B**) The subsequent angiogram, taken 10 minutes later, indicated a patent blood vessel with a focal hyperintensity observed at the distal end of the M1 segment, implying the development of an iatrogenic dissection, without any contrast agent retention

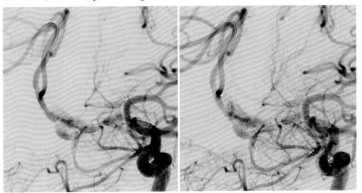

Fig. 6.4.13 The angiogram showed arterial rupture

术后第 1 日复查头颅 CT 提示蛛网膜下腔出血，部分对比剂渗出（图 6.4.16）。

术后 6 个月头颅 MRA 提示右大脑中动脉 M1 段血管通畅（图 6.4.17）。

（五）讨论

本例患者右大脑中动脉 M1 段串联重度狭窄，术中出现医源性血管破裂，及时给予球囊封堵。术后患者病情平稳，远期随访提示疗效尚可。

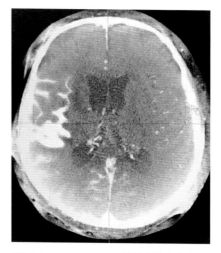

图 6.4.15　Dyna-CT 示蛛网膜下腔出血

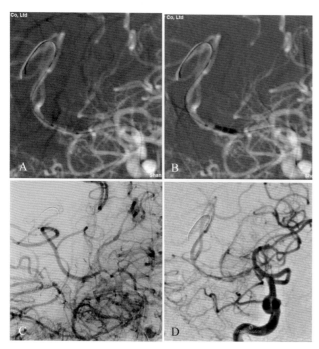

图 6.4.14　**A** 和 **B**. 将 Sino 球囊送至右大脑中动脉 M1 段末端，加压扩张；**C**. 球囊加压扩张后复查造影未见对比剂渗出；**D**. 术后即刻造影显示血管通畅，远端血管显影差

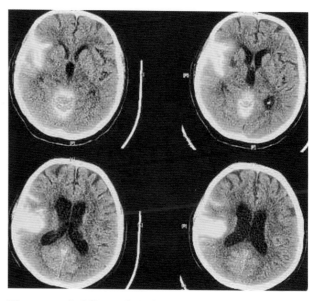

图 6.4.16　术后第 1 日复查头颅 CT 提示蛛网膜下腔出血，部分对比剂渗出

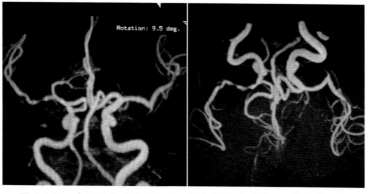

图 6.4.17　术后 6 个月头颅 MRA 示右大脑中动脉 M1 段血管通畅

（水新俊　蒯东）

On the first day after the procedure, Repeat CT scans revealed the occurrence of the subarachnoid hemorrhage with some contrast agent extravasation (Fig. 6.4.16).

The follow-up MRA conducted six months after the procedure demonstrated the M1 segment of the right middle cerebral artery was unobstructed (Fig. 6.4.17).

5. Comments

In this case, the patient presented with severe stenosis of the M1 segment of the right middle cerebral artery. During the procedure, an iatrogenic arterial rupture occurred, which was promptly managed through balloon occlusion. The patient's condition after the procedure remained stable, and long-term follow-up indicated satisfactory therapeutic outcomes.

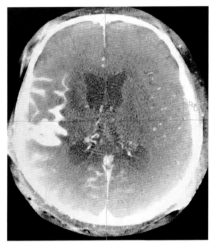

Fig. 6.4.15 The Dyna-CT scan showed the presence of subarachnoid hemorrhage

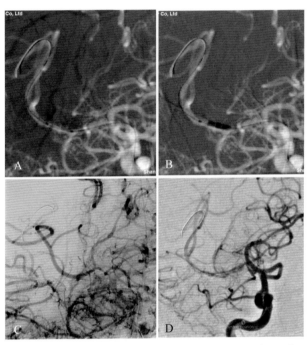

Fig. 6.4.14 (**A, B**) A 2.0 mm×10 mm Sino balloon was advanced to the distal end of the right M1 segment for pressurized dilation (**C**) The Subsequent angiogram showed without any contrast agent exudation. (**D**) The angiogram revealed an unobstructed vessel, albeit with limited visualization of the distal branches

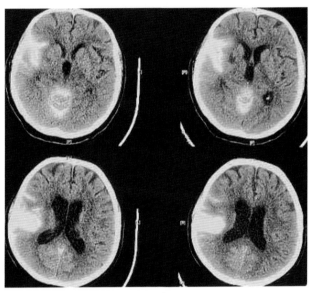

Fig. 6.4.16 On the first day after the procedure, Repeat CT scans revealed the occurrence of the subarachnoid hemorrhage with some contrast agent extravasation

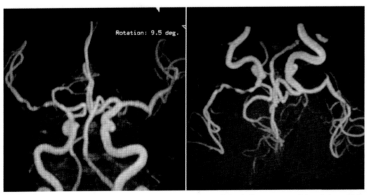

Fig. 6.4.17 The follow-up MRA conducted six months after the procedure demonstrated the M1 segment of the right middle cerebral artery was unobstructed

(Translated by Rongrong Cui, Revised by Zhikai Hou)

病例 43　右大脑中动脉 M1 段闭塞再通术中血管破裂

（一）临床病史及影像分析

患者，男性，60 岁，主因"头晕伴左侧肢体无力 2 个月"入院。

既往史：右上肢骨折病史。

查体：神经系统查体无阳性体征。

头部 MRI 示急性脑梗死，MRA 示右大脑中动脉 M1 段闭塞（图 6.4.18）。

头部 CTP：右大脑中动脉供血区域低灌注（图 6.4.19）。

DSA：右大脑中动脉闭塞，右颈内动脉交通段动脉瘤（图 6.4.20），左颈动脉系统造影未见明显异常（图 6.4.21 A 和 B），后循环系统造影未见明显异常（图 6.4.21 C 和 D）。

高分辨率 MRI：右大脑中动脉 M1 段闭塞（图 6.4.22）。

入院后给予双联抗血小板（阿司匹林 100 mg 1 次 / 日 + 氯吡格雷 75 mg 1 次 / 日）及降脂（阿托伐他汀 20 mg 1 次 / 日）。

（二）诊断

症状性右大脑中动脉 M1 段闭塞。

（三）术前讨论

结合患者病史及相关影像学检查，考虑右大脑中动脉闭塞为责任病变，拟行右大脑中动脉血管内

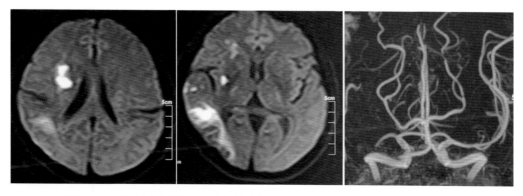

图 6.4.18　头颅磁共振 DWI 示急性脑梗死，MRA 示右大脑中动脉 M1 段闭塞

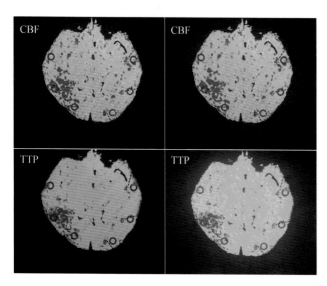

图 6.4.19　头部 CTP 示右大脑中动脉供血区域低灌注

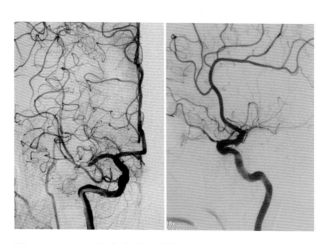

图 6.4.20　DSA 示右大脑中动脉闭塞，右颈内动脉交通段（C7 段）动脉瘤

Case 43 Arterial rupture during endovascular treatment of a right middle cerebral artery M1 segment occlusion

1. Clinical presentation and radiological studies

A 60-year-old male patient was admitted to the hospital due to dizziness and left-sided hemiplegia for two months.

The patient had a medical record of a fracture in the right upper limb.

Upon admission, the physical examination indicated intact neurological function.

The MRI results revealed acute cerebral infarction. And the MRA revealed the presence of occlusion in the M1 segment of the right middle cerebral artery (Fig. 6.4.18).

The CT perfusion scan showed hypoperfusion in the region supplied by the right middle cerebral artery (Fig. 6.4.19).

DSA imaging demonstrated occlusion of the right middle cerebral artery, along with the detection of an aneurysm in the C7 segment of the right internal carotid artery (Fig. 6.4.20). No significant anomalies were observed in the left carotid artery

system or the posterior circulation system. (Fig. 6.4.21 A–D).

The high-resolution MRI revealed complete occlusion in the M1 segment of the right middle cerebral artery (Fig. 6.4.22).

Upon admission, the patient was prescribed a dual-antiplatelet regimen consisting of a daily dose of 100 mg of Aspirin and 75 mg of Clopidogrel daily, along with statin therapy with a daily dose of 20 mg of Atorvastatin.

2. Diagnosis

Symptomatic occlusion in the M1 segment of the right middle cerebral artery.

3. Treatment schedule

Based on the patient's clinical presentation and relevant imaging examinations, the M1 segment of the right middle cerebral artery was identified as the culprit artery. Endovascular

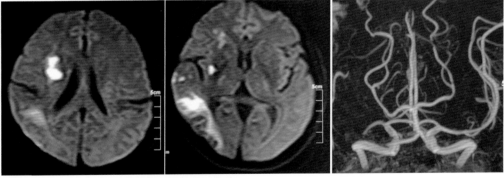

Fig. 6.4.18 The MRI results revealed acute cerebral infarction. The MRA revealed occlusion in the M1 segment of the right middle cerebral artery

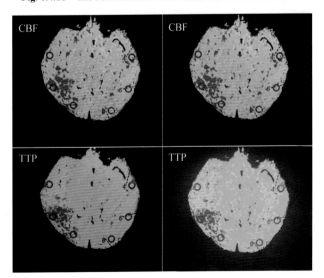

Fig. 6.4.19 The CT perfusion scan showed hypoperfusion in the region supplied by the right middle cerebral artery

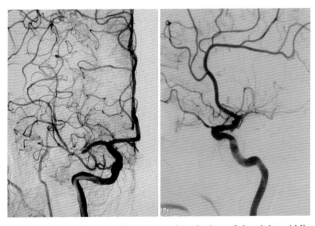

Fig. 6.4.20 Angiogram demonstrated occlusion of the right middle cerebral artery, along with the detection of an aneurysm in the C7 segment of the right internal carotid artery

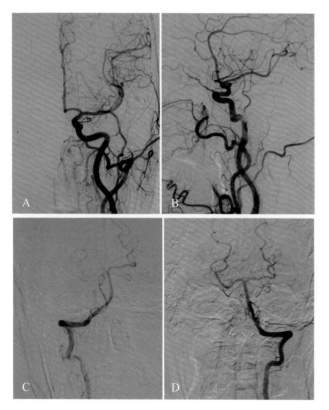

图 6.4.21 DSA 示左颈动脉系统未见明显异常（**A** 和 **B**），后循环系统未见明显异常（**C** 和 **D**）

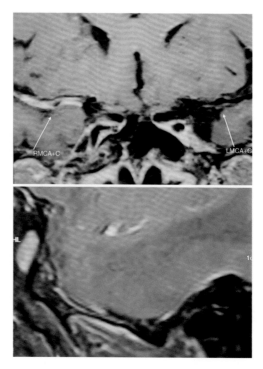

图 6.4.22 高分辨率 MRI 示右大脑中动脉 M1 段闭塞

治疗。相关风险包括栓子脱落、医源性夹层、动脉破裂、穿支事件、急性血栓形成等。

（四）治疗过程及随访

全麻下右股动脉穿刺入路，置入 8F 鞘，将 8F 导引导管内套 6F Navien 导管（115 cm）送至右颈内动脉 C2 段，造影明确右大脑中动脉 M1 段闭塞（图 6.4.23 A），

沿导引导管送入 Synchro 微导丝（0.014 in，200 cm）及 Echelon-10 微导管，在路径图下微导丝携微导管小心通过病变处至右大脑中动脉 M2 段（图 6.4.23 B 和 C），撤出 Synchro 微导丝，沿微导管送入 Transend 微导丝（0.014 in，300 cm），撤出微导管，沿微导丝送入赛诺球囊（1.5 mm×10 mm），加压扩张（图 6.4.24 A 和 B）。观察 10 min，再次造影血管通畅，无血栓形成，欲结束手术，回撤导丝，牵拉血管，导致出血（图 6.4.24 C 和 D）。立即给予鱼精蛋白中和肝素，沿 Transend 微导丝将 TREK 球囊（2.0 mm×8 mm）送至右大脑中动脉 M1 段近端，以 10 atm 压力扩张球囊，手推造影见右大脑中动脉 M1 段以远未见显影，持续扩张球囊 5 min 后复查造影见对比剂外渗明显减少（图 6.4.25 A 和 B）。再次以 10 atm 压力扩张球囊 5 min 后，复查造

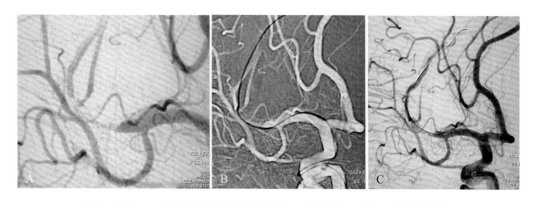

图 6.4.23 **A**. 术前造影示右大脑中动脉 M1 段闭塞；**B** 和 **C**. 微导丝到位

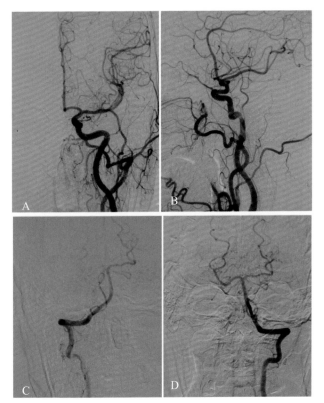

Fig. 6.4.21 No significant anomalies were observed in the left carotid artery system (**A**, **B**) or the posterior circulation system. (**C**, **D**)

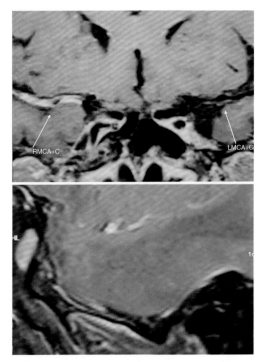

Fig. 6.4.22 The high-resolution MRI revealed complete occlusion in the M1 segment of the right middle cerebral artery

therapy was indicated. Potential risks associated with the procedure encompassed emboli dislodgement, iatrogenic dissection, arterial rupture, perforating arteries occlusion, and acute in-stent thrombosis.

4. Treatment and follow-up

Under general anesthesia, an 8F guiding catheter, along with a 6F Navien catheter (115 cm) inserted within it, was positioned at the C2 segment of the right internal carotid artery. The angiogram confirmed the presence of occlusion of the M1 segment of the right middle cerebral artery (Fig. 6.4.23 A).

A Synchro microwire (0.014 in, 200 cm) and an Echelon-10 microcatheter successfully advanced through the lesion to the M2 segment of the right middle cerebral artery (Fig. 6.4.23 B, C). The Synchro microwire was replaced by a

Transend microwire (0.014 in, 300 cm). A 1.5 mm×10 mm Sino balloon was delivered along the Transend microwire to dilate the lesion (Fig. 6.4.24 A, B). The subsequent angiogram showed that the vessel lumen was patent without signs of thrombus formation. While retracting the microwire, an iatrogenic arterial rupture occurred as a result of a vascular avulsion injury (Fig. 6.4.24 C, D). Prompt administration of protamine was undertaken to counteract the effects of heparin. A TREK balloon (2.0 mm×8 mm) was used to dilate the M1 segment of the right middle cerebral artery at a pressure of 10 atm. The angiogram showed that the distal end of the right middle cerebral artery M1 segment was not visualized. Following a continuous five-minute balloon dilation, the subsequent angiogram revealed a significant reduction in contrast agent extravasation. (Fig. 6.4.25 A, B). Following an additional five minutes of balloon dilatation at a pressure of 10 atm, no evidence of contrast agent extravasation was observed. The trunk and division of the right middle

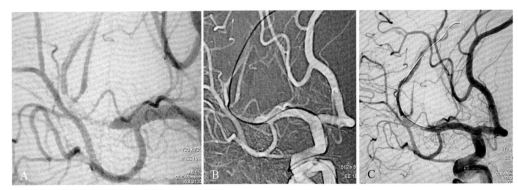

Fig. 6.4.23 (**A**) The angiogram confirmed the presence of occlusion of the M1 segment of the right middle cerebral artery. (**B**, **C**) A Synchro microwire (0.014 in, 200 cm) and an Echelon-10 microcatheter successfully advanced through the lesion to the M2 segment of the right middle cerebral artery

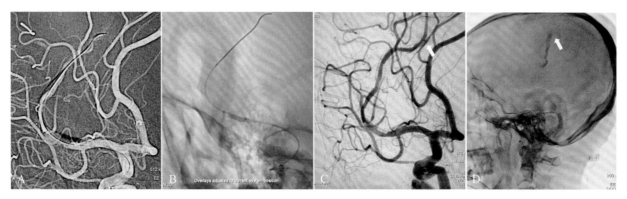

图 6.4.24　**A** 和 **B**.赛诺球囊扩张病变；**C** 和 **D**.球囊扩张后回撤导丝时牵拉血管导致出血（箭头）

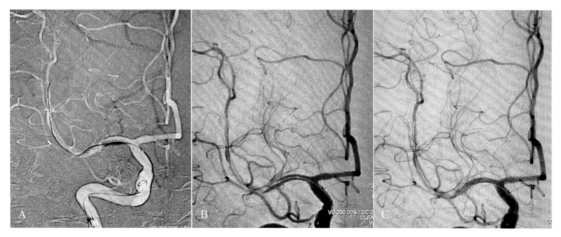

图 6.4.25　**A** 和 **B**.球囊加压止血 5 min 后造影见对比剂外渗明显减少；**C**.再次球囊加压止血 5 min 后造影未见对比剂外渗

影未见对比剂外渗，右大脑中动脉主干及分支血流通畅（图 6.4.25 C）。

术后予以镇静、镇痛、呼吸机辅助呼吸，查体双侧瞳孔等大等圆，直径约 2 mm，右侧肢体刺激可动，左侧肢体无活动。

术后第 1 日复查头部 CT 提示蛛网膜下腔出血以及脑室内出血（图 6.4.26），并予以侧脑室血肿

穿刺引流术，患者神志逐渐恢复，左侧肢体肌力较前好转。术后 15 天患者神志清楚，左侧肢体肌力4-级，转入康复医院进行肢体康复训练。

术后 3 个月患者左侧肢体肌力 5-级。CTA 提示右大脑中动脉 M1 段管腔通畅（图 6.4.27）。

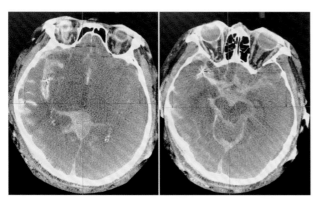

图 6.4.26　术后第 1 日复查头部 CT 提示蛛网膜下腔以及脑室内出血

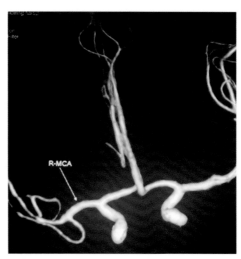

图 6.4.27　术后 3 个月复查头部 CTA 提示右大脑中动脉 M1 段管腔通畅（箭头）

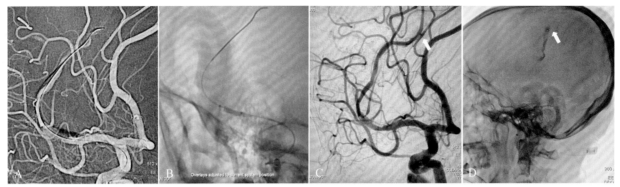

Fig. 6.4.24   The lesion was dilated with a Sino balloon (**A, B**). While retracting the microwire, an iatrogenic arterial rupture occurred as a result of a vascular avulsion injury (arrow) (**C, D**)

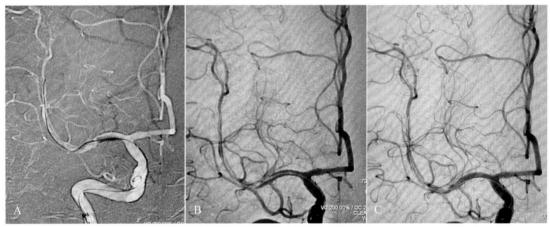

Fig. 6.4.25   (**A, B**) Following a continuous five-minute balloon dilation, the subsequent angiogram revealed a significant reduction in contrast agent extravasation. (**C**) Following an additional five minutes of balloon dilatation at a pressure of 10 atm, no evidence of contrast agent extravasation was observed

cerebral artery were patent (Fig. 6.4.25 C).

Postoperatively, sedation, analgesia, and mechanical ventilation were provided. Physical examination revealed equal and round pupils bilaterally, with a diameter of approximately 2 mm. The right extremities demonstrated responsiveness to stimulation, while the left extremities showed no movement.

On the first day following the procedure, the repeated CT scans showed the presence of subarachnoid hemorrhage and intraventricular hemorrhage (Fig. 6.4.26). The patient underwent lateral ventricular puncture drainage, leading to a gradual restoration of consciousness and improved muscle strength in the left-sided limbs. Fifteen days later, the patient had an alert state of consciousness and displayed a grade 4 level of muscle strength in the left extremities. The patient was then moved to a rehabilitation hospital for specialized limb rehabilitation training.

Three months after the procedure, the physical examination showed the muscle strength in the patient's left limbs was graded at 5. The CTA result revealed the M1 segment in the right middle cerebral artery was patent (Fig. 6.4.27).

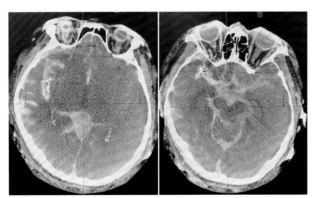

Fig. 6.4.26   On the first day following the procedure, the repeated CT scan showed the presence of subarachnoid hemorrhage and intraventricular hemorrhage

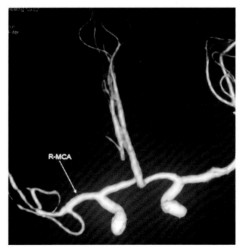

Fig. 6.4.27   The CTA result showed the M1 segment in the right middle cerebral artery was patent (arrow)

（五）讨论

本例患者右大脑中动脉闭塞，治疗过程中牵拉血管导致血管破裂出血，及时予以降低血压、鱼精蛋白中和肝素、球囊临时阻断大脑中动脉等治疗。

复查造影未见对比剂外渗，术后予以镇静、血肿穿刺引流等一系列补救治疗，患者症状逐步恢复。后期随访患者恢复良好，且右大脑中动脉管腔通畅。

（王玉峰　蒯东）

病例 44　左大脑中动脉 M1 段重度狭窄血管内治疗术中血管破裂

（一）临床病史及影像分析

患者，男性，25 岁，主因"发作性右侧肢体无力伴言语不利 1 年"入院。

当地医院完善头部 MRI 未见急性梗死灶，完善 TCD 提示左大脑中动脉 M1 段重度狭窄。为求血管内治疗转入我院。

既往史：否认高血压、糖尿病及心脏病等病史。吸烟 10 余年。

查体：神经系统查体无明显异常。

入院后完善 HRMRI：左大脑中动脉 M1 段管腔重度狭窄，管壁增厚，以腹侧壁为主（图 6.4.28）。

病后一直口服阿司匹林（100 mg 1 次 / 日）、氯吡格雷（75 mg 1 次 / 日）治疗。

（二）诊断

症状性左大脑中动脉 M1 段重度狭窄。

（三）术前讨论

结合患者病史及相关影像学检查，考虑左大脑中动脉 M1 段重度狭窄系本次发病的责任病变，有血管内介入治疗指征。相关风险包括医源性夹层、急性血栓形成、动脉破裂等。

（四）治疗过程及随访

全麻下右股动脉穿刺入路，置入 6F 导引导管送至左颈内动脉 C1 段，造影显示左大脑中动脉 M1 段重度狭窄（图 6.4.29 A）。Transend 微导丝（0.014 in，300 cm）携 Gateway 球囊（2.5 mm × 15 mm）送至左大脑中动脉 M1 段狭窄段（图 6.4.29 B），球囊扩张后造影，见 M1 段狭窄段对比剂外溢（图 6.4.29 C），将球囊回撤至出血点附近，再次缓慢充盈球囊，加压止血，约 20 min 后造影未见出血，左大脑中动脉各分支显影良好（图 6.4.29 D），右颈内动脉及左椎动脉造影见代偿良好。遂结束治疗。

术后头部 CT 见蛛网膜下腔出血及双侧侧脑室血肿形成。行双侧侧脑室穿刺引流术（图 6.4.30）。

术后第 5 天患者意识障碍较前加重，呈昏睡状，完善头部 MRI 提示左侧额、顶、颞叶皮质及皮质下、左侧基底节区、右侧丘脑急性梗死灶（图

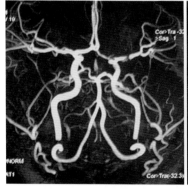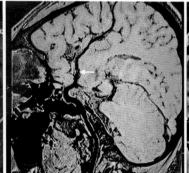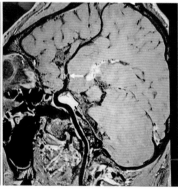

图 6.4.28　HRMRI 提示左大脑中动脉 M1 段重度狭窄伴管壁增厚（以腹侧壁为主）

5. Comments

This case involved a patient with right middle cerebral artery occlusion. During the treatment process, there was a vascular rupture and subsequent bleeding due to vessel traction. Prompt interventions were undertaken, including blood pressure reduction, neutralization of heparin with protamine sulfate, and temporary balloon occlusion of the middle cerebral artery. No contrast agent extravasation was observed in the follow-up angiography. The patient received a series of remedial treatments after the procedure, including sedation and hematoma aspiration. Gradually, the patient's symptoms improved. In the later stages of follow-up, the patient's recovery was satisfactory, and the lumen of the right middle cerebral artery remained unobstructed.

(Translated by Rongrong Cui, Revised by Zhikai Hou)

Case 44   Arterial rupture during endovascular treatment of a severe stenosis of the left middle cerebral artery M1 segment

1. Clinical presentation and radiological studies

A 25-year-old male patient presented with paroxysmal weakness in the right-sided limbs and dysphasia for one year.

The MRI results showed the absence of acute infarction. Transcranial Doppler (TCD) revealed significant stenosis in the M1 segment of the left middle cerebral artery.

The patient had been cigarette smoking for over 10 years.

Upon admission, the physical examination indicated intact neurological function.

The high-resolution MRI displayed the thickening of the M1 segment of the left middle cerebral artery, specifically in the ventral wall (Fig. 6.4.28).

Since the onset of symptoms, the patient has been prescribed a dual-antiplatelet regimen, which entails a daily administration of 100 mg of aspirin combined with a dose of 75 mg of clopidogrel.

2. Diagnosis

Symptomatic severe stenosis in the M1 segment of the left middle cerebral artery.

3. Treatment schedule

Based on the patient's clinical presentation and relevant imaging examinations, the M1 segment of the left middle cerebral artery was identified as the culprit artery. Endovascular treatment was indicated. Potential risks associated with the procedure included iatrogenic dissection, acute in-stent thrombosis, arterial rupture, etc.

4. Treatment and follow-up

Under general anesthesia, a 6F guide catheter was positioned at the C1 segment of the left internal carotid artery. The angiogram showed severe stenosis in the M1 segment of the left middle cerebral artery (Fig. 6.4.29 A). A 2.5 mm×15 mm Gateway balloon was advanced along the Transend microwire (0.014 in, 300 cm) to the M1 segment of the left middle cerebral artery (Fig. 6.4.29 B). The post-balloon dilation angiogram showed the contrast agent extravasation in the M1 segment of the left middle cerebral artery (Fig. 6.4.29 C). Subsequently, the balloon was carefully retracted to the proximity of the site of the hemorrhage and gradually inflated to manage the bleeding. Approximately 20 minutes later, the angiogram revealed no indications of recurrent bleeding. The branches of the left middle cerebral artery were adequately visualized (Fig. 6.4.29 D).

The postprocedural CT scan indicated the presence of subarachnoid hemorrhage and lateral ventricular hemorrhage. Consequently, bilateral drainage of the lateral ventricles was carried out (Fig. 6.4.30).

Post the fifth day of the procedure, the patient's level of consciousness exhibited a greater decline compared to previous

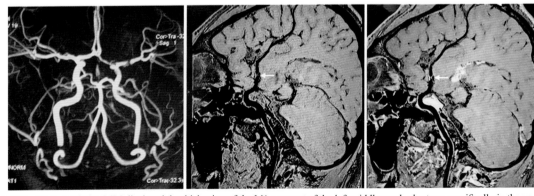

Fig. 6.4.28   High-resolution MRI displayed the thickening of the M1 segment of the left middle cerebral artery, specifically in the ventral wall

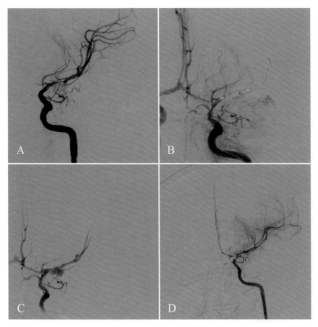

图 6.4.29 **A**. 术前造影提示左大脑中动脉 M1 段重度狭窄；**B**. Transend 微导丝携 Gateway 球囊到位于左大脑中动脉 M1 段；**C**. 球囊扩张后对比剂外溢；**D**. 球囊加压止血后造影显示出血停止，左大脑中动脉各分支显影良好

6.4.31）。继续给予镇静、脱水降颅压、预防血管痉挛以及抗癫痫等积极治疗，仍遗留有运动性失语及右侧肢体无力。

术后 1 年复查头部 MRA 发现左大脑中动脉 M1 段囊状动脉瘤（图 6.4.32）。

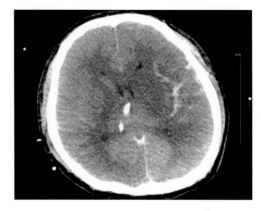

图 6.4.30 术后头部 CT 提示蛛网膜下腔出血及双侧侧脑室血肿形成

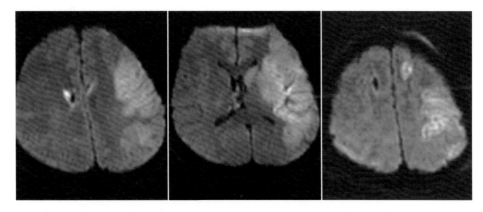

图 6.4.31 术后第 5 天头部 MRI 提示左侧额、顶、颞叶皮质及皮质下、左侧基底节区以及右侧丘脑急性梗死灶

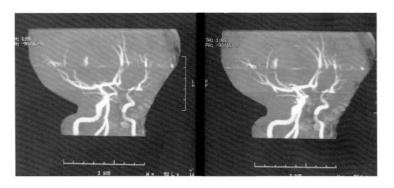

图 6.4.32 术后 1 年头部 MRA 示左大脑中动脉 M1 段囊状动脉瘤

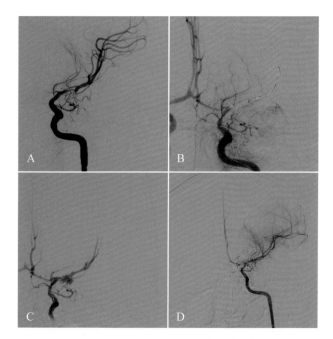

Fig. 6.4.29 (**A**) The preprocedural angiogram showed severe stenosis in the M1 segment of the left middle cerebral artery. (**B**) A Gateway balloon was navigated into the M1 segment of the left middle cerebral artery. (**C**) The post-balloon dilation angiogram showed the contrast agent extravasation. (**D**) the angiogram revealed no indications of recurrent bleeding. The branches of the left middle cerebral artery were adequately visualized

assessments. The MRI result showed acute infarction in the left frontal, parietal, and temporal lobes, as well as left basal ganglia and right thalamus (Fig. 6.4.31). Efforts were made to administer sedatives, reduce intracranial pressure through dehydration, prevent vascular spasms, and provide anticonvulsant treatment. Despite these proactive measures, the patient continued to experience motor aphasia and weakness in the right limbs.

The subsequent MRA conducted one year after the procedure revealed the presence of a saccular aneurysm located in the M1 segment of the left middle cerebral artery (Fig. 6.4.32).

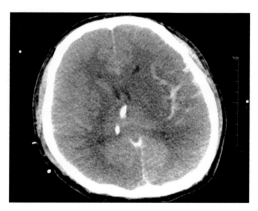

Fig. 6.4.30 Postprocedural CT scan showed subarachnoid hemorrhage and lateral ventricular hemorrhage

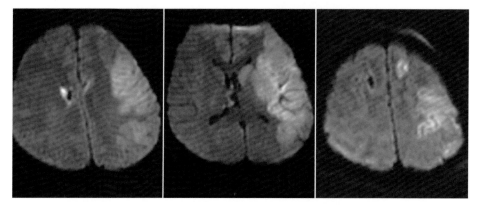

Fig. 6.4.31 The MRI result showed acute infarction in the left frontal, parietal, and temporal lobes, as well as left basal ganglia and right thalamus

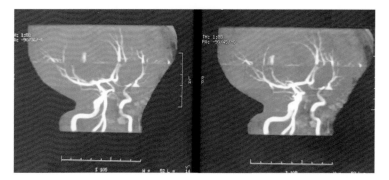

Fig. 6.4.32 The subsequent MRA revealed the presence of a saccular aneurysm located in the M1 segment of the left middle cerebral artery

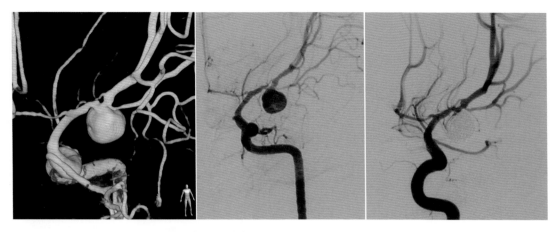

图 6.4.33 术后 1 年 DSA 示左大脑中动脉 M1 段假性动脉瘤形成，并给予支架辅助弹簧圈栓塞术

复查 DSA 提示左大脑中动脉 M1 段假性动脉瘤形成，同期给予支架辅助弹簧圈栓塞术（图 6.4.33）。

（五）讨论

本例乃青年卒中患者，因血管狭窄行血管成形术，术中血管破裂致蛛网膜下腔出血与侧脑室血肿形成，及时给予球囊加压止血后出血得到控制。患者术后 5 天发生急性脑梗死，考虑与出血后继发血管痉挛相关。给予积极对症以及康复治疗 1 年后，临床症状逐渐好转，原狭窄部位假性动脉瘤形成。

（毛更生 聂庆彬）

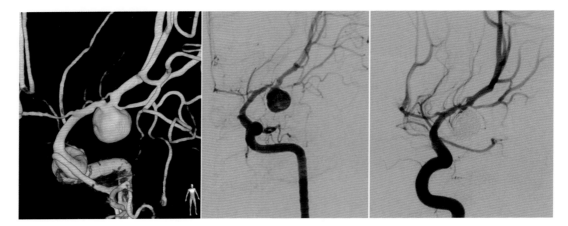

Fig. 6.4.33   The angiogram demonstrated the development of a pseudoaneurysm in the M1 segment of the left middle cerebral artery. The stent-assisted coiling procedure was performed

The angiogram demonstrated the development of a pseudoaneurysm in the M1 segment of the left middle cerebral artery. Simultaneously, the stent-assisted coiling procedure was performed (Fig. 6.4.33).

5. Comments

In this particular scenario, percutaneous transluminal angioplasty was conducted to address the significant stenosis of the M1 segment of the left middle cerebral artery. Unfortunately, an unintended vascular rupture occurred during the procedure, leading to the occurrence of subarachnoid hemorrhage and lateral ventricle hemorrhage. To manage the bleeding, a balloon occlusion procedure was implemented. However, five days after the intervention, the patient experienced an acute cerebral infarction, which suspected to be a consequence of vasospasm resulting from the previous hemorrhage. Over the course of one year, the clinical symptoms gradually ameliorated, however, a pseudoaneurysm developed at the site of the initial stenosis.

(Translated by Rongrong Cui, Revised by Zhikai Hou)

第七章

支架内再狭窄的处理

第一节　单纯球囊扩张成形术治疗支架内再狭窄

病例 45　左颈内动脉 C6 段支架内再狭窄

（一）临床病史及影像分析

患者，女性，主因"发作性右侧肢体无力9个月，言语不清及口角歪斜28天"入院。

9个月前患者出现发作性右侧肢体无力。当地医院头部CTA提示左颈内动脉C6段支架内再狭窄（图7.1.1）。给予双联抗血小板（阿司匹林及氯吡格雷）及他汀类药物（瑞舒伐他汀）调脂等治疗后，肢体无力未再发作。

28天前出现言语不清和口角歪斜。头部CT提示脑梗死（图7.1.2）。予以强化内科药物治疗仍有症状反复。患者为行血管内治疗来我院就诊。

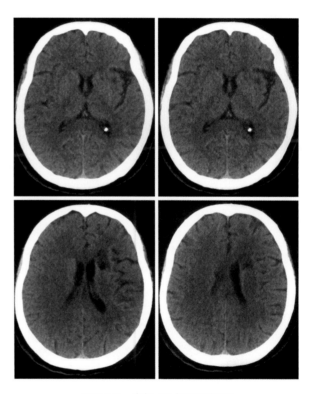

图 7.1.2　头部 CT 提示脑梗死

既往史：高血压病史6年。脑梗死病史2年（图7.1.3），同期行"左颈内动脉C6段支架置入术"（图7.1.4和图7.1.5）。

支架术后7个月复查DSA提示左颈内动脉C6段再狭窄（中度）（图7.1.6），考虑患者无症状，未予以血管内治疗。

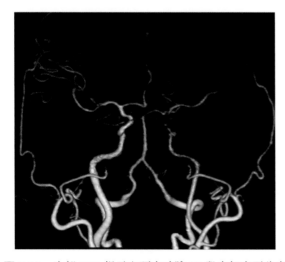

图 7.1.1　头部 CTA 提示左颈内动脉 C6 段支架内再狭窄

Chapter 7

In-stent Restenosis

Section 1　Primary Balloon Angioplasty for In–stent Restenosis

Case 45　In-stent restenosis after left internal carotid artery C6 segment stenting

1. Clinical presentation and radiological studies

A female patient was admitted to the hospital due to episodes of paroxysmal weakness in the right-sided limbs for nine months, companied by dysarthria and mouth deviation for 28 days.

Approximately nine months ago, the patient exhibited paroxysmal weakness in the right-sided limbs. The CT angiography (CTA) results showed the presence of restenosis in the stent of the left C6 segment (Fig. 7.1.1). The patient was prescribed a dual-antiplatelet regimen consisting of the Aspirin and Clopidogrel, as well as statin therapy with Rosuvastatin. The episodes of weakness in the right-sided limbs were alleviated.

She developed dysarthria and mouth deviation 28 days ago. The follow-up CT scan revealed the presence of cerebral infarction (Fig. 7.1.2). Despite receiving aggressive medical

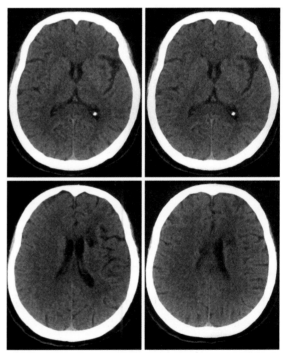

Fig. 7.1.2　The CT scan revealed the presence of cerebral infarction

treatment, the symptoms persisted and recurred.

The patient had a six-year history of hypertension. Additionally, two years prior, due to an incidence of cerebral infarction (Fig. 7.1.3). A stenting procedure was performed in the C6 segment of the left internal carotid artery (Fig. 7.1.4 and Fig. 7.1.5).

The follow-up angiogram, conducted seven months after the stent implantation, showed the presence of moderate restenosis within the stent located in the left C6 segment. However, the patient remained asymptomatic with no signs of ischemia. Consequently, further endovascular treatment was not performed (Fig. 7.1.6).

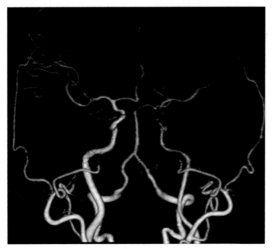

Fig. 7.1.1　The CTA indicated restenosis within the stent located in the C6 segment of the left internal carotid artery

322

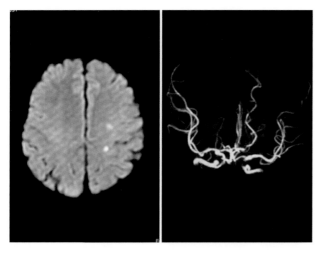

图 7.1.3 既往头部 MRI 提示左侧顶叶梗死灶，头部 MRA 提示左颈内动脉 C6 段严重狭窄

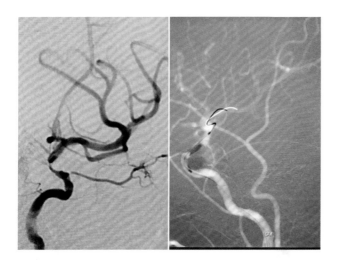

图 7.1.4 既往支架置入前造影

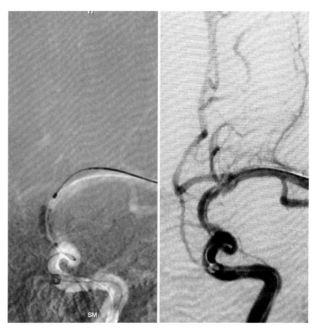

图 7.1.5 既往支架置入后造影

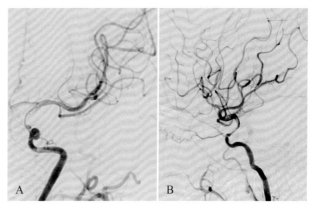

图 7.1.6 支架术后 7 个月复查 DSA 示左颈内动脉 C6 段再狭窄（中度）

查体：近记忆力减退，右侧中枢性面瘫，右侧肢体轻瘫试验（＋）。

甘油三酯（TG）：1.82 mmol/L；低密度脂蛋白胆固醇（LDL-C）：1.98 mmol/L。

入院后给予双联抗血小板（阿司匹林 100 mg 1 次 / 日＋氯吡格雷 75 mg 1 次 / 日）、降脂（瑞舒伐他汀 20 mg 1 次 / 日）等治疗。

（二）诊断

左颈内动脉 C6 段支架术后再狭窄。

（三）术前讨论

患者 9 个月内反复出现左颈内动脉系统缺血症状，内科药物治疗无效，有血管内介入治疗指征。

左颈内动脉 C6 段支架内再狭窄，拟行单纯球囊扩张，如弹性回缩明显再考虑放置支架。相关风险包括高灌注综合征、动脉夹层、血管破裂、急性或亚急性支架内血栓形成等。

（四）治疗过程

全麻下右股动脉入路，将 6F 导引导管放置在左颈内动脉 C4 段近端，术前造影示左颈内动脉 C6 段重度狭窄（图 7.1.7 A）。

路径图下沿导引导管送入 Pilot 微导丝（0.014 in，190 cm）与 Gateway 球囊（2.25 mm×15 mm）同轴，微导丝越过狭窄病变置于左大脑中动脉 M1 段，球囊到位后在狭窄处扩张一次（图 7.1.7 B）。扩张后

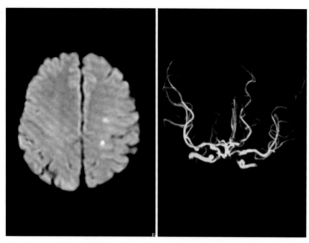

Fig. 7.1.3　The MRI conducted two years ago showed acute multiple cerebral infarctions in the left parietal lobe. The MRA results showed severe stenosis in the C6 segment of the left internal carotid artery

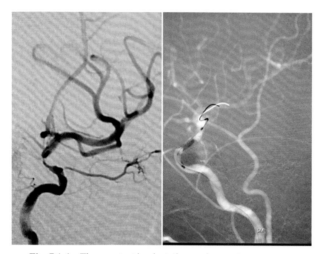

Fig. 7.1.4　The pre-stent implantation angiogram two years ago

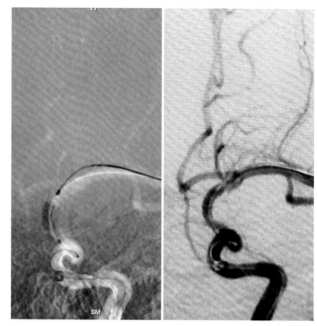

Fig. 7.1.5　The post-stent implantation angiogram two years ago

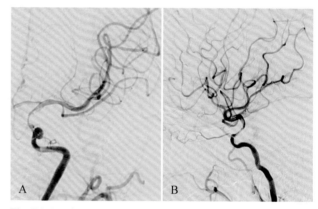

Fig. 7.1.6　The angiogram, conducted seven months after the stent implantation, showed the presence of moderate restenosis within the stent located in the left C6 segment

Physical examination showed short-term memory impairment and right-sided central facial paralysis. The hemiparesis test in the right-sided limbs was positive.

The serum concentration of the triglyceride and LDL cholesterol (LDL-C) was measured at 1.82 mmol/L and 1.98 mmol/L, respectively.

Upon admission, She was prescribed a dual antiplatelet regimen consisting of a daily dose of 100 mg of Aspirin and 75 mg of Clopidogrel, as well as statin therapy with a daily dose of 20 mg of Rosuvastatin.

2. Diagnosis

In-stent restenosis within the C6 segment of the left internal carotid artery.

3. Treatment schedule

The patient exhibited recurrent symptoms of ischemic events within the left carotid artery system. Despite the intensive medical intervention, the symptoms of ischemia persisted and recurred. Endovascular treatment was indicated for her. The balloon angioplasty will be carried out to address the in-stent restenosis in the left LC6. If there was a significant elastic recoil, stent implantation would be taken into consideration. Potential risks associated with the procedure include hyperperfusion syndrome, arterial dissection, vessel rupture, and acute/ subacute in-stent thrombosis.

4. Treatment

Under general anesthesia, a 6F guiding catheter was positioned at the C4 segment of the left internal carotid artery. The angiogram confirmed severe stenosis in the C6 segment of the left internal carotid artery (Fig. 7.1.7 A).

Under the roadmap, A Pilot microwire (0.014 in, 190 cm) successfully navigated through the stenotic segment to reach the M1 segment of the left middle cerebral artery. A Gateway balloon (2.25 mm×15 mm) was delivered along the microwire and dilated the lesion (Fig. 7.1.7 B). The post-

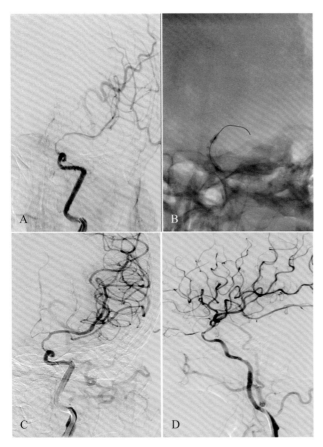

图 7.1.7　**A**. 术前造影示左颈内动脉 C6 段重度狭窄；**B**. Gateway 球囊扩张病变；**C** 和 **D**. 球囊扩张后造影

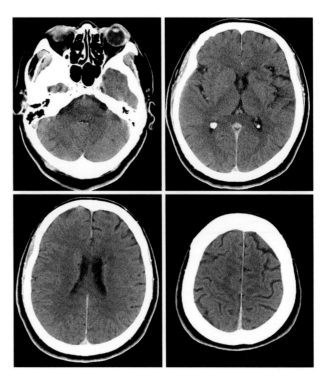

图 7.1.8　术后头部 CT 未见出血

造影显示残余狭窄率约 40%，前向血流 mTICI 分级 3 级（图 7.1.7 C 和 D）。

术后头部 CT 未见出血（图 7.1.8）。

术后 CTA：左颈内动脉颅内段及左大脑中动脉显影较术前明显改善（图 7.1.9）。

（五）讨论

颈内动脉颅内段较颅内其他部位更易发生支架内再狭窄，相较于无症状性再狭窄，症状性再狭窄的狭窄程度更重。处理再狭窄时一般选择单纯球囊扩张，若效果不好再考虑放置支架，如路径好，可以考虑放置药物涂层支架。本例因再狭窄程度重，为预防高灌注综合征，未选择更大直径的球囊。

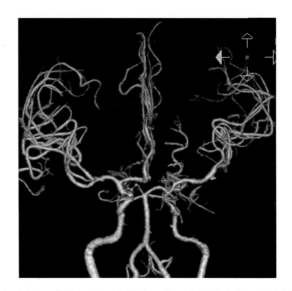

图 7.1.9　术后 CTA 示左颈内动脉颅内段及左大脑中动脉显影较前改善

（杨炯　张义森　姜鹏　马宁）

7.1　手术操作视频
（病例 **45**）

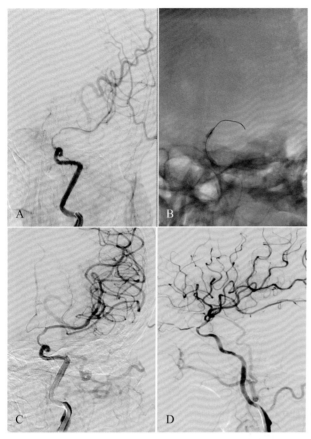

Fig. 7.1.7 (**A**) The preprocedural angiogram showed severe stenosis in the C6 segment of the left internal carotid artery. (**B**) A Gateway balloon was utilized to dilate the lesion. (**C, D**) The post-balloon balloon dilation angiogram

balloon dilation angiogram showed residual stenosis of approximately 40%, accompanied by antegrade blood flow in mTICI grade 3 (Fig. 7.1.7 C, D).

Post-procedural CT scan showed no signs of intracranial hemorrhage (Fig. 7.1.8).

The post-procedural CTA revealed enhanced visualization of both the intracranial segment of the left internal carotid artery and the left middle cerebral artery compared to the pre-procedure scans (Fig. 7.1.9).

5. Comments

The incidence of in-stent restenosis in the intracranial segment of the internal carotid artery was more prevalent compared to other intracranial arteries. Moreover, the stenosis degree of symptomatic in-stent restenosis was more significant compared to asymptomatic cases. Primary balloon angioplasty was the common treatment approach for addressing in-stent restenosis. Stent implantation was reserved only for cases of significant elastic recoil while drug-eluting stents were considered as an alternative option if the access approach was smooth. In this case, the patients had severe in-stent restenosis, and the use of a large-diameter balloon angioplasty was avoided to prevent hyperperfusion syndrome.

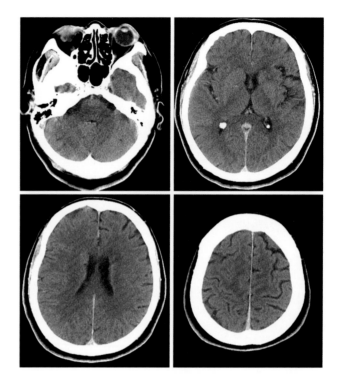

Fig. 7.1.8 The postprocedural CT scans showed no signs of intracerebral hemorrhage

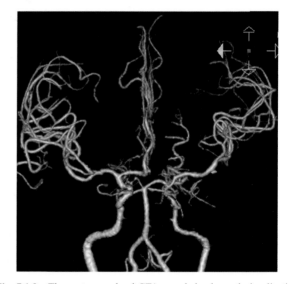

Fig. 7.1.9 The post-procedural CTA revealed enhanced visualization of both the intracranial segment of the left internal carotid artery and the left middle cerebral artery compared to the pre-procedure scans

(Translated by Rongrong Cui, Revised by Zhikai Hou)

7.1   Video of endovascular therapy (Case 45)

病例 46 基底动脉支架内再狭窄

（一）临床病史及影像分析

患者，男性，57 岁，因"发作性头晕 2 个月"入院。

6 年前头部 CTA：基底动脉中段重度狭窄，右椎动脉 V4 段重度狭窄，左椎基底动脉交界区中度狭窄（图 7.1.10）。

6 年前 DSA：基底动脉中段重度狭窄（图 7.1.11 A 和 B）。于狭窄处置入 Apollo 球囊扩张式支架一枚（2.5 mm×8 mm），支架置入术后残余狭窄率约10%（图 7.1.11 C 和 D）。

术后患者头晕症状完全缓解，分别于术后 1 个月复查头部 CTA（图 7.1.12 A 和 B）、术后 6 个月复查头颈部 CTA（图 7.1.12 C 和 D）、术后 1 年复查

DSA（图 7.1.13），均提示基底动脉无明显再狭窄。

2 个月前，患者突发头晕，复查头部 CTA 提示基底动脉支架内再狭窄（图 7.1.14）。头颅 CT 提示右枕叶陈旧性梗死（图 7.1.15）。患者为进一步治疗，再次入院。

既往史：高血压病史 15 年。

查体：神经系统查体无明显异常。

患者第一次支架术后长期口服阿司匹林，并行降压治疗，再次发病后加用了氯吡格雷 75 mg 1 次 / 日。

（二）诊断

症状性基底动脉支架内再狭窄。

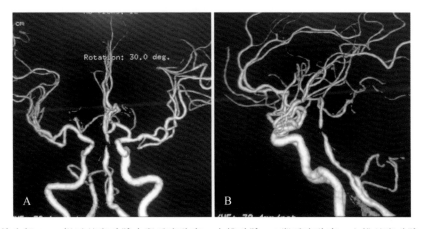

图 7.1.10 6 年前头部 CTA 提示基底动脉中段重度狭窄，右椎动脉 V4 段重度狭窄，左椎基底动脉交界区中度狭窄

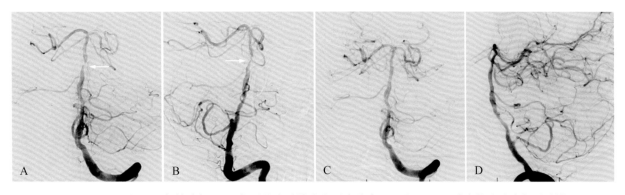

图 7.1.11 **A** 和 **B**.6 年前头部 DSA 提示基底动脉中段重度狭窄；**C** 和 **D**.置入球囊扩张式支架后造影

Case 46　In-stent restenosis after the basilar artery stenting

1. Clinical presentation and radiological studies

A 57-year-old male patient was admitted to the hospital due to episodes of paroxysmal dizziness for two months.

The CTA examination conducted six years ago showed severe stenosis in both the mid-basilar artery and the V4 segment of the right vertebral artery, along with moderate stenosis at the junction of the left vertebro-basilar artery (Fig. 7.1.10).

The angiogram conducted six years ago revealed severe stenosis of the mid-basilar artery (Fig. 7.1.11 A, B). A balloon-mounted Apollo stent (2.5 mm×8 mm) was implanted in the mid-basilar artery, leaving approximately 10% of residual stenosis (Fig. 7.1.11 C, D).

The symptoms of dizziness were completely alleviated after the stent implantation. The follow-up CTA scans conducted at one month (Fig. 7.1.12 A, B), six months (Fig. 7.1.12 C, D), and the angiogram conducted after one year (Fig. 7.1.13) all indicated the absence of restenosis in the stented basilar artery.

A recurrence of dizziness episodes occurred two months ago. Subsequent CTA follow-up indicated the occurrence of restenosis in the stented basilar artery (Fig. 7.1.14). Additionally, a CT scan revealed the presence of an old infarction in the right occipital lobe (Fig. 7.1.15).

He had a medical history of hypertension for 15 years.

Upon admission, the physical examination indicated intact neurological function.

Following the implantation of the basilar artery stent, the patient was prescribed Aspirin and antihypertensive medication. In light of the recurrence of dizziness symptoms, a daily dose of 75 mg of Clopidogrel was added to the patient's treatment regimen.

2. Diagnosis

Symptomatic in-stent restenosis within the basilar artery.

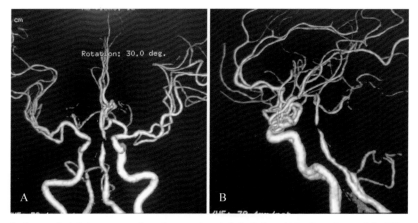

Fig. 7.1.10　The CTA examination conducted six years ago showed severe stenosis in both the mid-basilar artery and the V4 segment of the right vertebral artery, along with moderate stenosis at the junction of the left vertebro-basilar artery (**A**, **B**)

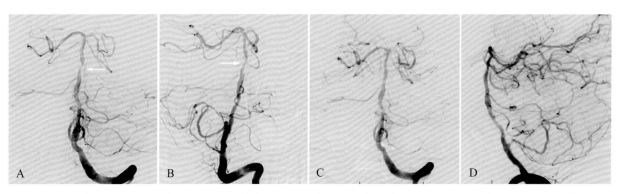

Fig. 7.1.11　The angiogram conducted six years ago revealed severe stenosis of the mid-basilar artery (**A**, **B**). A balloon-mounted Apollo stent was implanted in the mid-basilar artery (**C**, **D**)

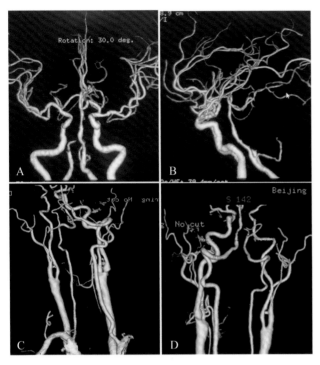

图 7.1.12　**A** 和 **B**. 术后 1 个月 CTA 未见支架内再狭窄；**C** 和 **D**. 术后 6 个月头颈部 CTA 未见支架内再狭窄

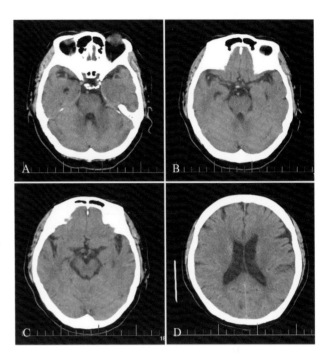

图 7.1.15　头部 CT 提示右枕叶陈旧性梗死

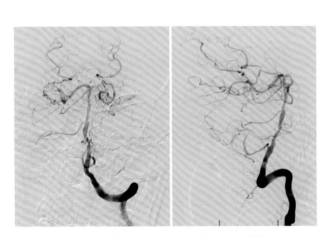

图 7.1.13　术后 1 年 DSA 未见支架内再狭窄

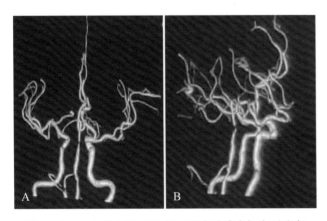

图 7.1.14　2 月前头部 CTA 提示基底动脉支架内再狭窄

（三）术前讨论

结合患者病史、临床症状及近期影像学检查，考虑基底动脉支架内再狭窄，拟采用单纯球囊扩张治疗，若弹性回缩明显或夹层形成再考虑置入支架。相关风险包括扩张病变困难、穿支动脉卒中、支架内血栓形成、医源性夹层等。

（四）治疗过程

全麻下右股动脉穿刺入路，将 6F 导引导管置于左锁骨下动脉近端造影显示，左椎动脉 V1 段重度狭窄（图 7.1.16 A），置入 Blue 球囊扩张式支架（5.0 mm×12 mm）（图 7.1.16 B）。经左椎动脉造影显示基底动脉支架术后再狭窄，狭窄程度约 90%，左椎基底动脉交界区中度狭窄（图 7.1.16 C 和 D）。

6F 导引导管跟进左椎动脉 V1 段支架略受阻，未做尝试，更换右椎动脉入路，将导引导管放置在右椎动脉 V2 段水平。将 Transend 微导丝（0.014 in，300 cm）结合 Gateway 球囊（2.5 mm×9 mm）越过病变，以命名压扩张病变一次（图 7.1.17 A 和 B）。撤出球囊及微导丝，造影显示原再狭窄处明

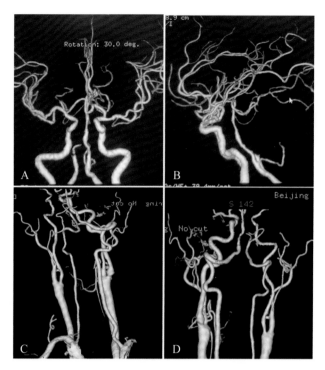

Fig. 7.1.12 The follow-up CTA scans at one month (**A**, **B**) and six months (**C**, **D**) revealed no evidence of restenosis in the stented basilar artery

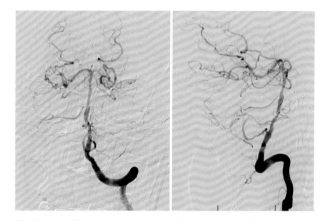

Fig. 7.1.13 The angiogram conducted at one year revealed the absence of the in-stent restenosis

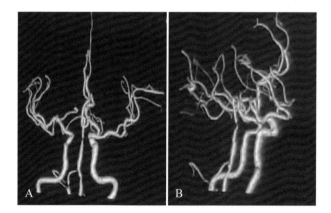

Fig. 7.1.14 The follow-up CTA indicated the occurrence of restenosis in the stented basilar artery

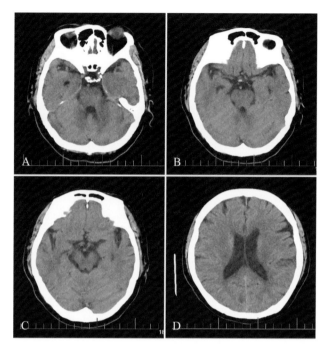

Fig. 7.1.15 The CT scans revealed the presence of an old infarction in the right occipital lobe

3. Treatment schedule

Based on the patient's clinical presentation and relevant radiological studies, the restenosis within the basilar artery stent was diagnosed. The approach to address the restenosis lesion was the primary balloon angioplasty. In cases where there was obvious elastic recoil or iatrogenic dissection, stent implantation was also considered. Potential risks associated with the procedure included difficulty in dilating the restenosis lesion, perforating artery occlusion, in-stent thrombosis, and iatrogenic dissection.

4. Treatment

Under general anesthesia, a 6F guide catheter was positioned at the proximal end of the left subclavian artery. The angiogram showed severe stenosis at the V1 segment of the left vertebral artery (Fig. 7.1.16 A). Subsequently, a Blue balloon-mounted stent (5.0 mm×12 mm) was implanted at the V1 segment of the left vertebral artery (Fig. 7.1.16 B). The angiogram of the left vertebral artery revealed a restenosis within the basilar artery stent, with a significant degree of stenosis at 90%. Additionally, there is a moderate stenosis observed at the junction of the left vertebro-basilar artery (Fig. 7.1.16 C, D).

The 6F guide catheter had difficulty advancing through the V1 segment of the left vertebral artery. Therefore, the right vertebral artery was selected as the treatment access. The guide catheter be positioned at the V2 segment of the right vertebral artery. A Gateway balloon (2.5 mm× 9 mm), in combination with a Transend microwire (0.014 in, 300 cm), navigated through the stenosis lesion. The lesion was dilated at a nominal pressure (Fig. 7.1.17 A, B).

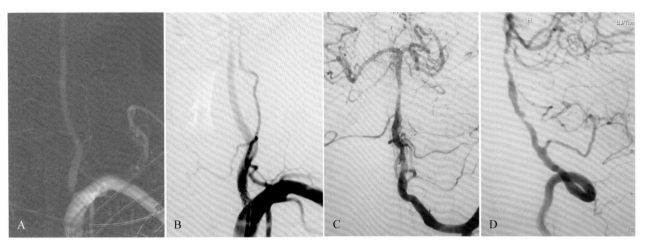

图 7.1.16　**A**. 术前造影提示左椎动脉 V1 段重度狭窄；**B**. 于左椎动脉 V1 段置入 Blue 球囊扩张式支架；**C** 和 **D**. 经左椎动脉造影显示基底动脉支架术后再狭窄，狭窄程度约 90%，左椎基底动脉交界区中度狭窄

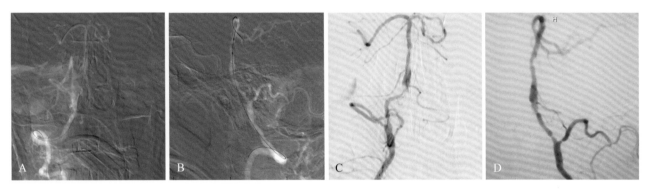

图 7.1.17　**A** 和 **B**. Gateway 球囊扩张狭窄病变；**C** 和 **D**. 球囊扩张后造影显示原再狭窄处明显改善，未见医源性夹层，残余狭窄率约 20%

显改善，未见医源性夹层，残余狭窄率约 20%（图 7.1.17 C 和 D）。观察 10 min，重复造影局部无变化后结束治疗。

术后患者头晕症状缓解。

（五）讨论

支架内再狭窄是颅内动脉粥样硬化狭窄患者支架置入术后常见的远期并发症之一。目前针对颅内动脉支架内再狭窄的处理策略如下：若为无症状性支架内再狭窄，可继续保守治疗；若为症状性支架内再狭窄，可考虑再次干预治疗，再次干预治疗一般选择单纯球囊扩张。但我们近期的研究结果表明，支架内再狭窄行单纯球囊扩张的效果似乎比再次置入支架的远期疗效差，这一结论还需要后续临床研究予以证实。此外，本例基底动脉支架内再狭窄可能与动脉粥样硬化进展有关（患者左椎动脉 V1 段出现新的狭窄）。再狭窄处理后依然有再次狭窄可能，有研究报道使用药物涂层球囊来治疗支架内再狭窄，我们期望未来能进行类似的临床尝试。

（尤吉栋　贾白雪　孙立倩　马宁）

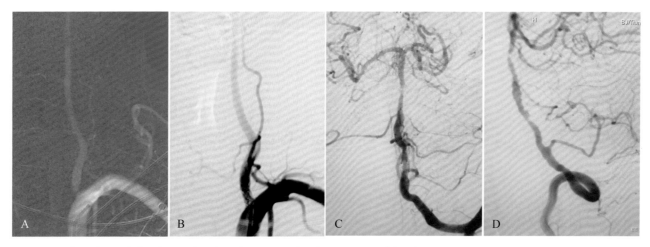

Fig. 7.1.16   The angiogram before the procedure showed severe stenosis at the V1 segment of the left vertebral artery (**A**). A Blue balloon-mounted stent was deployed at the V1 segment of the left vertebral artery (**B**). The angiogram of the left vertebral artery revealed a re-stenosis within the basilar artery stent, with a significant degree of stenosis at 90%. Additionally, there is a moderate stenosis observed at the junction of the left vertebro-basilar artery (**C, D**)

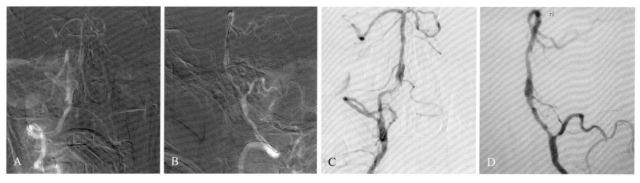

Fig. 7.1.17   A Gateway balloon was utilized to dilate the lesion (**A, B**). The subsequent angiogram demonstrated a residual stenosis of around 20%, with no indication of iatrogenic arterial dissection (**C, D**)

The subsequent angiogram demonstrated a residual stenosis of around 20%, with no indication of iatrogenic arterial dissection (Fig. 7.1.17 C, D). Following a-10 minutes of observation, the repeated angiogram showed no alteration in the stenosis lesion. Therefore the procedure was terminated.

The patient's dizziness was relieved post-operation.

5. Comments

In-stent restenosis is one of the common long-term complications in patients with intracranial atherosclerotic stenosis after stent implantation. The current management strategies for intracranial in-stent restenosis are as follows: for asymptomatic in-stent restenosis, conservative treatment can be continued. For symptomatic in-stent restenosis, repeat interventional therapy with balloon angioplasty is considered the preferred approach. However, our recent research findings indicated that the efficacy of primary balloon angioplasty for in-stent restenosis appeared to be inferior to the long-term benefits of re-stenting. This conclusion still requires confirmation in the subsequent clinical studies. Additionally, in this case of basilar artery instent restenosis, it may be associated with the progression of atherosclerosis (new stenosis observed in the patient's left vertebral artery V1 segment). It was noteworthy that the potential for recurrent stenosis still exists following endovascular treatment for restenosis. Studies have reported the use of drug-coated balloons for the treatment of in-stent restenosis, and we look forward to explore similar clinical approaches in the future.

(Translated by Rongrong Cui, Revised by Zhikai Hou)

第二节 支架置入治疗支架内再狭窄

病例 47 自膨式支架治疗基底动脉支架内再狭窄

（一）临床病史及影像分析

患者，男性，51 岁，主因"发作性视物模糊 7 个月，头晕、言语不清伴右侧肢体无力 23 天"入院。

患者 7 个月前发生脑梗死。头颅 MRI 示左大脑半球分水岭急性梗死灶（图 7.2.1）。头部 MRA 示左颈内动脉闭塞，基底动脉中段重度狭窄（图 7.2.2）。CTA 示左颈内动脉闭塞，基底动脉重度狭窄（图 7.2.3）。给予双联抗血小板（阿司匹林和氯吡格雷）以及他汀类药物（阿托伐他汀）等治疗后，双眼视物模糊仍反复发作。

DSA 示右颈内动脉未见明显狭窄（图 7.2.4），左颈内动脉闭塞（图 7.2.5），基底动脉中段重度狭窄（图 7.2.6），左后交通动脉向左大脑中动脉代偿供血（图 7.2.7）。同期于基底动脉狭窄处置入一枚 Apollo 支架（2.5 mm×8 mm）（图 7.2.8）。因患者痛风发作，

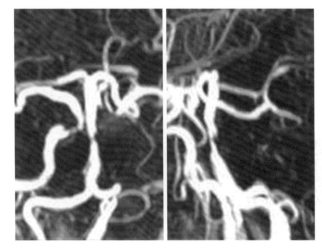

图 7.2.2 7 个月前头部 MRA 示左颈内动脉闭塞，基底动脉中段重度狭窄

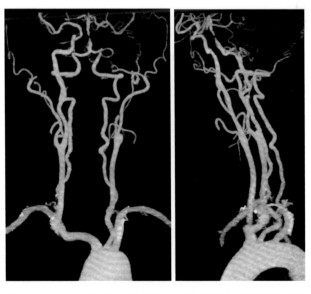

图 7.2.3 7 个月前 CTA 示左颈内动脉闭塞，基底动脉重度狭窄

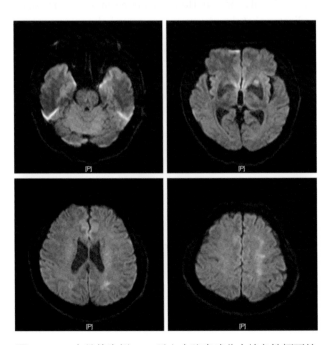

图 7.2.1 7 个月前头颅 MRI 示左大脑半球分水岭急性梗死灶

术后给予氯吡格雷＋西洛他唑抗血小板聚集治疗。

术后 3 个月 CTA 示基底动脉支架内再狭窄（图 7.2.9），CTP 提示后循环低灌注（图 7.2.10）。

Section 2 Stenting for In–stent Restenosis

Case 47 Self-expanding stenting for in-stent restenosis of the basilar artery

1. Clinical presentation and radiological studies

A 51-year-old man was admitted to the hospital because he had intermittent blurred vision for seven months and experienced dizziness, slurred speech, and weakness in his right limbs for 23 days.

The patient had a cerebral infarction seven months ago. Subsequent MRI indicated acute ischemic infarction in the left watershed area (Fig. 7.2.1). The MRA revealed the left internal carotid artery occlusion and significant narrowing of the mid-basilar artery (Fig. 7.2.2). The CTA revealed the occlusion of the left internal carotid artery and the severe stenosis of the mid-basilar artery (Fig. 7.2.3). Despite undergoing intensive medical treatment, he continued to experience recurring episodes of blurred vision.

The angiogram did not show any significant narrowing in the right internal carotid artery (Fig. 7.2.4). However, it revealed an occlusion in the left internal carotid artery (Fig. 7.2.5), as well as the detection of severe narrowing in the mid-basilar artery (Fig. 7.2.6). The territory of the left middle cerebral artery was compensated by the ipsilateral left posterior cerebral artery through the unobstructed posterior communicating artery

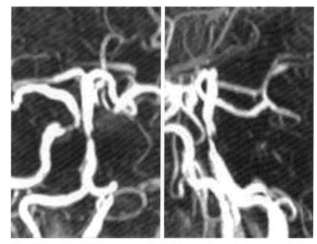

Fig. 7.2.2 The MRA revealed the left internal carotid artery occlusion and significant narrowing of the mid-basilar artery

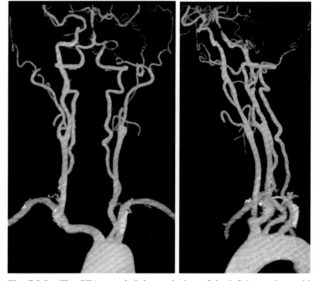

Fig. 7.2.3 The CTA revealed the occlusion of the left internal carotid artery and the severe stenosis of the mid-basilar artery

(Fig. 7.2.7). An Apollo stent (2.5 mm × 8 mm) was implanted the basilar artery stenosis (Fig. 7.2.8). Given the gout attack, Clopidogrel and Cilostazol were selected as the antiplatelet regimen following the procedure.

The subsequent CTA results, conducted three months post-procedure, revealed restenosis within the basilar artery stent (Fig. 7.2.9), accompanied by hypoperfusion in the posterior circulation as depicted by the CTP findings (Fig. 7.2.10).

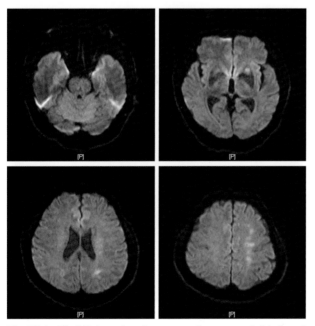

Fig. 7.2.1 The MRA conducted seven months ago revealed indicated the left internal carotid artery occlusion and significant narrowing of the mid-basilar artery

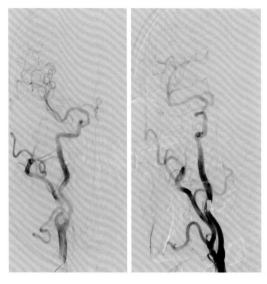

图 7.2.4 DSA 示右颈内动脉未见明显狭窄

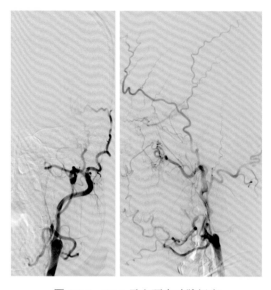

图 7.2.5 DSA 示左颈内动脉闭塞

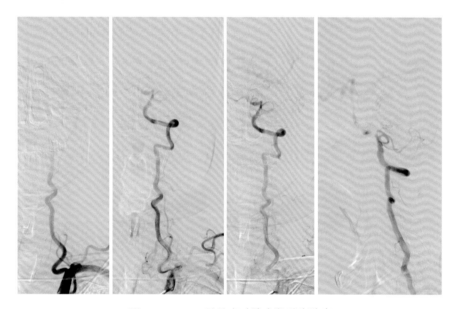

图 7.2.6 DSA 示基底动脉中段重度狭窄

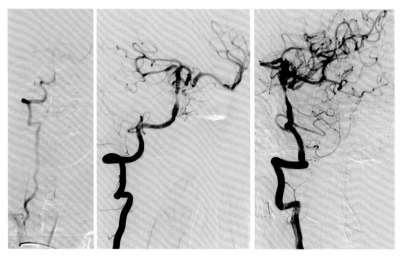

图 7.2.7 DSA 示左后交通动脉向左大脑中动脉代偿供血

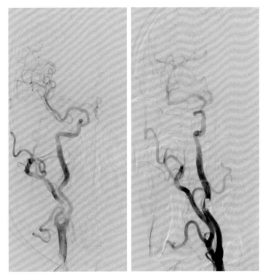

Fig. 7.2.4 The angiogram did not show any significant narrowing in the right internal carotid artery

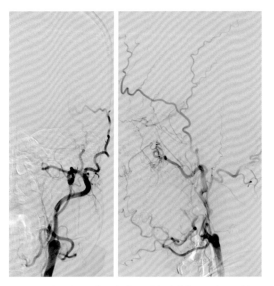

Fig. 7.2.5 DSA showed occlusion of the left internal carotid artery

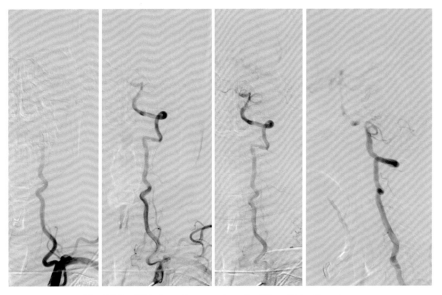

Fig. 7.2.6 DSA showed severe stenosis of the mid-basilar artery

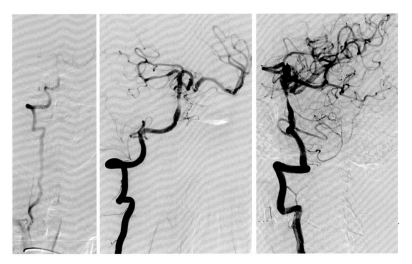

Fig. 7.2.7 The territory of the left middle cerebral artery was compensated by the ipsilateral left posterior cerebral artery through the unobstructed posterior communicating artery

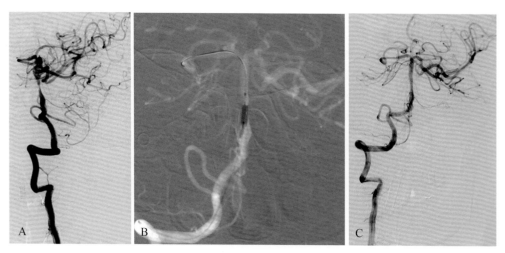

图 7.2.8 **A**. 术前造影提示基底动脉重度狭窄；**B**. 释放 Apollo 支架；**C**. 释放 Apollo 支架后造影

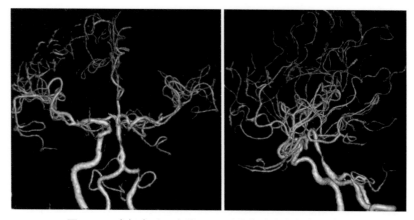

图 7.2.9 支架术后 3 个月 CTA 示基底动脉支架内再狭窄

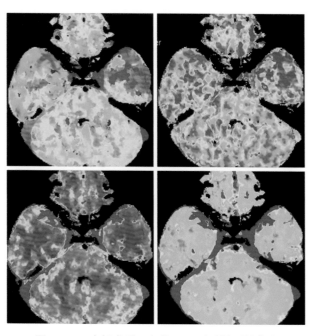

图 7.2.10 支架术后 3 个月 CTP 示后循环低灌注

23 天前患者再次出现头晕、言语不清伴右侧肢体无力。头颅 MRI 示脑桥梗死（图 7.2.11）。CTA 示基底动脉重度狭窄至闭塞（图 7.2.12）。DSA 确认基底动脉中段闭塞（图 7.2.13）。患者为进一步治疗再次入院。

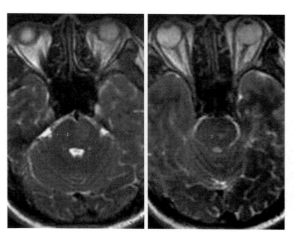

图 7.2.11 23 天前头颅 MRI 示脑桥梗死

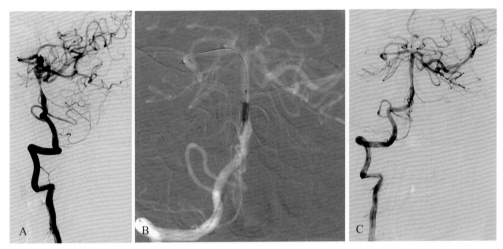

Fig. 7.2.8 (**A**) Preprocedural angiogram revealed severe stenosis of the basilar artery. (**B**) An Apollo stent was deployed. (**C**) The angiogram after deploying the Apollo stent

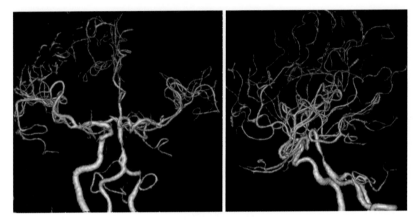

Fig. 7.2.9 CTA conducted three months post-procedure revealed restenosis within the basilar artery stent

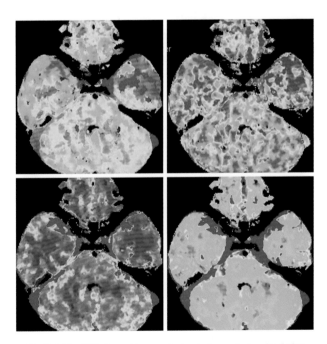

Fig. 7.2.10 CTP showed hypoperfusion in the posterior circulation

Twenty-three days ago, the patient presented with symptoms of dizziness, slurred speech, and weakness in the right extremities. The follow-up MRI revealed cerebral infarction in the pontine (Fig. 7.2.11). The CT angiography revealed the presence of severe stenosis or total occlusion of the basilar artery (Fig. 7.2.12). The angiogram confirmed the total occlusion at the middle segment of the basilar artery (Fig. 7.2.13).

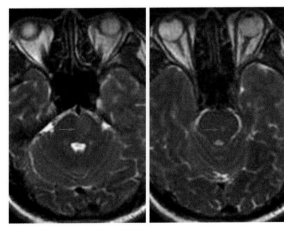

Fig. 7.2.11 The MRI results showed cerebral infarcts in the pontine

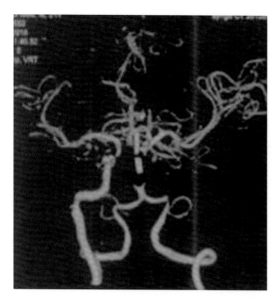

图 7.2.12　23 天前 CTA 示基底动脉重度狭窄，不除外闭塞可能

既往史：高血压、痛风病史，以及吸烟、饮酒史。

查体：构音障碍，右侧肢体肌力 4 级。NIHSS 评分 5 分，mRS 评分 3 分。

低密度脂蛋白胆固醇（LDL-C）：2.15 mmol/L。

血栓弹力图：ADP 抑制率 9.8%。

CYP2C19 基因检测：中等代谢型。

入院后给予双联抗血小板聚集（阿司匹林 100 mg 1 次 / 日＋替格瑞洛 90 mg 2 次 / 日）、降脂（瑞舒伐他汀 10 mg 1 次 / 日）及降压等治疗。

（二）诊断

基底动脉支架内再狭窄。

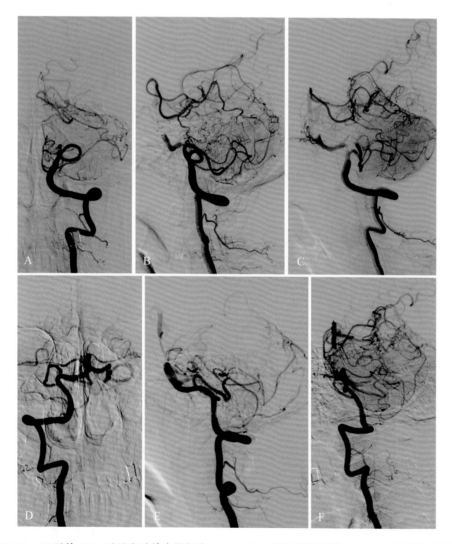

图 7.2.13　23 天前 DSA 示基底动脉中段闭塞。**A ～ C.** 左侧椎动脉造影；**D ～ F.** 右侧椎动脉造影

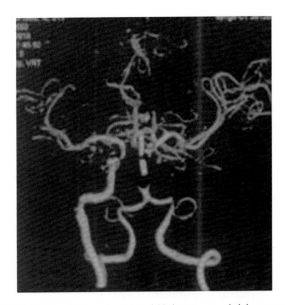

Fig. 7.2.12 The CTA result conducted 23 days ago revealed the presence of severe stenosis or total occlusion of the basilar artery

He has a medical history including hypertension, gout, cigarette smoking, and alcohol drinking.

The physical assessment exhibited dysarthria, with a muscle strength rating of 4 in the right extremities. The National Institutes of Health Stroke Scale (NIHSS) score was 5, and the modified Rankin Scale (mRS) score was 3.

The serum LDL-C concentration was determined to be 2.15 mmol/L.

The thromboelastography test indicated an ADP inhibition of 9.8%.

The CYP2C19 genotype indicated a moderate metabolizer status.

Upon admission, the patient was administered a dual antiplatelet regimen comprising a daily dose of 100 mg of Aspirin and twice daily doses of 90 mg of Ticagrelor, as well as statin therapy with a daily dose of 10 mg of Rosuvastatin.

2. Diagnosis

In-stent restenosis within the basilar artery.

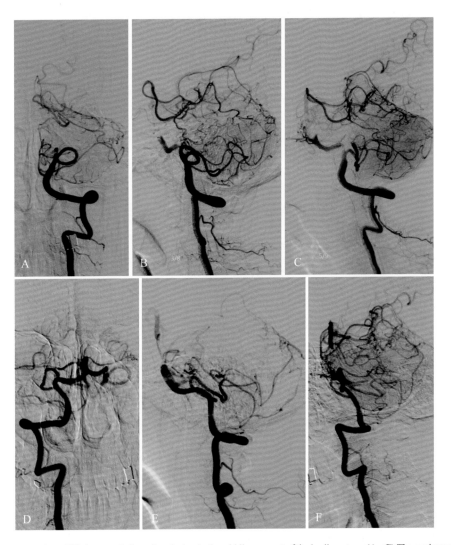

Fig. 7.2.13 The angiogram conducted 23 days ago indicated occlusion in the middle segment of the basilar artery. (**A**–**C**) The angiogram of the left vertebral artery. (**D**–**F**) The angiogram of the right vertebral artery

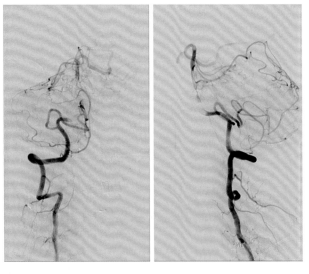

图 7.2.14 术前造影证实基底动脉中段闭塞

（三）术前讨论

患者基底动脉相关供血区域新发脑梗死，结合影像学检查，考虑基底动脉支架内再狭窄，有血管内治疗的指征。拟先行球囊扩张，再酌情考虑是否置入支架。相关风险包括急性或亚急性血栓形成、开通失败等。

（四）治疗过程

全麻下右股动脉入路，6F 导引导管至右椎动脉 V2 段远端，造影证实基底动脉中段闭塞（图7.2.14）。

路径图下沿导引导管送入 Pilot 50 微导丝（0.014 in，190 cm），在 Echelon-10 微导管辅助下通过基底动脉闭塞段至左大脑后动脉 P2 段远端（图 7.2.15 A 和 B），其后更换为 Transend 微导丝（0.014 in，300 cm）。沿 Transend 微导丝送入 SoloFlex 球囊（2.5 mm×15 mm）扩张 2 次，扩张后造影显示，基底动脉闭塞未见缓解（图 7.2.15 C 和 D）。更换 Rebar-18 微导管至基底动脉顶端，送入 Solitaire AB 支架（6.0 mm×30 mm），释放后前向血流改善（图 7.2.16 A 和 B）。经导引导管动脉内给予替罗非班 0.4 mg，观察 5 min 后造影示基底动脉及各分支通畅，支架贴壁良好，管腔较前光滑。撤出支架输送系统，观察 10 min 后反复多角度造影示基底动脉及各分支通畅，mTICI 分级 3 级，基底动脉中段残余狭窄率约 30%（图 7.2.16 C 和 D）。

术后头部 CT：未见脑出血、蛛网膜下腔出血

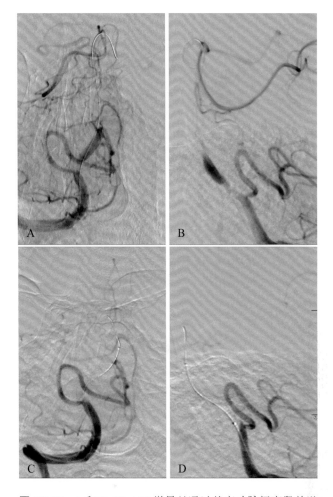

图 7.2.15 **A** 和 **B**. Pilot 50 微导丝通过基底动脉闭塞段并送至左大脑后动脉 P2 段；**C** 和 **D**. 球囊扩张 2 次后基底动脉闭塞未见缓解

（图 7.2.17）。

术后 CTA 示基底动脉支架内血流通畅（图7.2.18），CTP 示后循环灌注较前改善（图7.2.19）。

患者自述头脑较前清醒，言语较前清晰，右侧肢体活动较前灵活。

（五）讨论

颅内动脉支架内再狭窄的处理，一般选择单纯球囊扩张。若回缩明显，可考虑放置自膨式或者球囊扩张式支架（酌情考虑冠状动脉支架）。本例球囊扩张后基底动脉仍未开通，考虑局部斑块负荷大，有可能形成附壁血栓，但也不除外夹层可能，遂选择较长的 Solitaire 支架以覆盖病变，并动脉内联合静脉内给予替罗非班。支架置入后虽有一定的残余狭窄，但考虑局部斑块不稳定，未行后扩张。

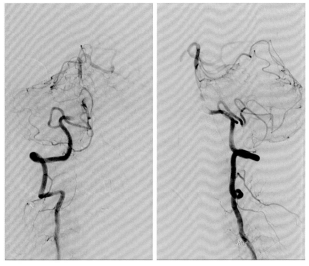

Fig. 7.2.14　The angiogram before the procedure confirmed occlusion in the middle segment of the basilar artery

3. Treatment schedule

Based on the patient's clinical manifestation and relevant radiological studies, it was determined that the patient displayed symptomatic in-stent restenosis of the basilar artery. Consequently, endovascular intervention was advised. Balloon angioplasty was scheduled as the chosen method for endovascular treatment. Stent deployment was considered if there was significant elastic recoil. Potential risks associated with the procedure included acute/subacute thrombosis and unsuccessful recanalization.

4. Treatment

Under general anesthesia, a 6F guiding catheter was positioned at the V2 segment of the right vertebral artery. The angiogram indicated occlusion at the middle segment of the basilar artery (Fig. 7.2.14).

Under the roadmap, A Pilot 50 microwire (0.014 in, 190 cm) and an Echelon-10 microcatheter coaxially navigated through the occlusion segment of the basilar artery to the P2 segment of the left posterior cerebral artery (Fig. 7.2.15 A, B). A SoloFlex balloon (2.5 mm×15 mm) was dilated the lesion twice. The post-balloon angioplasty angiogram showed the basilar artery remained occluded (Fig. 7.2.15 C, D). A self-expanding Solitaire AB stent (6.0 mm×30 mm) was released at the occlusion segment. The angiogram showed a notable enhancement in the antegrade blood flow (Fig. 7.2.16 A, B). A dosage of 0.4 mg of tirofiban was administered intravenously through the arterial route. Following 5 minutes, the angiogram revealed excellent stent wall apposition, ensuring the basilar artery and its branches were well visualized. The angiogram conducted 10 minutes later showed that the basilar artery and its branches were patent, with a grade 3 of antegrade blood flow. There was a residual stenosis of about 30% in the middle segment of the basilar artery (Fig. 7.2.16 C, D).

Postprocedural CT scan showed no signs of intracranial

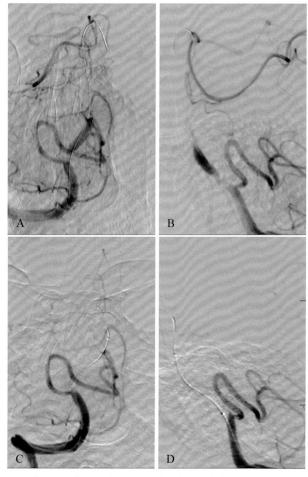

Fig. 7.2.15　A Pilot 50 microwire navigated through the occlusion segment of the basilar artery to the P2 segment of the left posterior cerebral artery (**A**, **B**). The post-balloon angioplasty angiogram showed the basilar artery remained occluded (**C**, **D**)

hemorrhage (Fig. 7.2.17).

The CT angiography performed after the procedure confirmed that the stent in the basilar artery was patent (Fig. 7.2.18). Additionally, the CTP scan demonstrated alleviation of hypoperfusion in the posterior circulation (Fig. 7.2.19).

Significant improvement was observed in the patient's dysarthria and weakness in the right limbs.

5. Comments

The management of intracranial in-stent restenosis typically involves the use of primary balloon angioplasty. If there is significant elastic recoil, the placement of selfexpanding or balloon-expandable stents may be considered (the coronary artery stenting can also be taken into account). In this case, despite balloon angioplasty, the basilar artery remained occluded, suggesting a high local plaque burden and the potential formation of mural thrombus, although the possibility of arterial dissection cannot be ruled out. Therefore, a longer Solitaire stent was chosen to cover the lesion, along with intraarterial and intravenous administration of tirofiban. Although residual stenosis was present after stent placement, the decision to postdilation was not made because of the focal plaque instability.

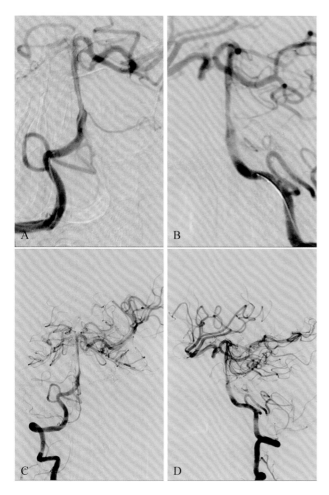

图 7.2.16　**A** 和 **B**. Solitaire AB 支架释放后，前向血流改善；**C** 和 **D**. 术后造影示基底动脉及各分支通畅，mTICI 分级 3 级，基底动脉中段残余狭窄率约 30%

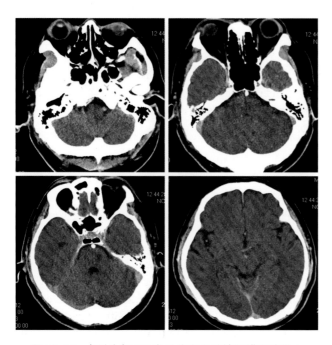

图 7.2.17　术后头部 CT 未见脑出血及蛛网膜下腔出血

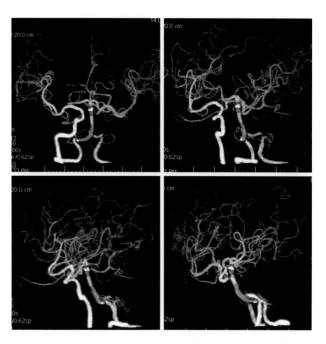

图 7.2.18　术后 CTA 示基底动脉支架内血流通畅

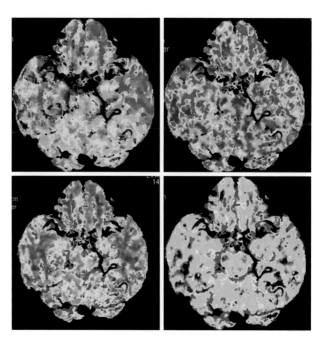

图 7.2.19　术后 CTP 示后循环灌注较前改善

（李新明　宋立刚　马宁）

7.2　手术操作视频
（病例 47）

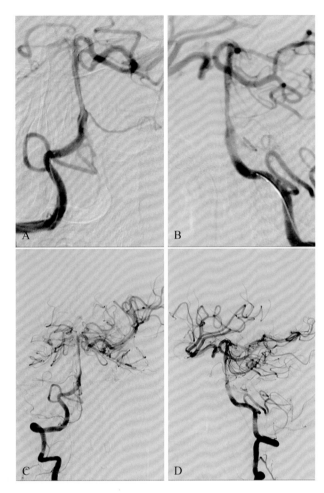

Fig. 7.2.16 A self-expanding Solitaire AB stent was released at the occlusion segment. The angiogram showed a notable enhancement in the antegrade blood flow (**A, B**). The final angiogram showed that the basilar artery and its branches were patent, with a grade 3 of antegrade blood flow. There was a residual stenosis of about 30% in the middle segment of the basilar artery (**C, D**)

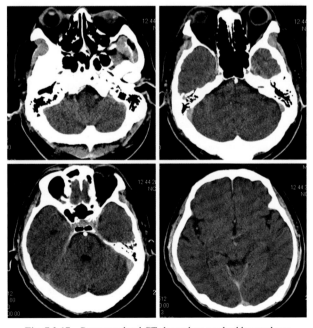

Fig. 7.2.17 Postprocedural CT showed no cerebral hemorrhage

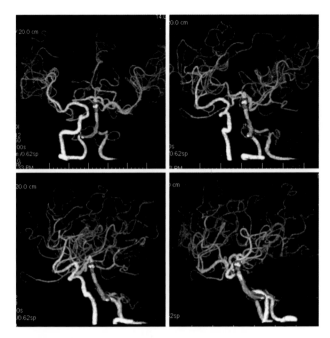

Fig. 7.2.18 Postprocedural CTA showed the basilar artery was patent

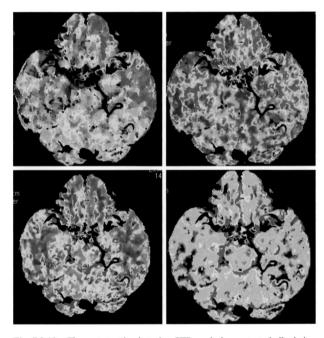

Fig. 7.2.19 The post-stent implantation CTP result demonstrated alleviation of hypoperfusion in the posterior circulation

(Translated by Rongrong Cui, Revised by Zhikai Hou)

7.2 Video of endovascular therapy (Case 47)

病例 48　药物涂层支架治疗基底动脉支架内再狭窄

（一）临床病史及影像分析

患者，男性，64 岁，主因"发作性头晕、视物模糊 5 年，视物重影 1 年"入院。

5 年前 DSA 示基底动脉重度狭窄（图 7.2.20 A 和 B），于狭窄处置入一枚 Apollo 支架（2.5 mm× 8 mm），术后残余狭窄率约 10%（图 7.2.20 C 和 D），术后患者头晕的发作程度和频率较术前改善。

术后 2 个月复查 DSA 示基底动脉支架内再狭窄（图 7.2.21 A 和 B），予以 Gateway 球囊（2.0 mm× 9 mm）扩张，术后残余狭窄率约 40%（图 7.2.21 C 和 D）。

1 年前患者出现发作性视物重影。头颅 MRI 未见急性脑梗死（图 7.2.22）。MRA 示基底动脉中段未显影（图 7.2.23）。CTA 示基底动脉支架内再狭窄程度显示不佳，支架远心段重度狭窄（图 7.2.24）。

半个月前上述症状再次发作。头部 MRI 示左侧脑桥急性梗死灶（图 7.2.25 A）。MRA 示基底动脉中段未显影（图 7.2.25 B）。现为进一步行血管内治疗收入我院。

既往史：高血压和脂蛋白代谢紊乱病史 15 年，糖尿病病史 5 年。3 年前因车祸外伤致脑出血、右侧锁骨骨折病史。饮酒 40 年。

查体：神经系统查体阴性。

血栓弹力图：AA 抑制率 0%，ADP 抑制率 0%。

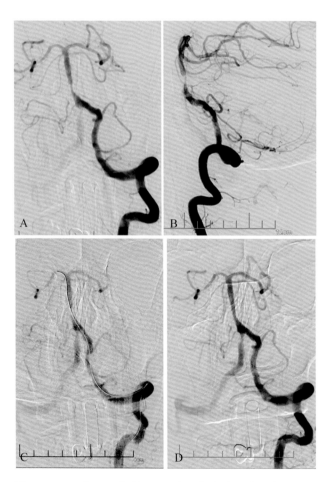

图 7.2.20　**A** 和 **B**. 5 年前 DSA 示基底动脉重度狭窄；**C** 和 **D**. 置入 Apollo 支架后造影显示残余狭窄率约 10%

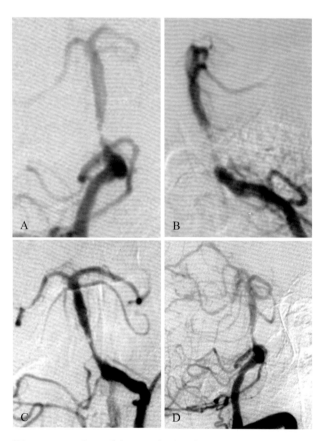

图 7.2.21　**A** 和 **B**. 支架置入术后 2 个月 DSA 示基底动脉支架内再狭窄；**C** 和 **D**. Gateway 球囊扩张后 DSA 示残余狭窄率约 40%

Case 48 Drug-eluting stenting for in-stent restenosis of the basilar artery

1. Clinical presentation and radiological studies

A 64-year-old male patient was admitted to the hospital due to episodes of paroxysmal dizziness and blurred vision for five years, accompanied by double vision for one year.

The angiogram conducted five years ago showed the presence of severe stenosis at the basilar artery (Fig. 7.2.20 A, B). A 2.5 mm×8 mm Apollo balloon-mounted stent was implanted at the basilar artery, with a residual stenosis of approximately 10% after the procedure (Fig. 7.2.20 C, D). After the procedure, the patient's symptoms of dizziness were alleviated.

The follow-up angiogram, conducted two months postprocedure, revealed the occurrence of in-stent restenosis within the basilar artery (Fig. 7.2.21 A, B). The stenosis lesion was dilated with a Gateway balloon (2.0 mm×9 mm), with a residual stenosis of approximately 40% following the balloon angioplasty (Fig. 7.2.21 C, D).

The patient developed episodes of paroxysmal diplopia one year ago. The MRI revealed no evidence of acute cerebral infarction (Fig. 7.2.22). The MRA demonstrated poor visualization at the middle segment of the basilar artery (Fig. 7.2.23). while the CT angiography revealed severe stenosis in the distal region of the stent within the basilar artery (Fig. 7.2.24).

The patient exhibited a recurring episode of diplopia two weeks ago. The repeated MRI results showed an acute infarction in the left pons (Fig. 7.2.25 A). The MRA did not show any visualization at the middle segment of the basilar artery (Fig. 7.2.25 B).

The patient had a 15-year history of hypertension and lipoprotein metabolism disorders, as well as a 5-year history of diabetes mellitus. Three years ago, he experienced a traumatic cerebral hemorrhage and right clavicle fracture due to a car accident. Additionally, he had been drinking for the past four decades.

The neurological examination was negative.

The thromboelastography test showed a 0% inhibition of AA and 0% inhibition of ADP.

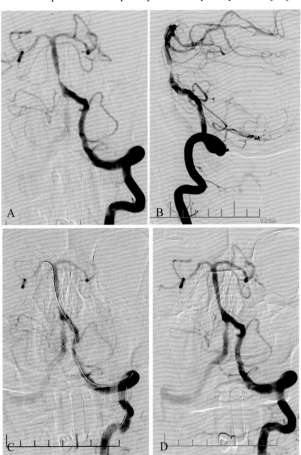

Fig. 7.2.20 The angiogram conducted five years ago showed the presence of severe stenosis at the basilar artery (**A, B**). A 2.5 mm×8 mm Apollo balloon-mounted stent was implanted at the basilar artery, with a residual stenosis of approximately 10% after the procedure (**C, D**)

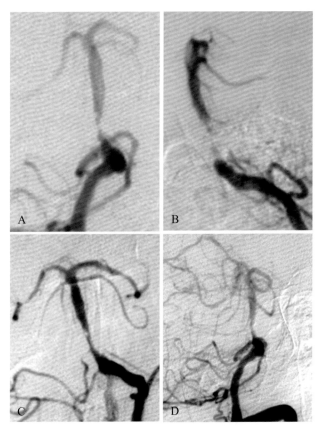

Fig. 7.2.21 The follow-up angiogram, conducted two months post-procedure, revealed the occurrence of in-stent restenosis within the basilar artery (**A, B**). The stenosis lesion was dilated with a Gateway balloon (2.0 mm×9 mm), with a residual stenosis of approximately 40% following the balloon angioplasty (**C, D**)

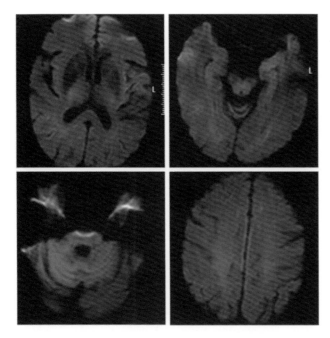

图 7.2.22　1 年前头颅 MRI 未见急性脑梗死

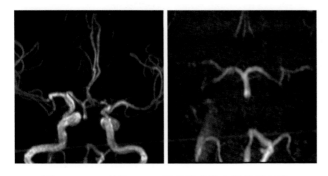

图 7.2.23　1 年前 MRA 示基底动脉中段显影不清

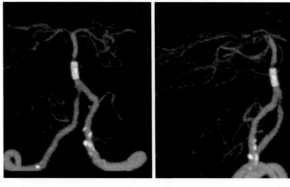

图 7.2.24　1 年前 CTA 示基底动脉支架内再狭窄程度显示不佳，支架远心段严重狭窄

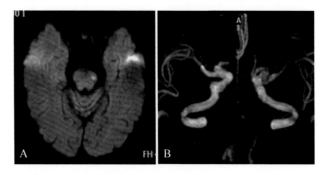

图 7.2.25　半月前复查头部 MRI 如下。**A.** MRI 示左侧脑桥急性梗死灶；**B.** MRA 示基底动脉中段显影不清

CYP2C19 基因检测：慢代谢型。

低密度脂蛋白胆固醇（LDL-C）：1.82 mmol/L。

入院后 DSA：右椎动脉造影显示右椎动脉 V1 段中度狭窄（图 7.2.26 A ～ C），左椎动脉造影显示基底动脉支架内再狭窄（图 7.2.26 D ～ F）。

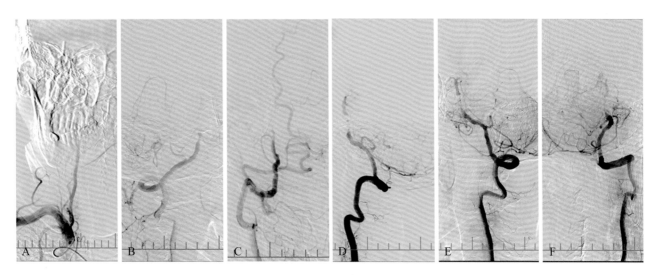

图 7.2.26　入院后复查 DSA 示：**A ～ C.** 右椎动脉造影显示右椎动脉 V1 段中度狭窄；**D ～ F.** 左椎动脉造影显示基底动脉支架内再狭窄

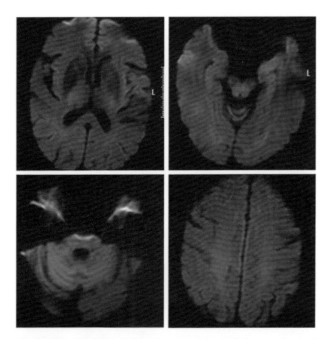

Fig. 7.2.22 The MRI conducted a year ago revealed no evidence of acute cerebral infarction

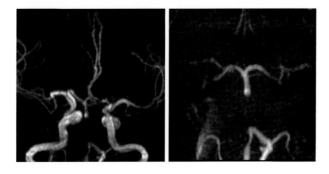

Fig. 7.2.23 The MRA conducted a year ago demonstrated poor visualization at the middle segment of the basilar artery

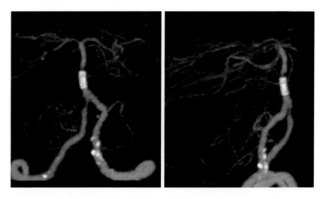

Fig. 7.2.24 The CT angiography conducted a year ago revealed severe stenosis in the distal region of the stent within the basilar artery

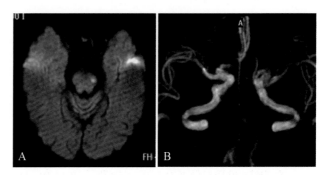

Fig. 7.2.25 Half a month ago, the MRI results showed acute infarcts in the left pons (**A**), and the MRA did not show any visualization at the middle segment of the basilar artery (**B**)

The CYP2C19 genotype showed a poor metabolizer status.

The serum LDL cholesterol (LDL-C) concentration was determined to be 1.82 mmol/L.

The angiogram conducted post-admission revealed moderate stenosis at the V1 segment of the right vertebral artery (Fig. 7.2.26 A–C), as well as restenosis within the stent in the basilar artery (Fig. 7.2.26 D–F).

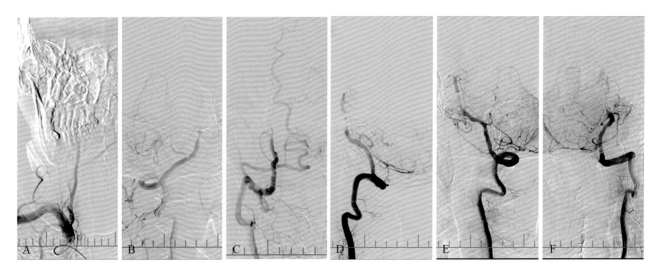

Fig. 7.2.26 The angiogram conducted post-admission revealed moderate stenosis at the V1 segment of the right vertebral artery (**A**–**C**), as well as restenosis within the stent in the basilar artery (**D**–**F**)

入院后给予双联抗血小板（替格瑞洛 90 mg 2 次 / 日 + 西洛他唑 100 mg 2 次 / 日）和降脂（阿托伐他汀 20 mg 1 次 / 日）等治疗。

（二）诊断

基底动脉支架内再狭窄。

（三）术前讨论

患者基底动脉支架术后 5 年，近一年有发作性头晕、视物重影，造影示基底动脉支架内再狭窄，有介入治疗指征。拟先予稍小直径球囊预扩张，再根据扩张效果看是否置入支架。相关风险包括扩张困难、穿支动脉闭塞、动脉夹层、急性或亚急性血栓形成等。

（四）治疗过程

全麻下右股动脉穿刺置入 8F 动脉鞘，6F 导引导管放至左椎动脉 V2 段远端，术前造影示基底动脉支架内再狭窄（图 7.2.27）。

路径图下沿导引导管送入 Pilot 50 微导丝（0.014 in，190 cm）携带 Echelon-10 微导管，Pilot 50 微导丝送至右大脑后动脉 P2 段，跟进 Echelon-10 微导管阻力大，无法越过病变。更换 Synchro 微导丝（0.014 in，300 cm）通过狭窄段，至右大脑后动脉 P2 段，沿微导丝分别送入 1.5 mm×15 mm、2.25 mm×15 mm Gateway 球囊（图 7.2.28）及 2.5 mm×15 mm SPL 冠状动脉球囊扩张病变，但残余狭窄率仍高（图

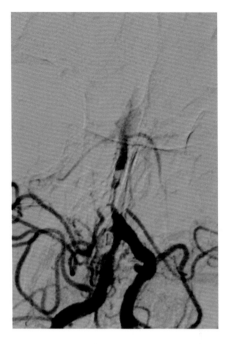

图 7.2.27 术前造影示基底动脉支架内再狭窄

7.2.29），将 Synchro 微导丝更换为 Transend 微导丝（0.014 in，300 cm）至右大脑后动脉 P2 段，送入 Resolute 冠状动脉支架（2.25 mm×14 mm）至狭窄处，扩张球囊释放支架，其后造影示支架贴壁良好，前向血流 mTICI 分级 3 级（图 7.2.30）。

术后即刻 CT：未见颅内出血（图 7.2.31）。

术后复查头颅 CTA：基底动脉支架内通畅（图 7.2.32）。

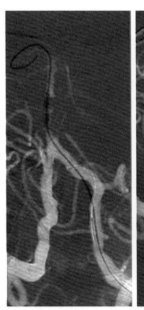
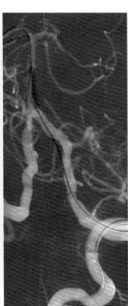
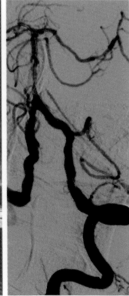

图 7.2.28 分别送入 1.5 mm×15 mm、2.25 mm×15 mm Gateway 球囊扩张狭窄病变

Upon admission, the patient was prescribed a dual antiplatelet regimen consisting of a twice-daily dose of 90 mg of Ticagrelor and a daily dose of 100 mg of Cilostazol, as well as statin therapy with a daily dose of 20 mg of Atorvastatin.

2. Diagnosis

Symptomatic in-stent restenosis within the basilar artery.

3. Treatment schedule

Five years ago, the patient was implanted with a stent in the basilar artery. However, the patient experienced recurrent episodes of dizziness and double vision in the past year. The follow-up angiography revealed the presence of restenosis within the basilar artery stent. Consequently, the patient exhibited a clear indication for undergoing endovascular treatment to address the issue of in-stent restenosis. The stenosis lesion was pre-dilated with a small-size balloon. Whether to implant the stent was based on the residual stenosis after the balloon dilation. Potential risks associated with the procedure included difficulty in balloon dilation, perforating artery occlusion, arterial dissection, and acute/subacute in-stent thrombosis.

4. Treatment

Under general anesthesia, a 6F guide catheter was positioned at the V2 segment of the left vertebral artery. The angiogram confirmed the presence of restenosis within the basilar artery stent (Fig. 7.2.27).

Under the roadmap, the Pilot 50 microwire (0.014 in, 190 cm) successfully navigated through the stenotic segment to reach the P2 segment of the right posterior cerebral artery. However, the attempts to advance the Echelon-10 microcatheter along the microwire through the lesion were unsuccessful. The Synchro microwire (0.014 in, 300 cm) was replaced and maneuvered through the lesion to the P2 segment of the right posterior cerebral artery. Subsequently, a 1.5 mm×15 mm, as well as a 2.25 mm×15 mm Gateway

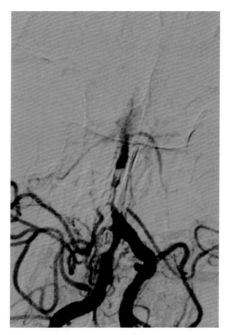

Fig. 7.2.27   The angiogram confirmed the presence of restenosis within the basilar artery stent

balloon (Fig. 7.2.28) and a 2.5 mm×15 mm SPL coronary artery balloon, were employed to dilate the stenosis lesion. However, despite these efforts, a significant degree of residual stenosis persisted (Fig. 7.2.29). The Synchro microwire was retracted. And a Transend microwire (0.014 in, 300 cm) was replaced and navigated through the lesion to the P2 segment of the right posterior cerebral artery. A Resolute coronary stent (2.25 mm×14 mm) was used to cover the lesion. The following angiogram showed an excellent stent wall apposition, with a grade 3 of antegrade blood flow (Fig. 7.2.30).

The postprocedural CT scan showed no indications of any intracranial hemorrhage (Fig. 7.2.31).

The postprocedural CTA revealed the stent in the basilar artery was patent (Fig. 7.2.32).

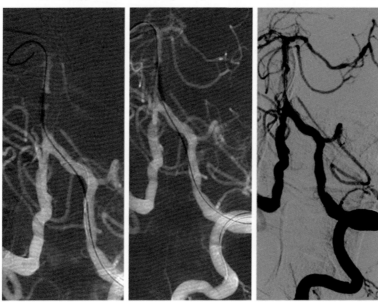

Fig. 7.2.28   A 1.5 mm×15 mm, as well as a 2.25 mm×15 mm Gateway balloon, were delivered to dilate the lesion, respectively

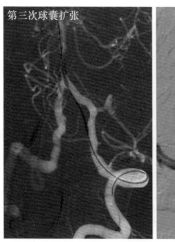
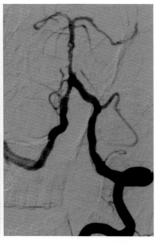

第三次球囊扩张

图 7.2.29 SPL 冠状动脉球囊扩张病变后，造影示残余狭窄率仍较高

（五）讨论

支架内再狭窄原因诸多，与术后残余狭窄程度、抗血小板药物的疗效、局部管壁的炎性反应等因素相关，但目前针对颅内支架再狭窄诱因及相关危险因素的研究尚少。支架内再狭窄是影响颅内支架远期疗效的重要因素。无症状的再狭窄可以选择继续保守治疗，而症状性狭窄就需要再次血管内介入治疗。治疗时首选单纯球囊扩张，如果扩张效果不满意，可以考虑再次置入支架。为预防再次狭窄，如病变及入路允许的话，可以考虑置入药物涂层支架。本例支架内再狭窄推测可能与抗血小板药物抵抗有关，故在用药方案上予以调整。

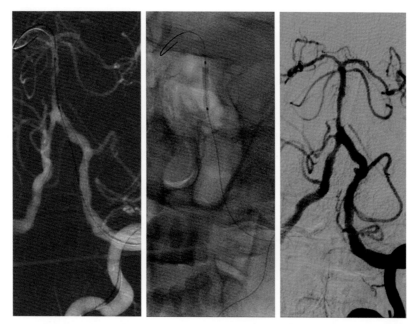

图 7.2.30 置入 Resolute 冠状动脉支架后造影示支架贴壁良好，前向血流 mTICI 分级 3 级

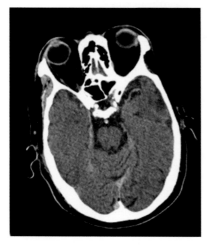

图 7.2.31 术后头颅 CT 未见出血

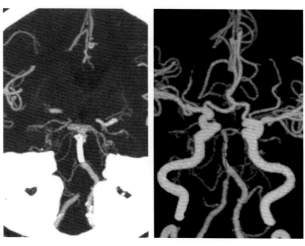

图 7.2.32 术后头颅 CTA 示基底动脉支架内通畅

（王天保 宋立刚 马宁）

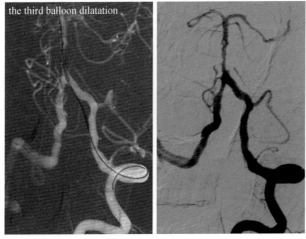

the third balloon dilatation

Fig. 7.2.29   A 2.5 mm×15 mm SPL coronary artery balloon, was employed to dilate the stenosis lesion. However, a significant degree of residual stenosis persisted

5. Comments

There are multiple causes for in-stent restenosis (ISR), including the degree of residual stenosis, the efficacy of antiplatelet medication, and inflammatory reactions within the focal vessel wall. However, there is limited research on the causes and risk factors of restenosis in intracranial stents. In-stent restenosis plays a crucial role in determining the longterm effectiveness of intracranial stenting. Asymptomatic restenosis may be managed conservatively, while symptomatic restenosis needed further endovascular intervention. The preferred first treatment option is primary balloon dilation. In cases of significant residual stenosis after balloon angioplasty, further stent implantation can be performed. To prevent recurrent restenosis, if the lesion and access permit, the use of drug-eluting stents can be considered. In this case, it is suspected that the in-stent restenosis may be related to resistance to antiplatelet medication, therefore adjustments to the medication regimen are warranted.

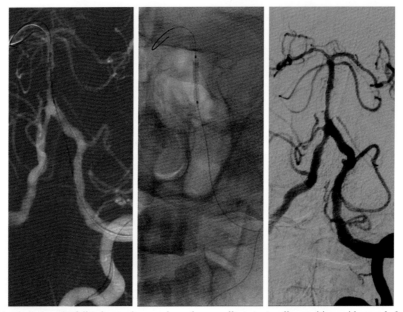

Fig. 7.2.30   After stent implantation, the following angiogram showed an excellent stent wall apposition, with a grade 3 of antegrade blood flow

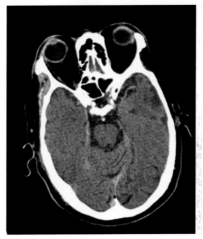

Fig. 7.2.31   The postprocedural CT scan showed no indications of any intracranial hemorrhage

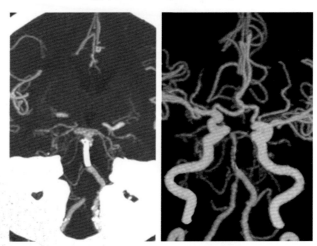

Fig. 7.2.32   The postprocedural CTA revealed the stent in the basilar artery was patent

(Translated by Rongrong Cui, Revised by Zhikai Hou)

第八章

围术期并发症的处理

第一节　穿支事件

病例 49　基底动脉重度狭窄围术期发生穿支卒中

（一）临床病史及影像分析

患者，男性，70岁，主因"视物不清20余天，加重伴一过性意识不清和右侧肢体无力3天"入院。

头部MRI：左侧枕叶、左侧侧脑室旁后角新发

梗死（图8.1.1 A）。

头颈部CTA：左椎动脉开口部重度狭窄，基底动脉远段重度狭窄，左侧大脑中动脉中度狭窄（图8.1.1 B～D）。

给予双联抗血小板及他汀类药物治疗。3天前再次发生缺血性脑血管事件，为求血管内治疗收入

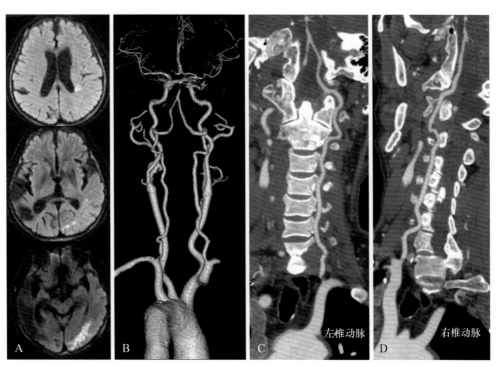

图8.1.1　**A**.头部MRI示左侧枕叶、左侧侧脑室旁后角新发梗死；**B**～**D**.头颈部CTA示左椎动脉开口部重度狭窄，基底动脉远段重度狭窄，左侧大脑中动脉中度狭窄

Chapter 8

Periprocedural Complication

Section 1　Perforating Artery Occlusion

Case 49　Periprocedural perforator stroke after the basilar artery stenting

1. Clinical presentation and radiological studies

A 70-year-old male patient was admitted to the hospital due to blurred vision for over 20 days, exacerbated by a recent episode of transient unconsciousness and weakness in the right limbs for three days.

The MRI findings unveiled acute infarctions localized in the left occipital lobe and left paraventricular posterior horn (Fig. 8.1.1 A).

The CT angiography exhibited pronounced stenosis at the origin of the left vertebral artery, as well as significant stenosis at the distal segment of the basilar artery. Additionally, a moderate stenosis was observed in the left middle cerebral artery (Fig. 8.1.1 B–D).

The patient was prescribed a dual antiplatelet regimen and statin therapy. However, despite undergoing intensive medical treatment, he experienced a recurrent ischemic stroke three days ago.

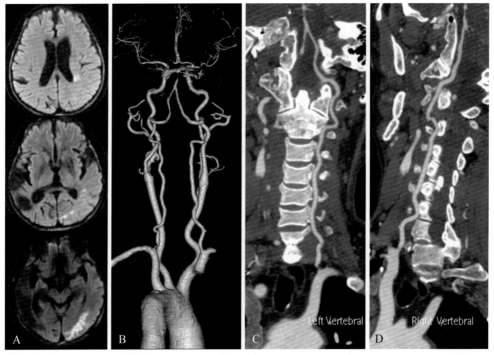

Fig. 8.1.1　The MRI findings unveiled acute infarctions localized in the left occipital lobe and left paraventricular posterior horn (**A**). The CT angiography exhibited pronounced stenosis at the origin of the left vertebral artery, as well as significant stenosis at the distal segment of the basilar artery. Additionally, a moderate stenosis was observed in the left middle cerebral artery (**B–D**)

354

我院。

既往史：高血压病史 20 余年，痛风病史 20 余年，脑梗死病史 3 年。

查体：右侧同向性偏盲，右下肢肌力 4 级。

入院后给予双联抗血小板（阿司匹林 100 mg 1 次 / 日＋氯吡格雷 75 mg 1 次 / 日）及降脂（阿托伐他汀 20 mg 1 次 / 日）等治疗。

（二）诊断

症状性基底动脉远端重度狭窄。

（三）术前讨论

结合患者病史以及影像学检查，考虑基底动脉为责任动脉，且规律内科药物治疗后仍有缺血事件复发，有血管内介入治疗指征。左椎动脉 V1 段开口部重度狭窄，远端血管走行迂曲，右椎动脉路径相对平直，拟先行左椎动脉 V1 段支架置入，后经右椎动脉入路行基底动脉介入治疗。因基底动脉远端富有穿支动脉，且 CTA 提示大脑后动脉导丝着陆区不理想，拟使用稍小球囊预扩张，再酌情放置自膨式或者球囊扩张式支架。相关风险包括穿支卒

中、急性或亚急性血栓形成、高灌注综合征、血管破裂以及血管夹层等。

（四）治疗过程

全麻下右股动脉入路，将 6F 导引导管头端置于左锁骨下动脉近段，造影显示左椎动脉 V1 段重度狭窄，狭窄率约 70%，狭窄长度约 10 mm（图 8.1.2 A）。沿导引导管送入 PT-2 微导丝（0.014 in，185 cm）通过左椎动脉开口狭窄处至 V2 段，沿导丝送入 Resolute 球囊扩张式支架（4.0 mm×15 mm）对位狭窄段后，以 12 atm 成功释放支架（图 8.1.2 B 和 C），复查造影示支架贴壁可，残余狭窄率小于 5%，前向血流良好（图 8.1.2 D）。

调整 6F 导引导管头端置于右椎动脉 V2 段远端，造影显示基底动脉远段重度狭窄，狭窄率约 90%，狭窄长度约 6 mm，大脑后动脉顺行显影欠佳（图 8.1.3）。SL-10 微导管在 Synchro-2 微导丝（0.014 in，200 cm）配合下，越过基底动脉狭窄段至右大脑后动脉，交换后更换导丝为 Transend 微导丝（0.014 in，300 cm），导丝头端置于右大脑后动脉 P1 段（图 8.1.4 A）。沿导丝送入 Legend 球囊

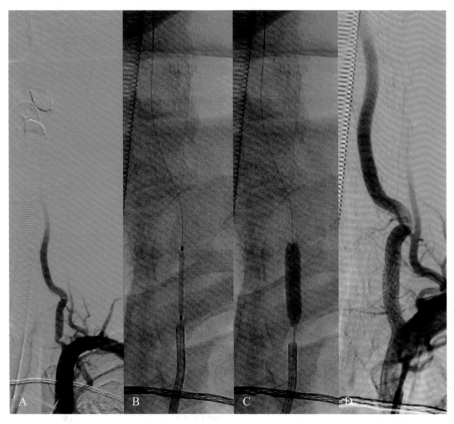

图 8.1.2　**A**. 术前造影显示左椎动脉 V1 段重度狭窄，狭窄率约 70%，狭窄长度约 10 mm；**B** 和 **C**. 释放 Resolute 球囊扩张式支架；**D**. 释放支架后造影显示支架贴壁可，残余狭窄率小于 5%，前向血流良好

The patient had a medical history of hypertension and gout for over 20 years. And three years ago, he suffered from an ischemic stroke.

The physical examination revealed the presence of right homonymous hemianopsia, along with a grade 4 muscle strength in the right lower limb.

After admission, he was prescribed a dual antiplatelet regimen consisting of a daily dose of 100 mg of Aspirin and a daily dose of 75 mg of Clopidogrel, as well as statin treatment with a daily dose of 20 mg of Atorvastatin.

2. Diagnosis

Symptomatic severe stenosis at the distal segment of the basilar artery.

3. Treatment schedule

Based on the patient's clinical presentation and radiological examinations, the basilar artery was identified as the culprit vessel. Despite receiving aggressive medical intervention, the patient experienced an ischemic stroke. Therefore, endovascular treatment was recommended. Notably, the left vertebral artery exhibited severe stenosis at its origin, with a tortuous course distal to the V1 segment. Conversely, the right vertebral artery displayed a relatively straight course. Consequently, the initial step involved the implantation of a stent in the V1 segment of the left vertebral artery, followed by stenting of the basilar artery via the access of the right vertebral artery. Due to the presence of abundant perforator arteries in the distal portion of the basilar artery and the suboptimal landing zone indicated by CTA in the posterior cerebral artery, it is proposed to perform pre-dilation using a slightly smaller balloon, followed by the placement of a self-expanding or balloon-expandable stent as deemed appropriate. Potential risks associated with the procedure include perforator stroke, acute/subacute in-stent thrombosis, hyperperfusion syndrome, vessel rupture, and arterial dissection.

4. Treatment

Under general anesthesia, a 6F guide catheter was positioned at the proximal segment of the left subclavian artery. The angiogram revealed significant stenosis at the V1 segment of the left vertebral artery, characterized by a 70% narrowing and a stenosis length of 10 mm (Fig. 8.1.2 A). A PT-2 microwire (0.014 in, 185 cm) was positioned at the V2 segment of the left vertebral artery and a 4.0 mm × 15 mm Resolute balloon-mounted stent was employed to cover the lesion (Fig. 8.1.2 B, C). The angiogram conducted after the stent implantation displayed a residual stenosis of less than 5% and demonstrated complete wall apposition of the stent (Fig. 8.1.2 D).

Subsequently, the 6F guide catheter was precisely positioned at the distal V2 segment of the right vertebral artery. The angiogram validated the presence of severe stenosis in the distal segment of the basilar artery, revealing a 90% narrowing along with a length of 6 mm. The visualization of both bilateral posterior cerebral arteries was found to be inadequate (Fig. 8.1.3). A Synchro-2 microwire (0.014 in, 200 cm) and an SL-

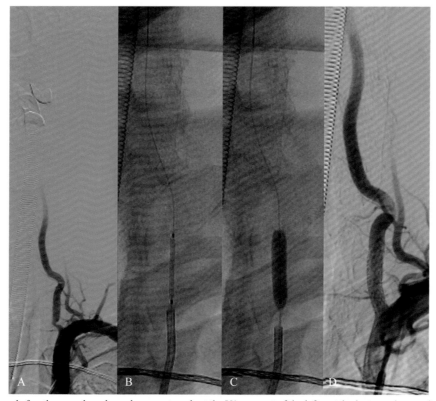

Fig. 8.1.2 The angiogram before the procedure showed severe stenosis at the V1 segment of the left vertebral artery, characterized by a 70% narrowing and a stenosis length of 10 mm (**A**). A 4.0 mm × 15 mm Resolute balloon-mounted stent was employed to cover the lesion (**B, C**). The angiogram conducted after the stent implantation displayed a residual stenosis of less than 5% and demonstrated complete wall apposition of the stent (**D**)

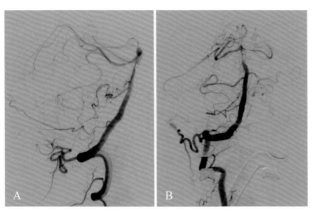

图 8.1.3 术前造影显示基底动脉远段重度狭窄，狭窄率约 90%，狭窄长度约 6 mm，大脑后动脉顺行显影欠佳

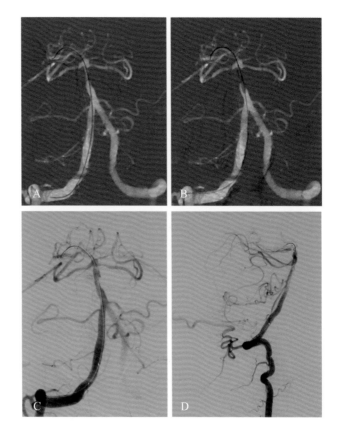

图 8.1.4 **A**. Transend 微导丝到位于右大脑后动脉 P1 段；**B**. Legend 球囊扩张狭窄病变；**C** 和 **D**. 球囊扩张后造影示狭窄程度较前好转，但局部可见夹层形成

（2.0 mm×10 mm），对位狭窄段后以 6 atm 缓慢预扩张一次（图 8.1.4 B）。再次造影显示基底动脉狭窄程度较前好转，但局部可见血管夹层征象（图 8.1.4 C 和 D）。因大脑后动脉导丝着陆区欠佳，考虑术中放置球囊扩张式支架。沿微导丝送入 Apollo 球囊扩张式支架（2.5 mm×8 mm），准确定位于狭窄处后缓慢扩张球囊至 7.0 atm，此时支架已释放贴壁，近远段扩张良好（图 8.1.5 A）。回撤微导丝及支架球囊，复查造影显示支架贴壁可，残余狭窄率小于 10%，基底动脉前向血流良好，大脑后动脉顺行显影较前好转（图 8.1.5 B 和 C）。

术后即刻复查头颅 CT 未见出血。

术后患者右侧肢体无力加重伴言语不清，头颅

MRI 提示脑桥左侧新发梗死（图 8.1.6），考虑术中球囊扩张及支架释放过程中，基底动脉斑块移位造成穿支动脉闭塞。

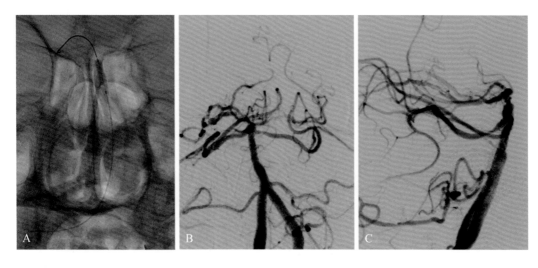

图 8.1.5 **A**. 于狭窄段释放 Apollo 球囊扩张式支架；**B** 和 **C**. 释放支架后造影显示支架贴壁良好，残余狭窄率小于 10%，前向血流良好，大脑后动脉顺行显影较前好转

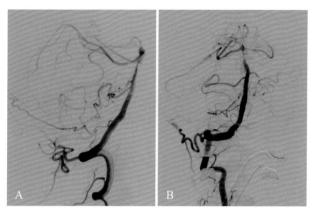

Fig. 8.1.3 The angiogram validated the presence of severe stenosis in the distal segment of the basilar artery, revealing a 90% narrowing along with a length of 6 mm. The visualization of both bilateral posterior cerebral arteries was found to be inadequate

10 microcatheter coaxially advanced the stenotic segment to the right posterior cerebral artery. Subsequently, a Transend microwire (0.014 in, 300 cm) was carefully exchanged and positioned at the P1 segment of the right posterior cerebral artery (Fig. 8.1.4 A). Following that, a 2 mm × 10 mm Legend balloon was successfully delivered to the stenosis lesion, aiming to dilate it (Fig. 8.1.4 B). The subsequent angiogram indicated an improvement in the degree of stenosis. However, it was also observed that an arterial dissection had occurred. (Fig. 8.1.4 C, D). Considering the suboptimal landing zone of the bilateral posterior cerebral arteries, the decision was made to proceed with the implantation of a balloon-mounted stent. An Apollo balloon-mounted stent (2.5 mm × 8 mm) was employed to cover the lesion (Fig. 8.1.5 A). The final angiogram revealed complete wall apposition of the stent, with a residual stenosis of less than 10%. The antegrade blood flow in the basilar artery was graded at 3. Furthermore, there was adequate visualization of the bilateral posterior cerebral arteries (Fig. 8.1.5 B, C).

The postprocedural CT scan revealed no evidence of cerebral hemorrhage.

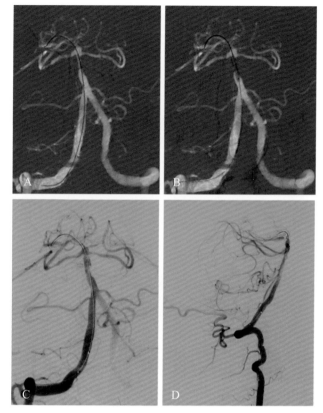

Fig. 8.1.4 A Transend microwire was carefully positioned at the P1 segment of the right posterior cerebral artery (**A**). The lesion was dilated with a Legend balloon (**B**). The subsequent angiogram indicated an improvement in the degree of stenosis. However, it was also observed that an arterial dissection had occurred (**C, D**)

Regrettably, there was a deterioration in the weakness observed in the right limb, accompanied by the onset of slurred speech. Subsequent MRI follow-up indicated the presence of new cerebral infarctions located within the left side of the pons (Fig. 8.1.6). The occurrence of the perforator stroke can be attributed to the displacement of plaque during the balloon dilation and stent deployment procedure.

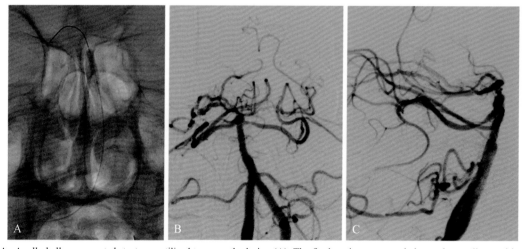

Fig. 8.1.5 An Apollo balloon-mounted stent was utilized to cover the lesion (**A**). The final angiogram revealed complete wall apposition of the stent, with a residual stenosis of less than 10%. The antegrade blood flow in the basilar artery was graded at 3. Furthermore, there was adequate visualization of the bilateral posterior cerebral arteries (**B, C**)

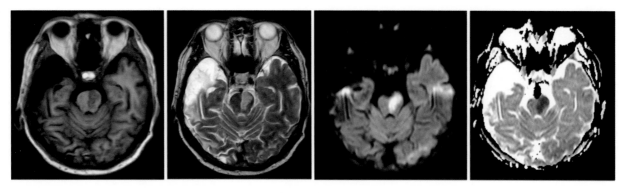

图 8.1.6 术后头部 MRI 提示脑桥左侧新发梗死

（五）讨论

本例基底动脉远段重度狭窄，属于颅内动脉富穿支区域，术前拟使用小球囊预扩张后再放置支架。因病变位置较高，且术前 CTA 及术中造影提示双侧大脑后动脉显影欠佳，导丝着陆区不理想，放置 Wingspan 支架或者经导管释放自膨式支架有潜在损伤大脑后动脉着陆区的风险，故选择 Apollo 球囊扩张式支架。患者术后出现右侧肢体肌力下降，影像学检查提示左侧脑桥新发梗死，考虑基底动脉背侧穿支开口受累闭塞所致。这可能与术中小球囊预扩张及支架释放过程中过于追求影像学完美有关，出现"雪梨效应"，导致基底动脉背侧斑块受挤压移位累及穿支开口。

（陈涵丰 计仁杰 俞妮妮 顾燕忠 徐子奇）

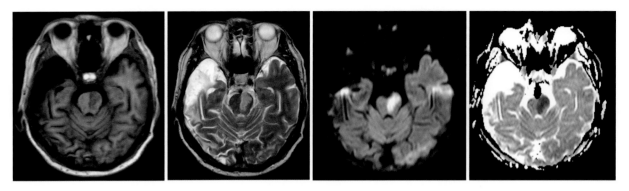

Fig. 8.1.6   Follow-up MRI indicated the presence of new cerebral infarctions located within the left side of the pons

5. Comments

In this particular instance, the patient presented with a significant constriction in the distal portion of the basilar artery, which falls within the territory of abundant perforating vessels of the intracranial arteries. To address the stenosis lesion, a small-size balloon was utilized to pre-dilate the stenosis lesion before stent implantation. However, due to the high location of the lesion and the suboptimal landing zone of the bilateral posterior cerebral arteries for the guidewire, there were concerns about the risk of compromising the posterior cerebral arteries by using the Wingspan stent or deploying a self-expanding stent through a catheter.

Therefore, an Apollo balloon-expandable stent was chosen. After the procedure, the patient experienced a decrease in muscle strength on the right side, and imaging studies revealed a new pontine infarction on the left side. The occurrence of the perforator stroke can be attributed to the displacement of plaque during the balloon dilation and stent deployment, a phenomenon known as the Snow-plow effect. This effect results in the obstruction of the origins of the perforator arteries due to the compression and displacement of the plaque within the basilar artery.

(Translated by Rongrong Cui, Revised by Zhikai Hou)

第二节　高灌注综合征

病例 50　右椎动脉 V4 段重度狭窄血管内治疗后高灌注出血

（一）临床病史及影像分析

患者，男性，51 岁，主因"发作性头晕、行走不稳 6 个月"入院。

当地医院头部 MRI 示右侧颞叶内侧急性梗死灶（图 8.2.1）。头部 CTA 示右椎动脉优势，右椎动脉 V4 段重度狭窄（图 8.2.2）。给予阿司匹林、氯吡格雷、他汀类药物等治疗后症状仍有发作。为求血管内治疗收入我院。

既往史：高血压、脂蛋白代谢紊乱病史以及吸烟史。

查体：神经系统查体无阳性定位体征。

血栓弹力图：AA 抑制率 100%，ADP 抑制率 66.1%。

头颅 CT：双侧椎动脉颅内段和基底动脉未见明显钙化（图 8.2.3）。

CTA：右椎动脉 V4 段重度狭窄（图 8.2.4）。

高分辨率 MRI：右椎动脉颅内段局部管壁偏心性增厚，呈等 T1 信号，管腔狭窄。增强后局部呈点状强化。考虑右椎动脉颅内段局部斑块形成（图 8.2.5）。

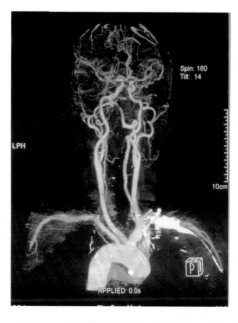

图 8.2.2　头部 CTA 示右椎动脉优势，右椎动脉 V4 段重度狭窄

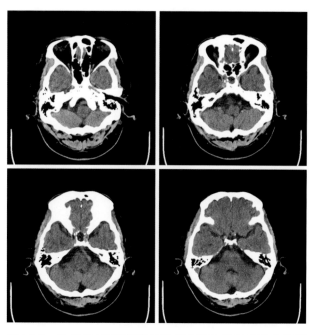

图 8.2.3　头颅 CT 示双侧椎动脉颅内段和基底动脉未见明显钙化

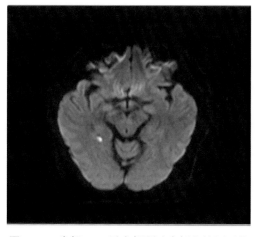

图 8.2.1　头部 MRI 示右侧颞叶内侧急性梗死灶

Section 2   Hyperperfusion Syndrome

Case 50   Periprocedural hyperperfusion syndrome after stenting for the V4 segment of the right vertebral artery

1. Clinical presentation and radiological studies

A 51-year-old male patient was admitted to the hospital due to episodes of paroxysmal dizziness and unsteady gait for six months.

The MRI findings revealed an acute infarction in the medial temporal lobe on the right side (Fig. 8.2.1). Additionally, the CT angiography demonstrated significant stenosis at the V4 segment of the dominant right vertebral artery (Fig. 8.2.2). Despite undergoing extensive medical intervention, the patient continued to experience symptoms of ischemia.

The patient had a medical history including hypertension, lipoprotein metabolism disorders, and a history of smoking.

He was neurologically intact on admission.

The thromboelastography test indicated a 100% inhibition of AA and a 66.1% inhibition of ADP.

The non-contrast CT scan revealed the absence of notable calcification in the intracranial portions of both bilateral vertebral arteries as well as the basilar artery (Fig. 8.2.3).

The CT angiography revealed severe stenosis at the V4 segment of the right vertebral artery (Fig. 8.2.4).

The high-resolution MRI demonstrated eccentric thickening of the vascular wall in the intracranial segment of the right vertebral artery, exhibiting an isointense signal on T1-weighted images with luminal stenosis. There were focal enhancements in the respective area after contrast administration, suggesting the formation of a localized plaque in the intracranial segment of the right vertebral artery (Fig. 8.2.5).

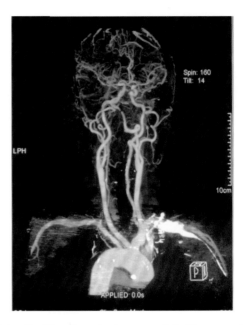

Fig. 8.2.2   The CT angiography demonstrated significant stenosis at the V4 segment of the dominant right vertebral artery

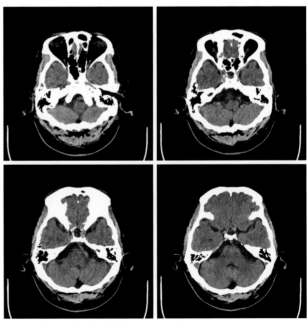

Fig. 8.2.3   The non-contrast CT scan revealed the absence of notable calcification in the intracranial portions of both bilateral vertebral arteries as well as the basilar artery

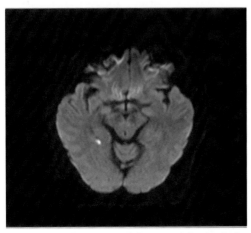

Fig. 8.2.1   The MRI findings revealed an acute infarction in the medial temporal lobe on the right side

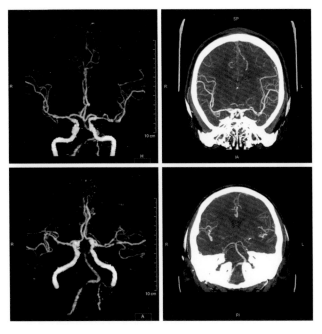

图 8.2.4　CTA 示右椎动脉 V4 段重度狭窄

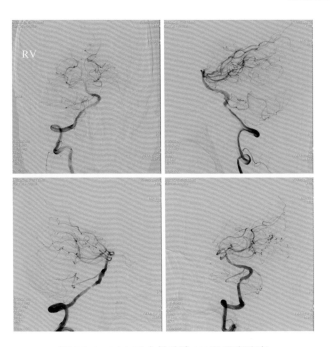

图 8.2.6　DSA 示右椎动脉 V4 段重度狭窄

DSA：右椎动脉 V4 段重度狭窄（图 8.2.6），左椎动脉发出左小脑后下动脉后闭塞，左小脑后下动脉通过软脑膜支代偿左小脑前下动脉（图 8.2.7）。未见前循环向后循环代偿（图 8.2.8）。

入院后给予双联抗血小板（阿司匹林 100 mg 1 次 / 日 ＋氯吡格雷 75 mg 1 次 / 日）、降脂（阿托伐他汀 20 mg 1 次 / 日）治疗。

（二）诊断

症状性右椎动脉 V4 段重度狭窄。

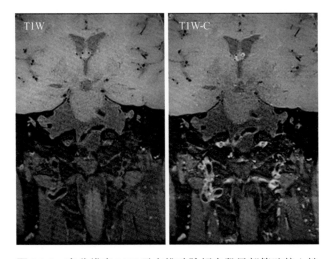

图 8.2.5　高分辨率 MRI 示右椎动脉颅内段局部管壁偏心性增厚，呈等 T1 信号，管腔狭窄，增强后局部呈点状强化

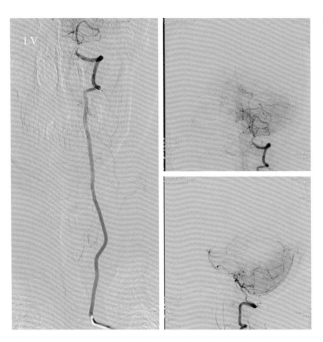

图 8.2.7　DSA 示左椎动脉发出左小脑后下动脉后闭塞，左小脑后下动脉通过软脑膜支代偿左小脑前下动脉

（三）术前讨论

患者左椎动脉 V4 段闭塞，右椎动脉 V4 段重度狭窄，双联抗血小板治疗后仍有症状发作，有介入治疗指征。病变狭窄程度重，但病变较直，拟在小球囊预扩张基础上置入球囊扩张式支架。相关风险包括高灌注综合征和穿支卒中。

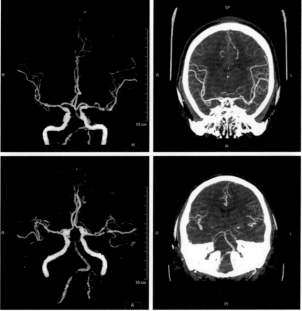

Fig. 8.2.4 The CT angiography revealed severe stenosis at the V4 segment of the right vertebral artery

The digital subtraction angiography (DSA) indicated significant stenosis at the V4 segment of the right vertebral artery (Fig. 8.2.6). Additionally, the left vertebral artery was found to be occluded distal to the origin of the posterior inferior cerebellar artery (PICA). Compensatory blood flow from the left PICA was redirected towards the left anterior inferior cerebellar artery (AICA) through the pial collaterals (Fig. 8.2.7). However, there was no compensatory blood flow observed from the anterior circulation to the posterior circulation (Fig. 8.2.8).

Upon admission, the patient was prescribed a dual antiplatelet regimen consisting of a daily dosage of 100 mg of Aspirin and 75 mg of Clopidogrel. In addition, statin therapy was given with a daily dosage of 20 mg of Atorvastatin.

2. Diagnosis

Symptomatic severe stenosis at the V4 segment of the right vertebral artery.

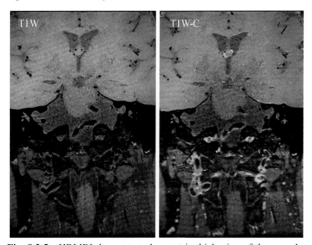

Fig. 8.2.5 HRMRI demonstrated eccentric thickening of the vascular wall in the intracranial segment of the right vertebral artery, exhibiting an isointense signal on T1-weighted images with luminal stenosis. There were focal enhancements in the respective area after contrast administration

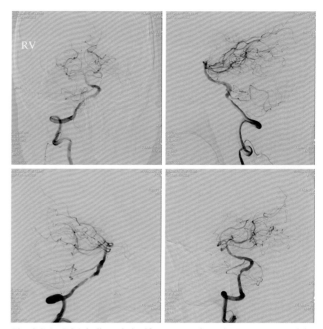

Fig. 8.2.6 DSA indicated significant stenosis at the V4 segment of the right vertebral artery

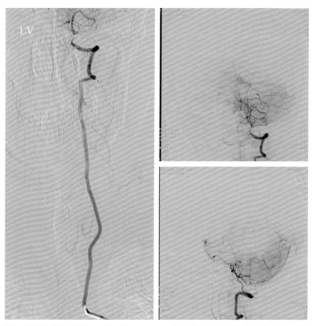

Fig. 8.2.7 The left vertebral artery was found to be occluded distal to the origin of the posterior inferior cerebellar artery (PICA). Compensatory blood flow from the left PICA was redirected towards the left anterior inferior cerebellar artery (AICA) through the pial collaterals

3. Treatment schedule

The patient experienced occlusion of the V4 segment of the left vertebral artery and significant stenosis of the V4 segment of the right vertebral artery. Despite receiving intensive medical intervention, the patient's condition persisted. Therefore, it was deemed necessary to consider endovascular intervention. A relatively straight lesion at the V4 segment of the right vertebral artery was pre-dilated using a small-size balloon, followed by the implantation of a balloon-mounted stent. Potential risks associated with the procedure included hyperperfusion syndrome and perforating artery occlusion.

（四）治疗过程

全麻下右股动脉穿刺置入 6F 动脉鞘，6F 导引导管置于右椎动脉 V2 段远端，造影示右椎动脉 V4 段重度狭窄（图 8.2.9）。Pilot 微导丝（0.014 in，190 cm）与微导管同轴通过狭窄段置于右大脑后动脉 P1 段，Sprinter Legend 球囊（2.5 mm×15 mm）预扩张后放置 Apollo 支架（3.0 mm×13 mm）（图 8.2.10），释放后支架贴壁良好，前向血流 mTICI 分级 3 级（图 8.2.11）。

术后即刻头颅 CT 示右侧小脑半球高密度影（图 8.2.12）。

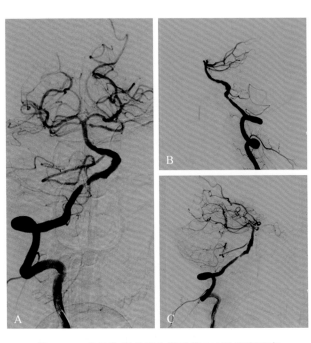

图 8.2.8　DSA 未见前循环向后循环代偿

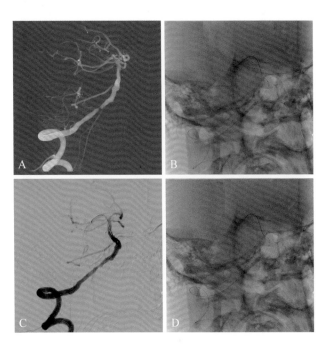

图 8.2.10　**A**. Pilot 微导丝置于右大脑后动脉 P1 段；**B**. Sprinter Legend 球囊预扩张；**C**. 球囊预扩张后造影；**D**. 置入 Apollo 支架

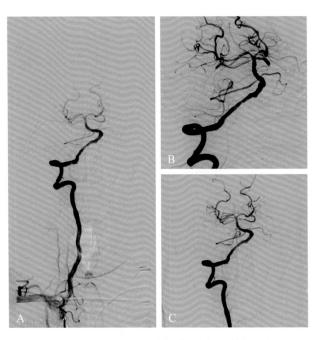

图 8.2.9　术前造影显示右椎动脉 V4 段重度狭窄

图 8.2.11　支架释放后造影示支架贴壁良好，前向血流 mTICI 分级 3 级

4. Treatment

Under general anesthesia, a 6F guide catheter was positioned at the V2 segment of the right vertebral artery. The angiogram confirmed severe stenosis at the V4 segment of the right vertebral artery (Fig. 8.2.9). A Pilot microwire (0.014 in, 190 cm) and a microcatheter coaxially navigated through the lesion to the P1 segment of the right posterior cerebral artery.

A 2.5 mm×15 mm Sprinter Legend balloon was utilized to predilate the stenosis lesion. Subsequently, a 3.0 mm×13 mm Apollo stent was employed to cover the lesion (Fig. 8.2.10). The final angiogram showed an excellent stent wall apposition, with a grade 3 of antegrade blood flow (Fig. 8.2.11).

The post-procedure non-contrast CT showed the presence of a high-density area in the right cerebellar hemisphere (Fig. 8.2.12).

Fig. 8.2.8 There was no compensatory blood flow observed from the anterior circulation to the posterior circulation

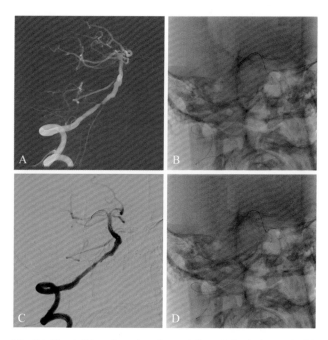

Fig. 8.2.10 A Pilot microwire advanced through the lesion to the P1 segment of the right posterior cerebral artery (**A**). A Sprinter Legend balloon was used to dilate the lesion (**B**, **C**). After the balloon dilation, an Apollo stent was used to cover the lesion (**D**)

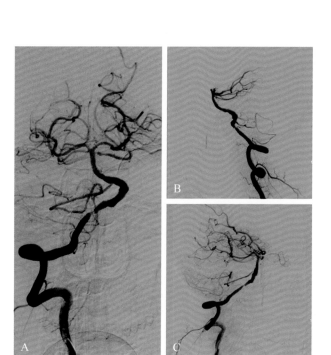

Fig. 8.2.9 The angiogram before the procedure showed severe stenosis at the V4 segment ofthe right vertebral artery

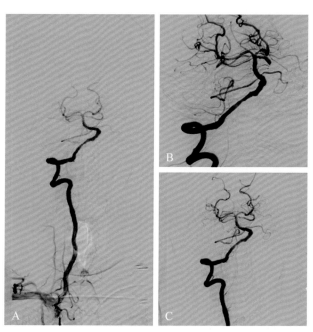

Fig. 8.2.11 The final angiogram showed an excellent stent wall apposition, with a grade 3 of antegrade blood flow

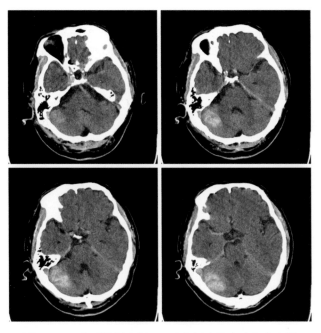

图 8.2.12　术后即刻头颅 CT 示右侧小脑半球高密度影

术后 3 天复查 CT 示右侧小脑半球血肿（图 8.2.13），患者病情逐渐加重，自行出院。

（五）讨论

本例患者发生术后出血的原因考虑为高灌注，虽然后循环的高灌注较前循环发生率低，但也不能忽视其存在，术中及术后应该严格控制血压。对于后循环幕下高灌注出血的处理包括：暂时停用抗血小板药物，根据患者具体情况决定是否去骨瓣减压或者脑室穿刺引流。

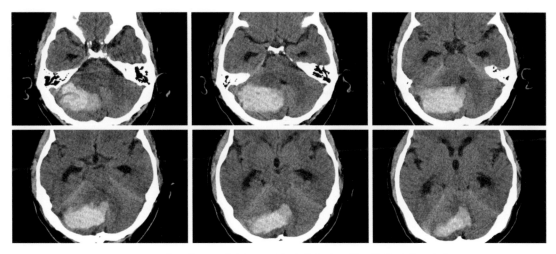

图 8.2.13　术后第 3 日头颅 CT 示右小脑半球血肿，较前无明显变化

（吴岩峰　王现旺　李红闪　韩明

杨海华　马宁）

病例 51　右大脑中动脉 M1 段支架术后高灌注

（一）临床病史及影像分析

患者，女性，62 岁，主因"发作性左侧肢体无力伴构音障碍 1 年"入院。

1 年前当地医院行头部 MRI 示右侧基底节、额顶叶新发脑梗死（图 8.2.14）。头部 CTA 示右大脑中动脉 M1 段重度狭窄（图 8.2.15）。给予患者口服阿司匹林、氯吡格雷以及阿托伐他汀等治疗。

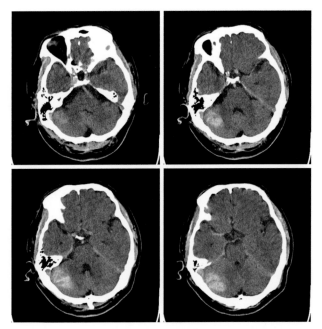

Fig. 8.2.12 The post-procedure non-contrast CT showed the the presence of a high density area in the right cerebellar hemisphere

The non-contrast CT scan conducted three days after the procedure indicated the existence of a hematoma in the right cerebellar hemisphere (Fig. 8.2.13). The patient's condition deteriorated gradually, resulting in voluntary discharge from the hospital.

5. Comments

In this case, the patient experienced hyperperfusion hemorrhage following the stent implantation. While the occurrence of hyperperfusion hemorrhage in the posterior circulation was less frequent compared to the anterior circulation, its significance should not be underestimated. Strict blood pressure control during and after the procedure is crucial in preventing hyperperfusion hemorrhage. If hyperperfusion hemorrhage occurs in the posterior circulation, antiplatelet medication will be stopped. Whether to proceed with decompressive craniectomy or ventricular puncture drainage will depend on the specific conditions of the patient.

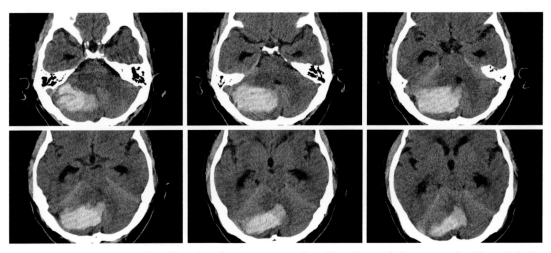

Fig. 8.2.13 The non-contrast CT scan conducted three days after the procedure indicated the existence of a hematoma in the right cerebellar hemisphere

(Translated by Rongrong Cui, Revised by Zhikai Hou)

Case 51 Periprocedural hyperperfusion syndrome after stenting for the M1 segment of the right middle cerebral artery

1. Clinical presentation and radiological studies

A 62-year-old woman was admitted to the hospital due to episodes of paroxysmal weakness in the left limbs with dysarthria for one year.

The MRI findings from one year ago indicated the presence of acute infarctions in the right basal ganglia and frontoparietal lobe (Fig. 8.2.14). Additionally, CT angiography (CTA) revealed significant stenosis in the M1 segment of the right middle cerebral artery (Fig. 8.2.15). The patient received intensive medical treatment.

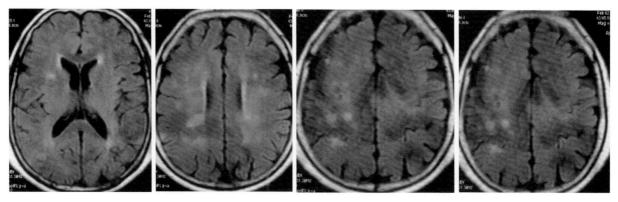

图 8.2.14 1 年前头部 MRI 示右侧基底节、额顶叶新发脑梗死

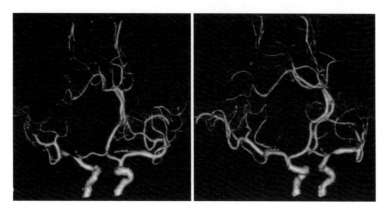

图 8.2.15 1 年前头部 CTA 示右大脑中动脉 M1 段重度狭窄

5 个月前患者再次出现上述症状。头部 MRI 示右侧侧脑室旁急性脑梗死（图 8.2.16）。头部 MRA 示右大脑中动脉 M1 段重度狭窄（图 8.2.17）。继续给予双联抗血小板治疗。

2 个月前上述症状再次发作。头部 MRI 示右侧颞顶叶急性脑梗死（图 8.2.18）。CTP 示右大脑中动脉供血区域低灌注（图 8.2.19）。DSA 示右颈总动脉起始处稍迂曲（图 8.2.20 A），右大脑中动脉 M1 段重度狭窄（图 8.2.20 B 和 C），前交通动脉开放（图 8.2.20 D 和 E），左侧椎动脉未见明显异常（图

8.2.21 A 和 B），未见明显后循环向前循环代偿（图 8.2.21 C 和 D）。患者为行血管内治疗收入我院。

既往史：脂蛋白代谢紊乱病史。

查体：左侧中枢性面瘫，左侧肢体肌力 4 级。TG 2.84 mmol/L，LDL-C 2.02 mmol/L。

血栓弹力图：AA 抑制率 100%，ADP 抑制率 5.1%。

入院后给予双联抗血小板（阿司匹林 100 mg 1 次 / 日＋氯吡格雷 75 mg 1 次 / 日）及降脂（阿托伐他汀 20 mg 1 次 / 日）等治疗。

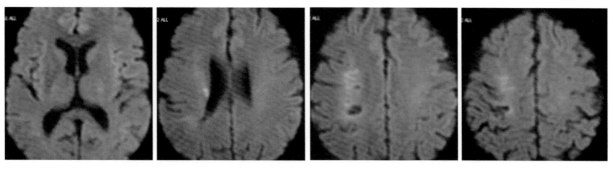

图 8.2.16 5 个月前头部 MRI 示右侧侧脑室旁急性脑梗死

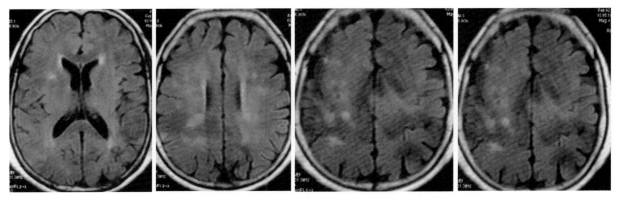

Fig. 8.2.14   The MRI findings from one year ago indicated the presence of acute infarctions in the right basal ganglia and frontoparietal lobe

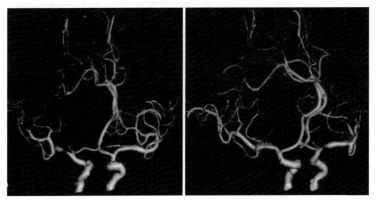

Fig. 8.2.15   The CTA revealed significant stenosis in the M1 segment of the right middle cerebral artery

Five months ago, the patient continued to exhibit weakness in the right limb. The MRI findings showed the presence of acute cerebral infarction in the periventricular area (Fig. 8.2.16). Furthermore, the MRA revealed severe stenosis in the M1 segment of the right middle cerebral artery (Fig. 8.2.17). Dual antiplatelet therapy was maintained.

Two months prior, the patient experienced identical symptoms. The MRI displayed acute cerebral infarctions in the right temporoparietal lobe (Fig. 8.2.18). The CT perfusion indicated hypoperfusion in the territory of the right middle cerebral artery (Fig. 8.2.19). The digital subtraction angiography (DSA) indicated the presence of tortuous access at the origin of the right common carotid artery (Fig. 8.2.20 A) along with severe stenosis in the M1 segment of the right middle cerebral artery (Fig. 8.2.20 B, C). The anterior communicating artery remained unobstructed (Fig. 8.2.20 D, E). No abnormal stenosis

was observed at the left vertebral artery (Fig. 8.2.21 A, B). There was no obvious compensation from the posterior circulation to the anterior circulation (Fig. 8.2.21 C, D).

The patient had a medical history of lipoprotein metabolism disorder.

Physical examination showed left central facial paralysis, and the muscle strength in the left limbs was grade 4.

The serum concentration of TG (triglycerides) and LDL-C (low-density lipoprotein cholesterol) was recorded at 2.84 mmol/L and 2.02 mmol/L, respectively.

The thromboelastography result indicated a 100% inhibition of AA and a 5.1% inhibition of ADP.

Upon admission, the patient was administered with a dual-antiplatelet regimen consisting of a daily dosage of 100 mg of Aspirin and 75 mg of Clopidogrel. In addition, statin therapy was given with a daily dosage of 20 mg of Atorvastatin.

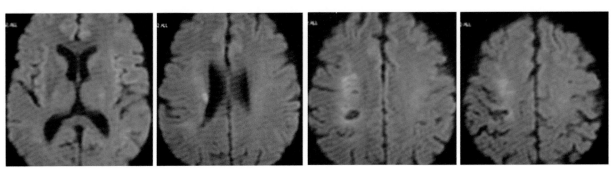

Fig. 8.2.16   The MRI findings showed the presence of acute cerebral infarction in the periventricular area

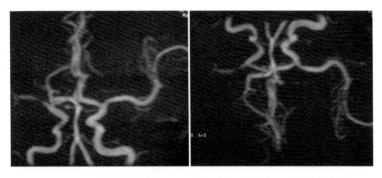

图 8.2.17　5 个月前头部 MRA 示右大脑中动脉 M1 段重度狭窄

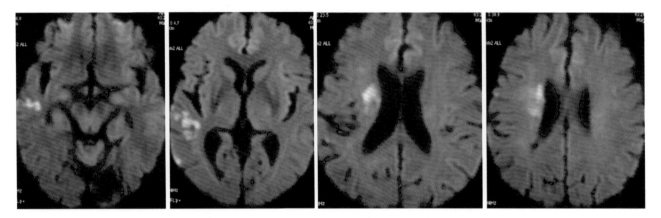

图 8.2.18　2 个月前头部 MRI 示右侧颞顶叶急性脑梗死

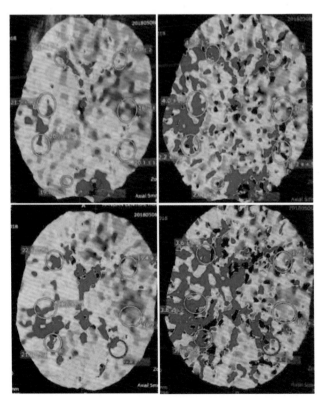

图 8.2.19　2 个月前 CTP 示右大脑中动脉供血区域低灌注

（二）诊断

症状性右大脑中动脉 M1 段重度狭窄。

（三）术前讨论

患者 1 年内反复出现右大脑中动脉供血区域脑梗死，CTP 提示相应区域低灌注，内科药物治疗无效，有介入治疗指征。右大脑中动脉 M1 段重度狭窄，狭窄远端毗邻外侧豆纹动脉组，拟球囊预扩张，再放置自膨式支架。右大脑中动脉狭窄远端分支稀疏，CTP 示相关区域低灌注明显，置入支架后有导致高灌注的可能，需严格控制血压。此外，还有动脉夹层、血管破裂、急性或亚急性支架内血栓形成等风险。

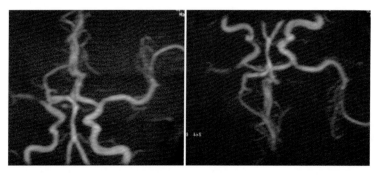

Fig. 8.2.17 The MRA revealed severe stenosis in the M1 segment of the right middle cerebral artery

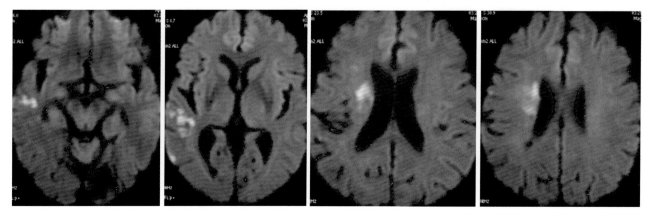

Fig. 8.2.18 The MRI displayed acute cerebral infarctions in the right temporoparietal lobe

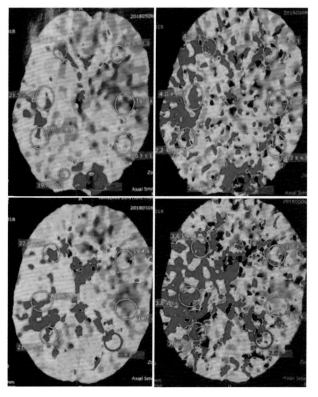

Fig. 8.2.19 The CT perfusion indicated hypoperfusion in the territory of the right middle cerebral artery

2. Diagnosis

Symptomatic severe stenosis in the M1 segment of the right middle cerebral artery.

3. Treatment schedule

The patient experienced recurrent cerebral infarctions within the territory of the right middle cerebral artery. The CT perfusion imaging revealed hypoperfusion in the affected region. Despite aggressive medical management, the patient experienced persistent recurrences. As a result, endovascular therapy was advised. The distal segment of the stenosis lesion was located near the lateral lenticulostriate arteries. The stenosis lesion was performed balloon angioplasty, followed by the implantation of a self-expandable stent. Given the limited distal branches beyond the stenosis and substantial hypoperfusion in the corresponding area, there is a high risk of hyperperfusion hemorrhage following the stent placement. Strict blood pressure control was imperative. Moreover, potential risks include arterial dissection, vessel rupture, and acute/subacute in-stent thrombosis.

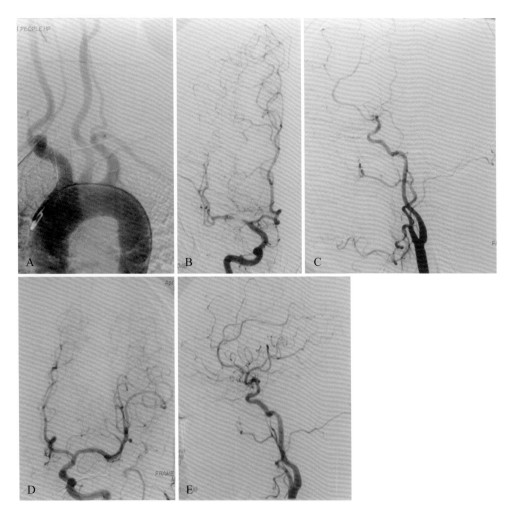

图 8.2.20　2 个月前 DSA 示右颈总动脉起始处稍迂曲（**A**），右大脑中动脉 M1 段重度狭窄（**B** 和 **C**），前交通动脉开放（**D** 和 **E**）

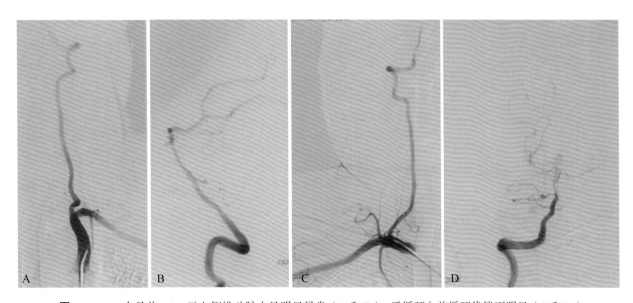

图 8.2.21　2 个月前 DSA 示左侧椎动脉未见明显异常（**A** 和 **B**），后循环向前循环代偿不明显（**C** 和 **D**）

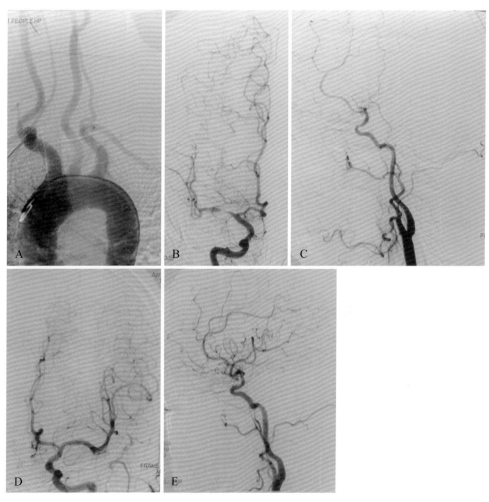

Fig. 8.2.20 The DSA conducted two months ago indicated the presence of tortuous access at the origin of the right common carotid artery (**A**), along with severe stenosis in the M1 segment of the right middle cerebral artery (**B, C**), The anterior communicating artery remained unobstructed (**D, E**)

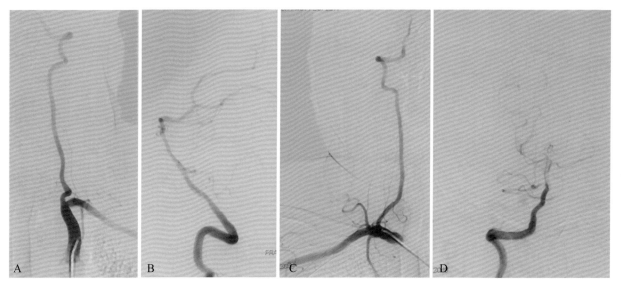

Fig. 8.2.21 No abnormal stenosis was observed at the left vertebral artery (**A, B**). There was no obvious compensation from the posterior circulation to the anterior circulation (**C, D**)

（四）治疗过程

全麻下右股动脉入路，6F 导引导管送至右颈内动脉 C1 段远端，术前造影示右大脑中动脉 M1 段重度狭窄（图 8.2.22）。路径图下沿导引导管送入 Transend 微导丝（0.014 in，300 cm）越过狭窄段放置在右大脑中动脉 M2 段以远，沿微导丝送入 Gateway 球囊（2 mm×9 mm）于狭窄处预扩张（图 8.2.23 A），撤出球囊导管，沿 Transend 微导丝送入 Wingspan 自膨式支架（3 mm×15 mm），造影提示支架贴壁良好，残余狭窄率约 5%（图 8.2.23 B 和 C）。

术后患者出现右颞部胀痛，立即复查头部 CT 未见出血（图 8.2.24）。

术后严格控制血压以及镇静治疗，患者仍诉头痛，分别于术后 5 h 和 24 h 复查头部 CT，未见出血（图 8.2.25 和图 8.2.26）。

复查 TCD：右大脑中动脉 M1 段血流速度 140 cm/s。

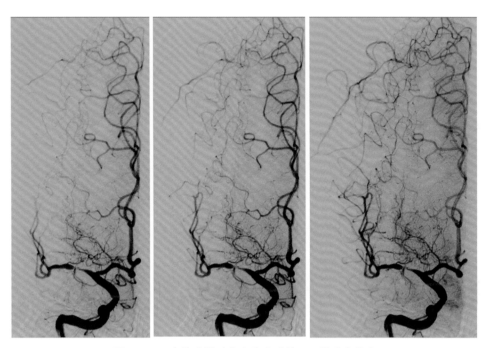

图 8.2.22 术前造影示右大脑中动脉 M1 段重度狭窄

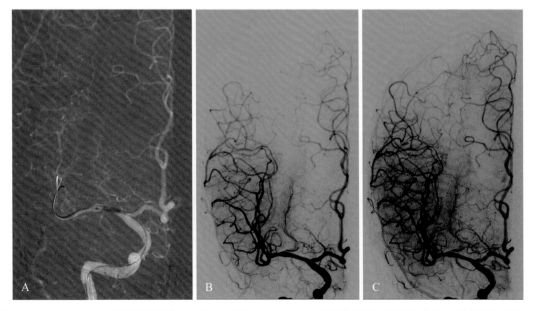

图 8.2.23 **A**. Gateway 球囊扩张病变；**B** 和 **C**. 释放 Wingspan 支架后造影示支架贴壁良好，残余狭窄率约 5%

4. Treatment

Under general anesthesia, a 6F guide catheter was positioned at the C1 segment of the right internal carotid artery. The angiogram indicated severe stenosis in the M1 segment of the right middle cerebral artery (Fig. 8.2.22). Under the roadmap, a Transend microwire (0.014 in, 300 cm) was navigated to the M2 segment of the right middle cerebral artery. And a 2 mm×9 mm Gateway balloon was delivered to pre-dilate the stenosis (Fig. 8.2.23 A). Following the balloon dilation, a 3 mm×15 mm Wingspan stent was utilized to cover the lesion. The post-stent implantation angiogram showed an excellent stent wall apposition, with a residual stenosis of approximately 5% (Fig. 8.2.23 B, C).

Post-procedure, the patient experienced headaches in the right temporal region. Subsequent CT scans revealed the absence of cerebral hemorrhage (Fig. 8.2.24).

The patient received strict blood pressure management and administration of sedatives. However, the patient continued to experience headaches. The CT scans conducted at 5 hours and 24 hours after the procedure did not reveal any signs of cerebral hemorrhage (Fig. 8.2.25 and Fig. 8.2.26).

The transcranial doppler (TCD) displayed a blood flow velocity of 140 cm/s in the M1 segment of the right middle cerebral artery.

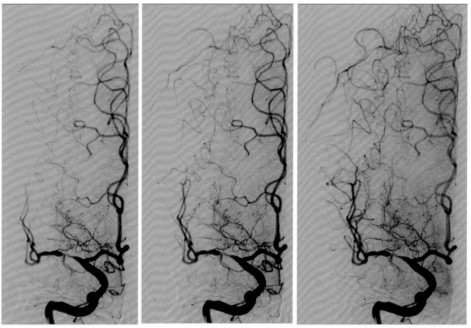

Fig. 8.2.22 The angiogram indicated severe stenosis in the M1 segment of the right middle cerebral artery

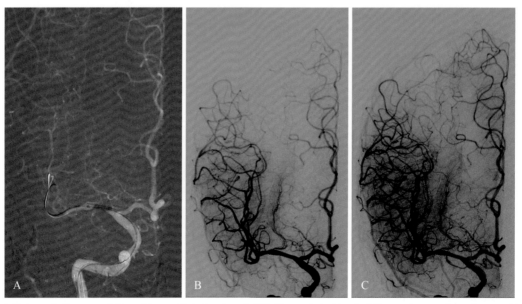

Fig. 8.2.23 A Gateway balloon was delivered to pre-dilate the stenosis (A). The post-stent implantation angiogram showed an excellent stent wall apposition, with residual stenosis of approximately 5% (B, C)

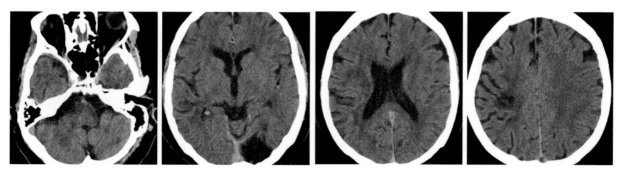

图 8.2.24　术后即刻头部 CT 未见出血

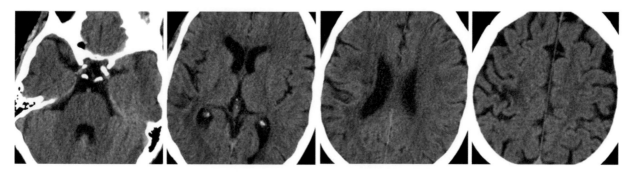

图 8.2.25　术后 5 h 头部 CT 未见出血

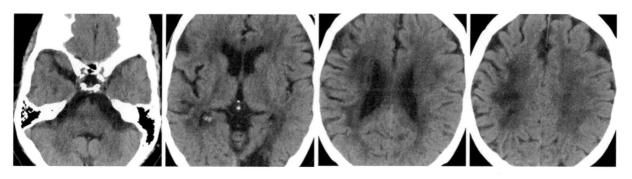

图 8.2.26　术后 24 h 头部 CT 未见出血

复查头部 CTA：右大脑中动脉支架内通畅（图 8.2.27）。

复查 CTP：右侧额、颞、顶区域低灌注较前明显改善（图 8.2.28）。

（五）讨论

本例系右大脑中动脉重度狭窄，血管内介入治疗后患者出现头痛，考虑乃血流改善后高灌注现象。术后严格控制血压（收缩压低于 120 mmHg），手术当晚给予镇静治疗，以防高灌注导致症状性出血的发生。术后高灌注出血一般发生在术后即刻和术后 24 h 内，超过 24 h 的高灌注出血病例相对少见。

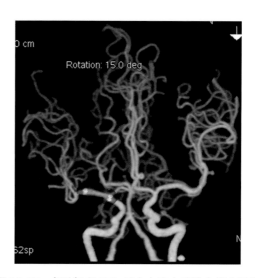

图 8.2.27　术后复查 CTA 示右大脑中动脉支架内通畅

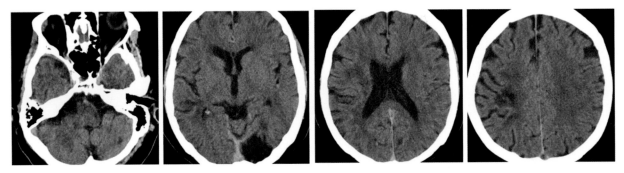

Fig. 8.2.24 The CT scans revealed the absence of cerebral hemorrhage

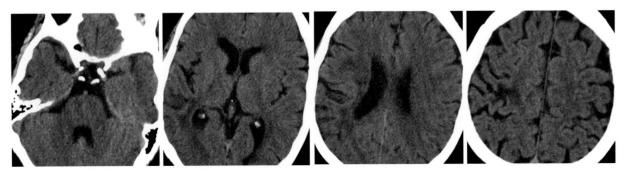

Fig. 8.2.25 The CT scans conducted 5 hours after the procedure did not reveal any signs of cerebral hemorrhage

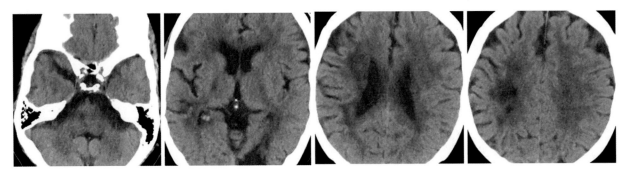

Fig. 8.2.26 The CT scans conducted 24 hours after the procedure did not reveal any signs of cerebral hemorrhage

The follow-up CTA revealed the stent in the right middle cerebral artery was patent (Fig. 8.2.27).

The CT perfusion scan unveiled a notable amelioration in the hypoperfusion observed in the right frontal, temporal, and parietal lobes (Fig. 8.2.28).

5. Comments

Following the stenting of the right middle cerebral artery, the patient experienced the emergence of headaches, indicative of hyperperfusion syndrome. To reduce the risk of symptomatic cerebral hemorrhage due to hyperperfusion, strict blood pressure control (maintaining systolic blood pressure below 120 mmHg) and administration of sedatives were implemented. Hyperperfusion hemorrhage typically manifests either immediately or within a 24-hour timeframe after the procedure. Instances of hyperperfusion hemorrhage occurring beyond this 24-hour window are relatively infrequent.

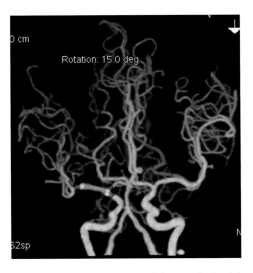

Fig. 8.2.27 The follow-up CTA revealed the stent in the right middle cerebral artery was patent

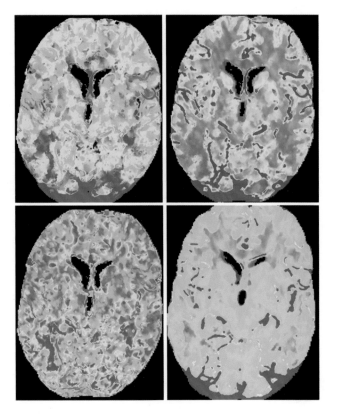

图 8.2.28　术后复查 CTP 示右侧额、颞、顶区域低灌注较前明显改善

（姚丽娜　李新明　宋立刚　马宁）

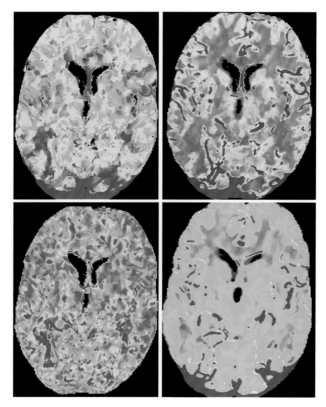

Fig. 8.2.28   The CT perfusion scan unveiled a notable amelioration in the hypoperfusion observed in the right frontal, temporal, and parietal lobes

(Translated by Rongrong Cui, Revised by Zhikai Hou)

第三节 术后急性血栓形成

病例 52 右椎基底动脉交界区支架术后急性血栓形成

（一）临床病史及影像分析

患者，男性，70 岁，主因"反复头晕 5 年，加重 2 个月"入院。

5 年前当地医院 TCD 提示基底动脉重度狭窄，给予阿司匹林和阿托伐他汀治疗之后仍有头晕反复发作。

2 个月前发作性头晕加重，伴有视物模糊、左上肢无力及行走不稳。当地医院头颅 MRA 提示基底动脉近端重度狭窄（图 8.3.1）。给予双联抗血小板（阿司匹林和氯吡格雷）和阿托伐他汀治疗后仍有症状发作。为行血管内治疗收入我院。

既往史：高血压病 30 年，糖尿病 10 余年，脂蛋白代谢紊乱 10 年，长期吸烟、饮酒史。

查体：左侧中枢性面瘫。

血栓弹力图：AA 抑制率 53.6%，ADP 抑制率 28.2%。

DSA：右椎基底动脉交界区重度狭窄（图 8.3.2），左椎动脉无明显狭窄（图 8.3.3），左颈动脉系统和右

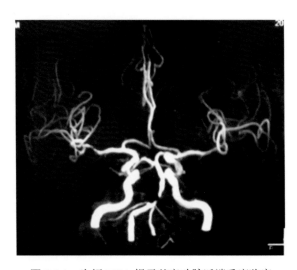

图 8.3.1 头颅 MRA 提示基底动脉近端重度狭窄

颈动脉系统无明显狭窄，未见明显前循环向后循环代偿（图 8.3.4）。

高分辨率 MRI 示右椎基底动脉交界区管壁斑块形成致管腔狭窄（图 8.3.5）。

入院后给予双联抗血小板（阿司匹林 100 mg

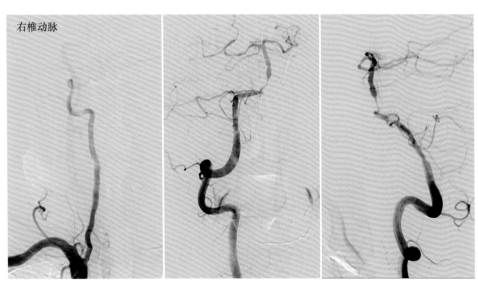

右椎动脉

图 8.3.2 DSA 示右椎基底动脉交界区重度狭窄

Section 3　Acute Thrombosis

Case 52　Acute thrombosis after right vertebro-basilar artery junction stenting

1. Clinical presentation and radiological studies

A 70-year-old male patient was admitted to the hospital due to episodes of paroxysmal dizziness for 5 years. And the symptoms have worsened over the past 2 months.

Five years ago, the transcranial doppler (TCD) examinations revealed a significant stenosis at the basilar artery. Despite being prescribed a regimen of aspirin and atorvastatin, the patient continued to endure episodes of dizziness.

Two months ago, the patient experienced worsening episodes of dizziness, accompanied by weakness in the left arm and blurred vision. The MRA results revealed a severe narrowing at the proximal segment of the basilar artery (Fig. 8.3.1). Despite aggressive medical treatment, the symptoms persisted.

The patient had a medical history including 30 years of hypertension, over 10 years of diabetes, a lipoprotein metabolism disorder lasting 10 years, and a prolonged habit of smoking and excessive alcohol consumption.

Physical examination showed left central facial paralysis.

The thromboelastography results indicated a 53.6% inhibition of AA and a 28.2% inhibition of ADP.

The digital subtraction angiography (DSA) demonstrated a significant narrowing at the junction of the right vertebro-basilar artery (Fig. 8.3.2). No significant narrowing was observed in the left vertebral artery (Fig. 8.3.3), as well as in the bilateral

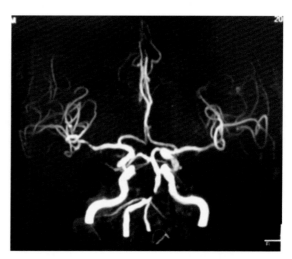

Fig. 8.3.1　MRA showed severe stenosis at the proximal segment of the basilar artery

carotid artery system. Moreover, there was no significant compensatory blood flow from the anterior circulation to the posterior circulation (Fig. 8.3.4).

The high-resolution MRI revealed the presence of plaque at the junction of the right vertebro-basilar artery, causing severe stenosis (Fig. 8.3.5).

Upon admission, the patient was administered with a

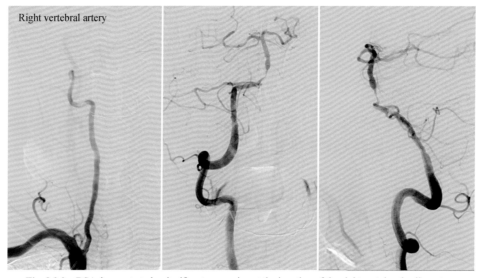

Right vertebral artery

Fig. 8.3.2　DSA demonstrated a significant narrowing at the junction of the right vertebro-basilar artery

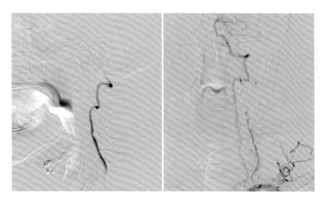

图 8.3.3　DSA 示左椎动脉无明显狭窄

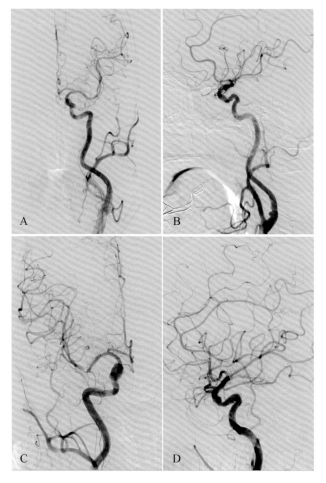

图 8.3.4　DSA 示左颈动脉系统和右颈动脉系统无明显狭窄，未见明显前循环向后循环代偿。**A** 和 **B**. 左颈动脉系统；**C** 和 **D**. 右颈动脉系统

1 次 / 日＋氯吡格雷 75 mg 1 次 / 日）以及强化降脂（阿托伐他汀 40 mg 1 次 / 日）等治疗。

（二）诊断

症状性右椎基底动脉交界区重度狭窄。

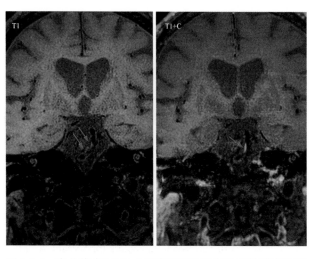

图 8.3.5　高分辨率 MRI 示右椎基底动脉交界区管壁斑块形成致管腔狭窄

（三）术前讨论

患者右椎基底动脉交界区重度狭窄，双联抗血小板治疗后仍有症状发作，有介入治疗指征。病变位于椎基底动脉交界区，虽然病变较直，但狭窄长度较长，粗测＞ 10 mm，拟采用球囊预扩张后置入自膨式支架覆盖狭窄段。相关风险包括穿支闭塞、急性或亚急性血栓形成以及高灌注综合征等。

（四）治疗过程

全麻下右股动脉穿刺置入 6F 动脉鞘，沿鞘送入 6F 导引导管至右椎动脉 V2 段远端，造影示基底动脉近端重度狭窄（图 8.3.6）。

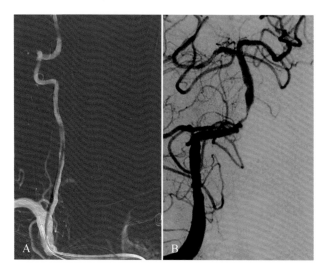

图 8.3.6　术前造影示基底动脉近端重度狭窄，前向血流 mTICI 分级 2b 级

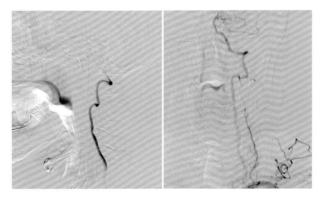

Fig. 8.3.3   DSA showed no significant stenosis in the left vertebral artery

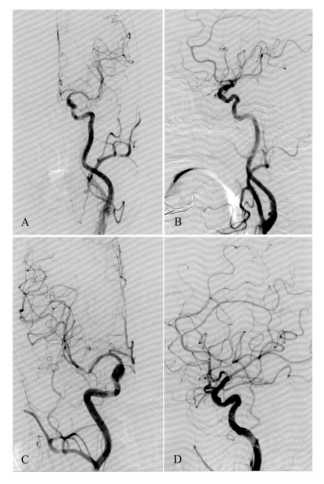

Fig. 8.3.4   No significant stenosis was observed in the bilateral carotid artery system. Moreover, there was no significant compensatory blood flow from the anterior circulation to the posterior circulation. (**A**, **B**) Left carotid artery system. (**C**, **D**) Right carotid artery system

dual-antiplatelet regimen consisting of a daily dose of 100 mg of Aspirin and 75 mg of Clopidogrel, as well as statin therapy with a daily dose of 40 mg of Atorvastatin.

2. Diagnosis

Symptomatic severe stenosis at the right vertebro-basilar artery junction.

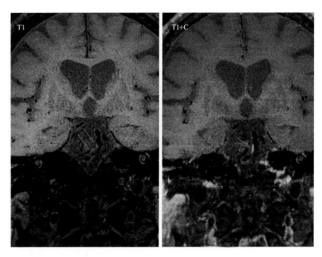

Fig. 8.3.5   HRMRI showed the presence of plaque at the junction of the right vertebro-basilar artery, causing a severe stenosis

3. Treatment schedule

The patient developed severe stenosis at the junction of the right vertebro-basilar artery. Despite receiving dual antiplatelet therapy, the clinical symptoms continue to recur and persist. Consequently, taking into account that the stenosis length exceeded 10 mm, the stenosis lesion was predilated with a small-size balloon, followed by the deployment of a self-expanding stent. Potential risks associated with the procedures included occlusion of the perforating arteries, acute or subacute in-stent thrombosis, and hyperperfusion syndrome.

4. Treatment

Under general anesthesia, a 6F guiding catheter was positioned at the V2 segment of the right vertebral artery. The angiogram confirmed severe stenosis at the proximal segment of the basilar artery (Fig. 8.3.6).

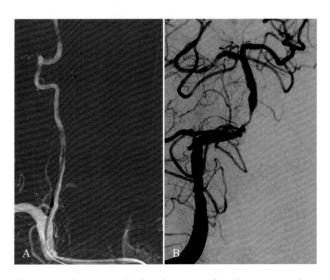

Fig. 8.3.6   The preprocedural angiogram confirmed severe stenosis at the proximal segment of the basilar artery

路径图下沿导引导管送入 Transend 微导丝（0.014 in，300 cm）至左大脑后动脉 P2 段。沿微导丝送入 Gateway 球囊（2.25 mm×15 mm）至狭窄段，定位准确后于狭窄处预扩张 1 次（图 8.3.7 A和 B）。沿 Transend 微导丝送入 Neuroform EZ 支架（3.5 mm×20 mm），释放后支架贴壁良好，前向血流 mTICI 分级 3 级（图 8.3.7 C）。

观察 5 min 后造影提示支架内可见数个充盈缺损，考虑急性血栓形成（图 8.3.8 A 和 B）。动脉内给予替罗非班 0.25 mg，结合微导丝头端塑形后在支架内轻柔旋转数次（图 8.3.8 C 和 D）。其后造影提示支架内管壁光整，遂结束治疗（图 8.3.9）。

术后 CTA：右椎基底动脉交界区支架内血流通畅（图 8.3.10）。

术后 CTP：左侧小脑半球 TTP 延长，MTT、CBF以及 CBV 无明显异常（图 8.3.11）。

术后复查血栓弹力图显示 ADP 抑制率 7.7%。将氯吡格雷调整为西洛他唑 100 mg 2 次 / 日。

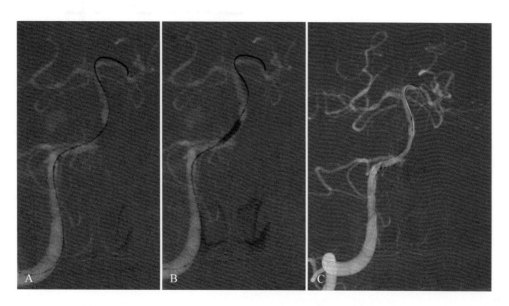

图 8.3.7　**A** 和 **B**. Gateway 球囊扩张狭窄病变；**C**. Neuroform EZ 支架释放后造影示支架贴壁良好，前向血流 mTICI 分级 3 级

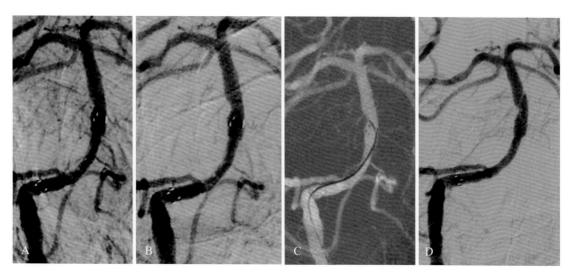

图 8.3.8　**A** 和 **B**. 观察 5 min 后造影提示支架内可见数个充盈缺损，考虑急性血栓形成；**C** 和 **D**. 微导丝头端塑形后在支架内轻柔旋转

Under the roadmap, a Transend microwire (0.014 inches, 300 cm) was positioned at the P2 segment of the left posterior cerebral artery. A 2.25 mm×15 mm Gateway balloon was deployed to dilate the stenosis (Fig. 8.3.7 A, B). After the balloon angioplasty, a 3.5 mm×20 mm Neuroform EZ stent was utilized to cover the lesion. The angiogram showed an excellent stent wall apposition, along with an antegrade blood flow graded as a level 3 (Fig. 8.3.7 C).

After an observation period of 5 minutes, the angiography revealed the presence of multiple filling defects within the stent, indicating acute thrombus formation (Fig. 8.3.8 A, B). An intravenous administration of 0.25 mg tirofiban was provided, accompanied by gentle rotations of the microwire within the stent after shaping its tip (Fig. 8.3.8 C, D). Subsequently, the angiography showed a smooth luminal surface within the stent (Fig. 8.3.9). The procedure concluded.

The follow-up CTA confirmed that the stent in the right vertebro-basilar artery junction remained unobstructed (Fig. 8.3.10).

The post-procedural CT perfusion scan indicated a prolonged time to peak (TTP) in the left cerebellar hemisphere without notable abnormalities in mean transit time (MTT), cerebral blood flow (CBF), and cerebral blood volume (CBV) (Fig. 8.3.11).

The follow-up thromboelastography test showed a 7.7% inhibition of ADP. Clopidogrel medication was replaced with a twice-daily dose of 100 mg of Cilostazol.

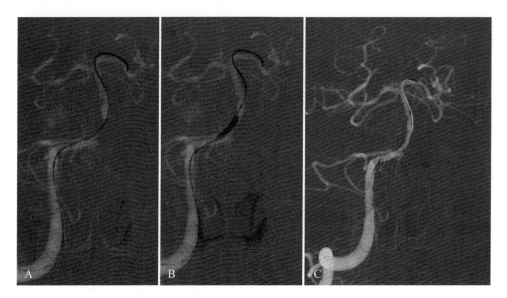

Fig. 8.3.7 A Gateway balloon was utilized to predilate the stenotic lesion (**A, B**). The post-stent implantation angiogram showed an excellent stent wall apposition, along with an antegrade blood flow graded as a level 3 (**C**)

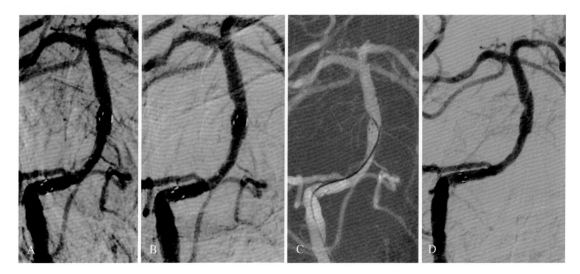

Fig. 8.3.8 After an observation period of 5 minutes, the angiography revealed the presence of multiple filling defects within the stent, indicating acute thrombus formation (**A, B**). The microwire rotated gently in the stent after its tip was shaped (**C, D**)

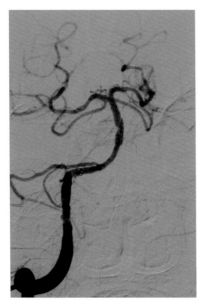

图 8.3.9 术后造影提示支架内管壁光整

（五）讨论

颅内动脉支架术后急性血栓形成发生率较低，一般考虑与抗血小板药物抵抗有关。对于长狭窄病变，置入的支架长度较长也易发生急性血栓形成。此外，如果支架置入后贴壁性不好，也容易导致急性血栓形成。目前尚没有循证医学证据支持的处理流程，主要以动脉内使用血小板糖蛋白Ⅱb/Ⅲa类受体拮抗剂，再结合微导丝或者球囊机械碎栓，一般都能迅速消除血栓。新发血栓若负荷量少且处理及时，患者术后一般不会形成新发症状。术后要酌情加大抗血小板聚集药物的用量或者调整用药方案，预防迟发血栓形成。

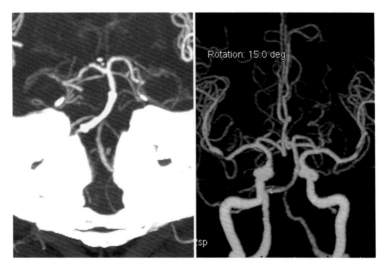

图 8.3.10 术后 CTA 示右椎基底动脉交界区支架内血流通畅

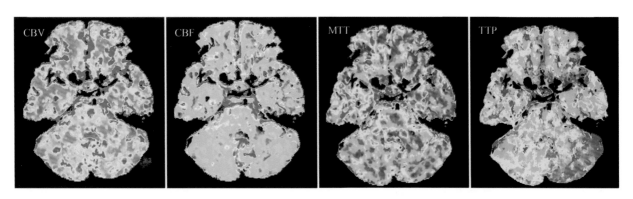

图 8.3.11 术后 CTP 示左侧小脑半球 TTP 延长，MTT、CBF 以及 CBV 无明显异常

（李红闪 李新明 董欢欢 杨海华 孙瑄 马宁）

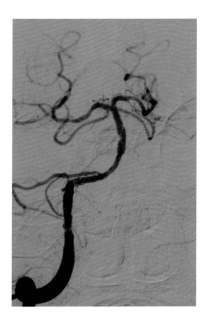

Figures 8.3.9   The angiography showed a smooth luminal surface within the stent

5. Comments

The incidence of acute thrombus formation after intracranial stenting is generally low, and it is commonly attributed to resistance to antiplatelet medication. Acute thrombus formation is more likely to occur with longer stents in cases of long stenotic lesions. Additionally, poor wall apposition of the stent can also contribute to acute thrombus formation. Currently, there is no evidence-based protocol for managing this condition. The primary approach involves the intra-arterial administration of glycoprotein II b/ III a receptor antagonists in combination with microwires or balloon mechanical thrombectomy, which can rapidly resolve the thrombus. If the low load of thrombus can be promptly treated, patients generally do not develop new neurological deficit symptoms. Adjustments in the dosage or treatment regimen of antiplatelet agents may be considered postoperatively to prevent delayed thrombus formation.

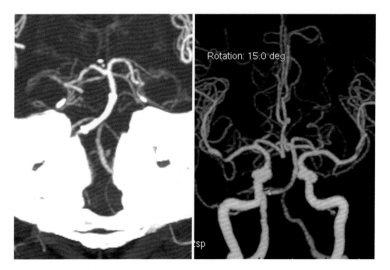

Fig. 8.3.10   The follow-up CTA confirmed that the stent in the right vertebro-basilar artery junction remained unobstructed

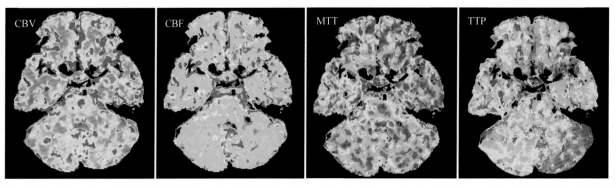

Fig. 8.3.11   The post-procedural CTP indicated a prolonged TTP in the left cerebellar hemisphere without notable abnormalities in MTT, CBF, and CBV

(Translated by Rongrong Cui, Revised by Zhikai Hou)

第四节 术后腹膜后血肿形成

病例 53 左大脑中动脉 M1 段支架术后腹膜后血肿形成

（一）临床病史及影像分析

患者，男性，70 岁，主因"发作性右侧肢体无力伴言语不利 6 个月"入院。

当地医院考虑诊断为短暂性脑缺血发作（TIA），给予阿司匹林、氯吡格雷和阿托伐他汀治疗。1 个月之后仍有症状反复发作。

完善头颅 MRI 提示左侧基底节以及额、颞、顶叶急性梗死灶（图 8.4.1）。DSA 提示右颈内动脉系统无明显异常，左大脑中动脉 M1 段重度狭窄，后循环系统未见明显异常（图 8.4.2）。

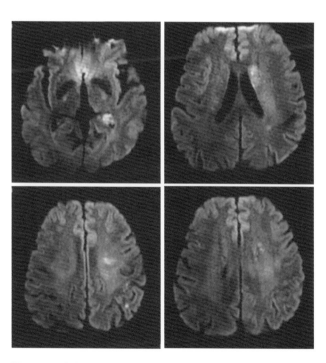

图 8.4.1 头颅 MRI 提示左侧基底节以及额、颞、顶叶急性梗死灶

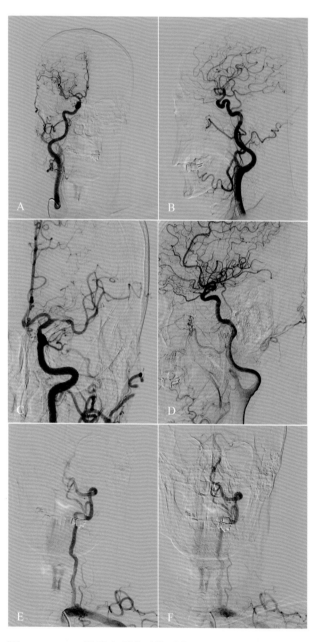

图 8.4.2 DSA 提示右颈内动脉系统无明显异常（**A** 和 **B**），左大脑中动脉 M1 段重度狭窄（**C** 和 **D**），后循环未见明显异常（**E** 和 **F**）

Section 4   Retroperitoneal Hematoma

Case 53   Retroperitoneal hematoma after stenting for the M1 segment of the left middle cerebral artery

1. Clinical presentation and radiological studies

A 70-year-old male patient was admitted to the hospital due to paroxysmal weakness in the right-sided limbs with dysarthria for six months.

The patient was diagnosed with a transient ischemic attack. And he was prescribed a combination treatment of Aspirin and Clopidogrel, as well as statin therapy with Atorvastatin. However, despite aggressive medical management, the patient continued to experience recurrent symptoms after one month.

The MRI findings depicted the presence of acute infarctions in the left basal ganglia, as well as in the frontal, temporal, and parietal lobes (Fig. 8.4.1). The digital subtraction angiography (DSA) displayed the absence of noteworthy abnormalities in the right internal carotid artery, severe stenosis in the M1 segment of the left middle cerebral artery, and no significant anomalies in the posterior circulation system (Fig. 8.4.2).

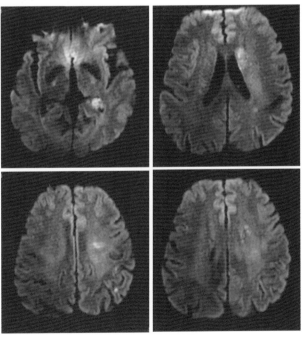

Fig. 8.4.1   The MRI findings depicted the presence of acute infarctions in the left basal ganglia, as well as in the frontal, temporal, and parietal lobes

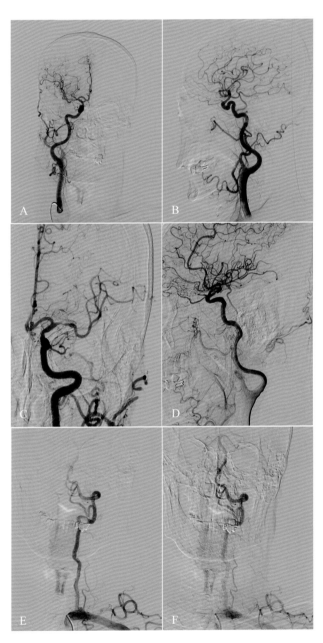

Fig. 8.4.2   DSA displayed the absence of noteworthy abnormalities in the right internal carotid artery (**A**, **B**), severe stenosis in the M1 segment of the left middle cerebral artery (**C**, **D**), and no significant anomalies in the posterior circulation system (**E**, **F**)

既往史：高血压病史 5 年余，长期吸烟和饮酒。

查体：神经系统查体未见明显异常。

甘油三酯（TG）：2.05 mmol/L；低密度脂蛋白胆固醇（LDL-C）：1.95 mmol/L。

血栓弹力图：ADP 抑制率 58.8%，AA 抑制率 100%。

入院后头部 CT：未见新发梗死（图 8.4.3）。

入院后 CTA 及 CTP：左大脑中动脉 M1 段重度狭窄（图 8.4.4 A），相关供血区域低灌注（图 8.4.4 B 和 C）。

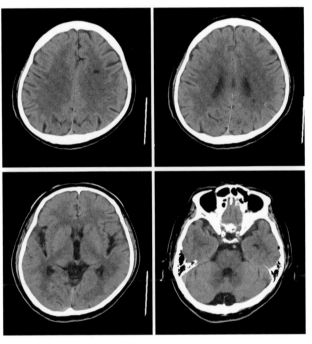

图 8.4.3　入院后头部 CT 未见新发梗死

入院后给予双联抗血小板（阿司匹林 100 mg 1 次 / 日＋氯吡格雷 75 mg 1 次 / 日）和降脂（阿托伐他汀 20 mg 1 次 / 日）等治疗。

（二）诊断

症状性左大脑中动脉 M1 段重度狭窄。

（三）术前讨论

患者 6 个月内反复出现左大脑中动脉供血区域脑梗死，CTP 提示相应区域低灌注，且内科药物治疗无效，有介入治疗指征。病变近端血管迂曲并且远端着陆区较短，且病变毗邻外侧豆纹动脉，治疗时拟用球囊预扩张，再放置自膨式支架。因手术入路迂曲，拟采用长鞘结合 Navien 导管以增加支撑力。相关风险包括高灌注综合征、动脉夹层、血管破裂、急性或亚急性支架内血栓形成等。

（四）治疗过程

全麻下右股动脉入路，7F 长鞘与 6F Navien 导管＋5F 多功能管同轴，将 6F Navien 导管放置在左颈内动脉 C4 段近端，造影示左大脑中动脉 M1 段重度狭窄（图 8.4.5 A）。路径图下沿导引导管送入 Transend 微导丝（0.014 in，300 cm）越过狭窄段至左大脑中动脉 M2 段以远，沿微导丝送入 Gateway 球囊（2 mm×9 mm）于狭窄处预扩张（图 8.4.5 B）。撤出球囊导管，沿 Transend 微导丝送入 Neuroform EZ 支架（3 mm×15 mm），造影

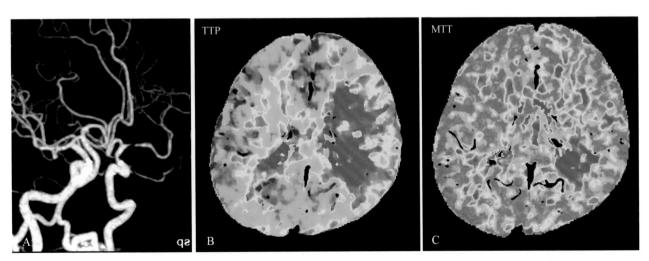

图 8.4.4　A. CTA 示左大脑中动脉 M1 段重度狭窄；B 和 C. CTP 示左大脑中动脉相关供血区域低灌注

The patient had a medical history of hypertension for over five years. Furthermore, he maintained a prolonged history of tobacco usage and alcohol consumption.

Upon admission, his neurological status displayed a state of intactness.

The serum levels of triglycerides and low-density lipoprotein cholesterol (LDL-C) were quantified at 2.05 mmol/L and 1.95 mmol/L, respectively.

The thromboelastography findings revealed a 58.8% inhibition of ADP-induced platelet function and complete inhibition of AA-induced platelet function.

The computed tomography (CT) scan conducted after admission exhibited the absence of any recent infarction (Fig. 8.4.3).

The CT angiography (CTA) revealed significant stenosis in the M1 segment of the left middle cerebral artery (Fig. 8.4.4 A). Additionally, the CT perfusion (CTP) depicted hypoperfusion in the corresponding territory (Fig. 8.4.4 B, C).

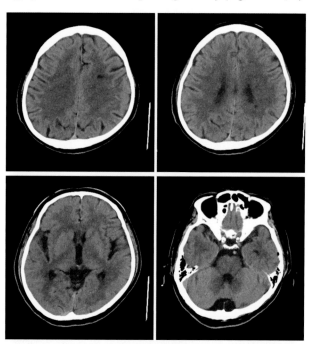

Fig. 8.4.3 The CT scan exhibited the absence of any recent infarction

Upon admission, the patient was prescribed a dual antiplatelet regimen of a daily of 100 mg of Aspirin and 75 mg of Clopidogrel, as well as statin therapy with a daily of 20 mg of Atorvastatin.

2. Diagnosis

Symptomatic severe stenosis in the M1 segment of the left middle cerebral artery.

3. Treatment schedule

The patient experienced recurrent ischemic strokes in the territory supplied by the left middle cerebral artery in the past 6 months. The CTP indicated hypoperfusion in the corresponding region. Furthermore, the patient did not respond to medical treatment. Consequently, the patient was indicated for endovascular treatment. The proximal arterial access exhibited tortuosity, while the distal landing zone was relatively short. Additionally, the lesion was adjacent to the lateral lenticulostriate artery. To address the lesion, the stenosis lesion was initially pre-dilated, followed by the implantation of a self-expanding stent. Due to the tortuous access route, a long sheath combined with a Navien guide catheter was considered to enhance support force. Potential risks associated with the procedure included hyperperfusion syndrome, arterial dissection, vessel rupture, and acute or subacute in-stent thrombosis.

4. Treatment

Under general anesthesia, the right femoral artery will serve as the access route. A 7F long sheath was coaxially combined with a 6F Navien guide catheter and a 5F multipurpose catheter. The 6F Navien guide catheter was placed at the proximal C4 segment of the left internal carotid artery. The angiogram demonstrated severe stenosis in the M1 segment of the left middle cerebral artery (Fig. 8.4.5 A). A Transend microwire (0.014 in, 300 cm) navigated through the stenosis segment to the M2 segment of the left middle cerebral artery. And a 2 mm×9 mm Gateway balloon was delivered to predilate the lesion (Fig. 8.4.5 B). Following the balloon dilation, a 3 mm×15 mm Neuroform EZ stent

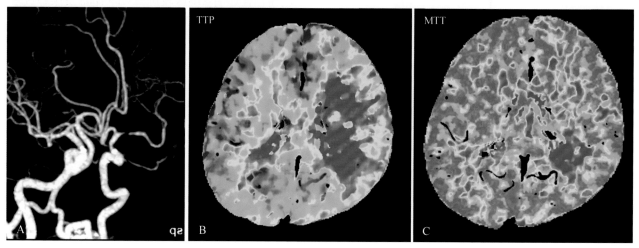

Fig. 8.4.4 The CTA revealed significant stenosis in the M1 segment of the left middle cerebral artery (**A**). CTP results depicted hypoperfusion in the corresponding territory (**B, C**)

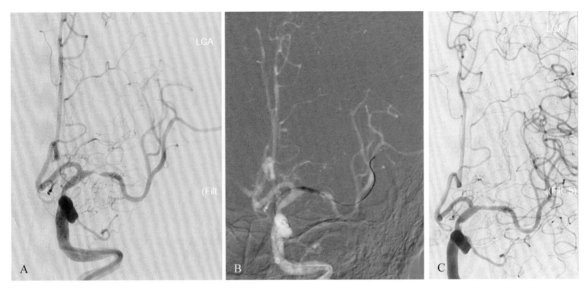

图 8.4.5　**A**.术前造影示左大脑中动脉 M1 段重度狭窄；**B**. Gateway 球囊预扩张；**C**.支架释放后造影

提示支架释放后贴壁良好，残余狭窄率约 20%（图 8.4.5 C）。

术后头颅 CT 未见出血。

术后头颅 CTA 示左大脑中动脉支架内通畅（图 8.4.6）。

患者术后出现腹膜后血肿（图 8.4.7），量约 100 ml，但生命体征平稳，经泌尿外科会诊予以保守治疗，血肿逐渐吸收后患者出院。

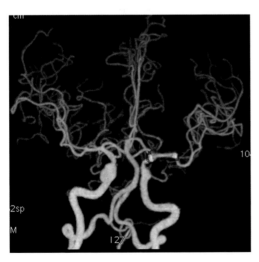

图 8.4.6　术后头颅 CTA 示左大脑中动脉支架内通畅

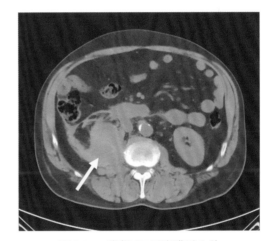

图 8.4.7　腹部 CT 示腹膜后血肿

（五）讨论

本例左大脑中动脉狭窄，病变短且局限，但路径迂曲，且远端着陆区较短，Wingspan 支架释放困难，故选择经导管释放的 Neuroform EZ 支架。由于后者的径向支撑力稍差，选择尺寸较长的支架有利于支架充分贴壁。腹膜后血肿是介入治疗的一个严重并发症，常见原因是穿刺针、导管、导丝等造成血管损伤。腹膜后血肿的处理包括密切监测生命体征，及时补液、输血，必要时介入栓塞靶血管或外科手术治疗。

（杨樟　张义森　姜鹏　马宁）

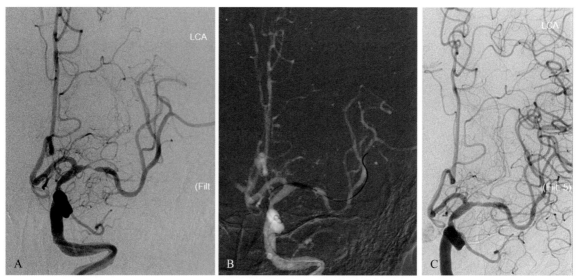

Fig. 8.4.5 (**A**) The angiogram before the procedure showed severe stenosis in the M1 segment of the left middle cerebral artery. (**B**) A Gateway balloon was used to predilate the lesion. (**C**) The post-stent implantation angiogram

was utilized to cover the lesion. The post-stent implantation angiogram revealed excellent stent wall apposition, with residual stenosis of approximately 20% (Fig. 8.4.5 C).

The postprocedural CT scans indicated the absence of intracerebral hemorrhage.

The postprocedural CTA showed the stent in the left middle cerebral artery was patent (Fig. 8.4.6).

Nonetheless, the patient experienced the emergence of a retroperitoneal hematoma (Fig. 8.4.7), with a volume of approximately 100 ml, after the procedure. Under the counsel of the Urologist, a conservative therapeutic approach was advised. Gradually, the retroperitoneal hematoma underwent absorption until the patient's discharge.

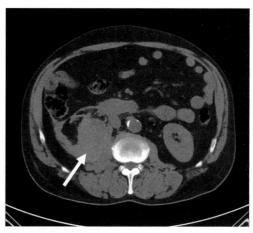

Fig. 8.4.7 The abdominal CT showed the retroperitoneal hematoma

5. Comments

In this particular case involving severe stenosis of the left middle cerebral artery, the stenotic lesion presented challenges due to its proximal tortuous access and limited landing zone. The successful deployment of a Wingspan stent proved to be difficult. Therefore, a Neuroform EZ stent was the alternative one, which was released via the microcatheter. Due to the slightly inferior radial support of the latter, opting for a longer-sized stent facilitates better wall apposition. Retroperitoneal hematoma is a serious complication of interventional treatment, commonly caused by vascular injury from puncture needles, catheters, guidewires, and other devices. Management of retroperitoneal hematoma involves close monitoring of vital signs, fluid infusion, and blood transfusion. If necessary, embolization of the target vessel or surgery was performed.

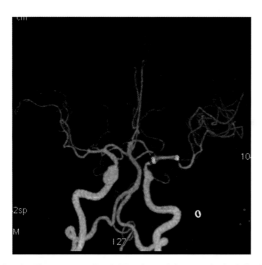

Fig. 8.4.6 The postprocedural CTA showed the stent in the left middle cerebral artery was patent

(Translated by Rongrong Cui, Revised by Zhikai Hou)

第九章

颅内动脉粥样硬化性慢性闭塞病变的外科治疗

病例 54 左颞浅动脉-大脑中动脉搭桥治疗左颈内动脉闭塞

（一）临床病史及影像分析

患者，男性，57岁，主因"突发言语不利伴右侧肢体无力8个月"入院。

8个月前患者行颈动脉彩超提示左颈内动脉闭塞伴右颈内动脉重度狭窄，药物治疗后症状无明显缓解，建议手术治疗。6个月前行右颈动脉内膜剥脱术，术后患者恢复良好，右侧肢体无力、言语不利症状好转，但仍有间断发作。完善脑动脉造影提示左颈内动脉闭塞，神经介入与神经外科联合诊疗，讨论认为血管内治疗再通可能性小，建议行颅外-颅内血运重建术改善颅内血流。

既往史：高血压病史6年。

查体：神经系统查体未见明显异常。

术前DSA：脑动脉造影提示左颈内动脉全程闭塞（图9.1.1 A和B），右颈内动脉经内膜剥脱术后血管通畅（图9.1.1 C）。

头部MRI：左侧额颞叶梗死灶（图9.1.2）。

头部CTP：左侧大脑半球低灌注（图9.1.3）。

（二）诊断

症状性左颈内动脉闭塞。

（三）术前讨论

患者系中老年男性，有动脉粥样硬化危险因素，影像学检查示右颈动脉重度狭窄、左颈动脉闭塞。内科药物治疗后仍间断出现右侧肢体力弱，CT灌注提示左侧脑组织灌注明显降低，考虑行血运重建

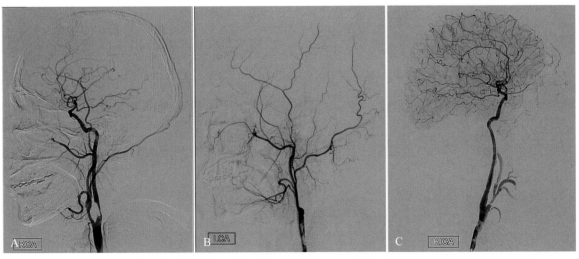

图9.1.1 A 和 B. 脑动脉造影提示左颈内动脉全程闭塞；**C.** 右颈内动脉经内膜剥脱术后血管通畅

Chapter 9

Surgical Therapy for Chronic Intracranial Atherosclerotic Occlusion

Case 54　Left superficial temporal artery-middle cerebral artery bypass for left internal carotid artery occlusion

1. Clinical presentation and radiological studies

A 57-year-old man was hospitalized for sudden episodes of dysarthria and weakness in his right limbs that had been present for eight months.

Carotid artery ultrasonography revealed occlusion of the left internal carotid artery and severe stenosis of the right internal carotid artery. Despite undergoing medical treatment, the patient's symptoms did not experience substantial relief. Therefore, vascular recanalization was indicated for this patient. The patient underwent a right carotid endarterectomy six months ago. While the procedure resulted in some improvement in the patient's symptoms of weakness in the right limbs and dysarthria, intermittent attacks continued to occur. Further examination using digital subtraction angiography (DSA) revealed occlusion of the left internal carotid artery. A multidisciplinary consultation between the neuro-interventional and neurosurgery departments concluded that endovascular treatment for the occlusion of the left internal carotid artery presented a challenge. As a result, it was recommended to undergo extracranial-intracranial revascularization to enhance intracranial blood flow.

He had a medical history of hypertension for six years.

Upon admission, the physical examination revealed intact neurological function.

DSA revealed total occlusion of the left internal carotid artery (Fig. 9.1.1 A, B), while the right internal carotid artery remained patent following the endarterectomy procedure (Fig. 9.1.1 C).

The MRI findings revealed the presence of cerebral infarctions in the left frontotemporal lobes (Fig. 9.1.2).

The CT perfusion indicated hypoperfusion in the left cerebral hemisphere (Fig. 9.1.3).

2. Diagnosis

Symptomatic occlusion of the left internal carotid artery.

3. Treatment schedule

The elderly male patient exhibited many atherosclerotic risk factors. Radiological examinations revealed significant stenosis in the right carotid artery and complete occlusion in the left carotid

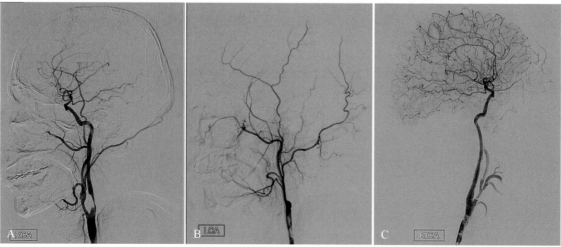

Fig. 9.1.1　DSA showed the left internal carotid artery was completely occluded (**A, B**), the right internal carotid artery was patent after endarterectomy (**C**)

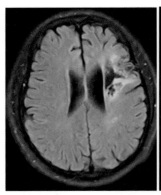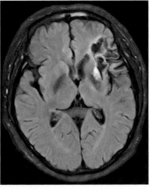

图 9.1.2　头部 MRI 提示左侧额颞叶梗死灶

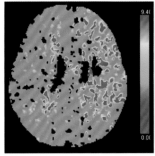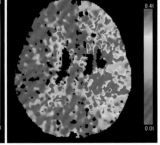

图 9.1.3　头部 CTP 提示左侧大脑半球低灌注

治疗。但患者左侧颈内动脉完全闭塞，成功再通概率低，遂行左颞浅动脉－大脑中动脉搭桥治疗。术后并发症主要包括高灌注综合征、颅内感染、癫痫等。

（四）治疗过程

患者全麻满意后平卧位头右偏，常规消毒铺巾。沿左侧颞浅动脉的走行 Y 型切开头皮，暴露、游离颞浅动脉前支和后支。临时阻断夹阻断颞浅动脉前支近端，锐性剪断前支远端，电灼残端止血。牵开皮瓣翻向两侧，T 型切开颞肌筋膜及颞肌，牵向两侧，暴露颅骨。颅骨钻 2 孔，铣刀铣下骨瓣约 5 cm×6 cm。显露脑膜中动脉及分支。硬脑膜四周悬吊后，弧形剪开硬脑膜，根部留于脑膜中动脉分支近端。脑组织张力中等。于外侧裂颞侧脑沟分离出一大脑中动脉 M4 分支，直径约 1.0 mm，罂粟碱棉条覆盖。分离处理颞浅动脉前支，吻合端直径

约 1.2 mm，处理外膜及内膜后，用肝素盐水冲洗管腔，2 枚临时阻断夹阻断暴露的大脑中动脉分支。纵行切开大脑中动脉分支约 1.2 mm，用肝素盐水冲洗管腔，10-0 线将颞浅动脉前支同大脑中动脉分支行端－侧吻合。先取下大脑中动脉分支的 2 枚临时阻断夹，颞浅动脉充盈良好，然后取下颞浅动脉的阻断夹，吻合口无渗血，止血纤维覆盖，动脉搏动好。将颞浅动脉后支表面筋膜与两侧硬脑膜缘间断缝合固定。创面止血，生理盐水冲洗清亮，脑组织搏动良好。硬脑膜翻转贴敷，间断缝合固定。充分止血后骨瓣复位固定，缝合颞肌、肌筋膜、皮下组织及皮肤。手术顺利。

术后 CTA 提示搭桥血管通畅，同侧脑灌注改善（图 9.1.4）。

（五）讨论

本患者双颈内动脉病变，右颈内动脉重度狭窄行右颈内动脉内膜剥脱术。左颈内动脉闭塞，左颈内动脉供血区明显低灌注，且患者有相应临床症状，神经介入与神经外科联合诊疗，评估后考虑血管内介入开通左颈内动脉难度大，治疗风险高，遂尝试行左侧颅外－颅内血运重建术，改善患者左侧大脑半球血流灌注情况。

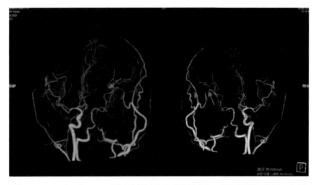

图 9.1.4　术后 CTA 提示搭桥血管通畅，同侧脑灌注改善（箭头）

（秦舒森　王嵘）

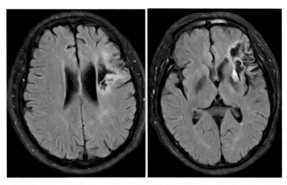

Fig. 9.1.2 The MRI showed cerebral infarctions in the left frontal and temporal lobes

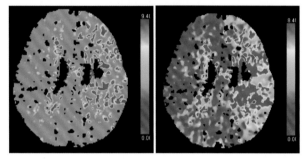

Fig. 9.1.3 The CTP showed hypoperfusion in the left cerebral hemisphere

artery. Despite receiving medical treatment, the patient continued to experience weakness in the right limbs. Additionally, CT perfusion indicated hypoperfusion in the left cerebral hemisphere, necessitating vascular recanalization. Due to the complete occlusion of the left carotid artery without any residual lumen, the likelihood of successful recanalization was deemed low. Therefore, it was recommended to proceed with a left superficial temporal artery-middle cerebral artery bypass. Potential complications associated with the procedure included hyperperfusion syndrome, intracranial infection, epilepsy, and so forth.

4. Treatment

Under general anesthesia, the patient was supine with the head tilted to the right. After disinfection, the anterior and posterior branches of the superficial temporal artery were exposed and isolated with a Y-shaped incision along the left superficial temporal artery. A temporary blocking clip blocked the proximal anterior branch of the superficial temporal artery, the distal end of the anterior branch was sharply clipped, and the residual end was burned with electrocautery for hemostasis. The flap was retracted and turned to both sides. The temporalis fascia and temporalis muscle were dissected in a T-shape and turned to both sides to expose the skull. Two holes were drilled into the skull, and the bone flap was cut about 5 cm×6 cm with a milling cutter. The middle meningeal artery and its branches were exposed. The dura was hung around and cut along a circular arc, and the root remained near the middle meningeal artery branch. Brain tissue tension was moderate. The M4 branch of the middle cerebral artery was isolated from the lateral fissure with a diameter of about 1.0 mm and covered with

a papaverine tampon. The anterior branch of the superficial temporal artery was separated with the diameter of an anastomotic end of about 1.2 mm, the lumen was rinsed with heparin saline after treating the outer membrane and intima. and the exposed middle cerebral artery branches were blocked with two temporary blocking clips. The middle cerebral artery branch was then longitudinally cut about 1.2 mm, the lumen was washed with heparin saline, and the anterior branch of the superficial temporal artery was anastomosed with the branch of the middle cerebral artery end-to-side by 10-0 suture. Two temporary blocking clips were removed from the middle cerebral artery branch and the superficial temporal artery was well filled. Then, the blocking clips of the superficial temporal artery were removed. The anastomotic site was observed without blood exudation, then covered with hemostatic fibers, and the artery pulsated well. The superficial fascia of the posterior branch of the superficial temporal artery was sutured intermittently with both dural borders. The wound was hemostatic and cleaned with normal saline, and brain tissue pulsation was well. The dura was reversed and fixed with intermittent suture. After adequate hemostasis, the bone flap was reduced and fixed. The temporalis, musculofascial, subcutaneous tissue, and skin were sutured. The operation was successful.

Postoperative CTA showed the bypass vessels were unobstructed, and the ipsilateral cerebral perfusion was improved (Fig. 9.1.4).

5. Comments

The patient presented with bilateral lesions in the internal carotid arteries. To address the severe stenosis in the right internal carotid artery, a right internal carotid endarterectomy was conducted. The left internal carotid artery was occluded, resulting in significant hypoperfusion in the corresponding brain region. Despite receiving medical treatment, the patient's ischemic symptoms persisted. Following a comprehensive consultation involving the neuro-interventional and neurosurgery departments, it was determined that endovascular treatment for the occluded left internal carotid artery posed a challenge with a high risk of complications. Consequently, a left extracranial-intracranial bypass procedure was performed to enhance perfusion in the left cerebral hemisphere.

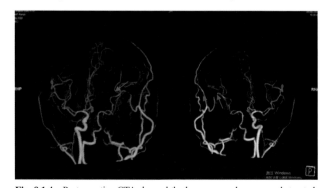

Fig. 9.1.4 Postoperative CTA showed the bypass vessels were unobstructed, and the ipsilateral cerebral perfusion was improved

(Translated by Shusen Qin, Revised by Zhikai Hou)

病例 55　右大脑中动脉闭塞颅外–颅内直接＋间接血运重建术

（一）临床病史及影像分析

患者，男性，58 岁，主因"突发头痛、头晕 2 个月"入院。

2 个月前当地医院头颅 CT 提示脑出血，CTA 提示右大脑中动脉闭塞，脑血管造影提示右大脑中动脉闭塞，当地医院给予药物保守治疗。为进一步诊治，转入我院。

既往史：脑梗死、脑出血及喉癌术后放疗史。饮酒、吸烟 30 年。

查体：构音障碍，余未见明显异常。

入院后完善头部 CTA + CTP：右大脑中动脉闭塞（图 9.2.1 A 和 B），右侧额、颞、顶、岛叶低灌注（图 9.2.1 C 和 D）。

（二）诊断

症状性右大脑中动脉闭塞。

（三）术前讨论

结合临床病史及影像学资料，考虑患者为动脉粥样硬化性右大脑中动脉闭塞–烟雾综合征（出血）。可行右侧颅外–颅内血管搭桥术，减少颅内末端血管代偿性扩张，降低缺血、出血发作风险。相关并发症有新发脑梗死、高灌注出血，可导致偏瘫、失语、癫痫等，极其严重者可能导致昏迷、死亡等。

（四）治疗过程及随访

患者全麻后取仰卧位，头偏向左侧，常规消毒后铺巾。沿颞浅动脉的走行 Y 型切开头皮，暴露、游离颞浅动脉后支及前支。牵开皮瓣翻向两侧，T 型切开颞肌筋膜及颞肌，牵向两侧，暴露颅骨。颅骨钻 2 孔，铣刀铣下骨瓣约 6 cm×5 cm。硬脑膜张力中等，显露脑膜中动脉及分支。硬脑膜四周悬吊后，弧形剪开硬脑膜。于外侧裂颞侧脑沟分离出一大脑中动脉 M4 分支，直径约 1.0 mm，用罂粟碱棉条覆盖。游离处理颞浅动脉前支，临时阻断近端，结扎远端，吻合端直径约 1.2 mm，处理外膜后，用肝素盐水冲洗管腔，2 枚临时阻断夹阻断目标 M4 分支。纵行切开大脑中动脉分支约 1.4 mm，用肝素盐水冲洗管腔，10-0 线将颞浅动脉前支同大脑中动脉分支行端–侧吻合（间断缝合 10 针）。先取下大脑中动脉分支的阻断夹，大脑中动脉及颞浅动脉充盈，然后取下颞浅动脉的阻断夹，吻合口少量出血，止血纤维覆盖后无活动性出血，动脉搏动好。颞浅动脉后支贴敷脑组织表面，硬脑膜翻转贴敷。硬脑膜未缝合，外覆免缝人工硬脑膜，充分止血后骨瓣复位、固定。逐层缝合颞肌、肌筋膜、皮下组织及皮肤。手术顺利。

术后 8 个月行 CTA + CTP 复查，见右侧开颅骨瓣区搭桥血管通畅（图 9.2.2 A 和 B），右侧额、颞、顶区缺血较前明显改善（图 9.2.2 C 和 D）。

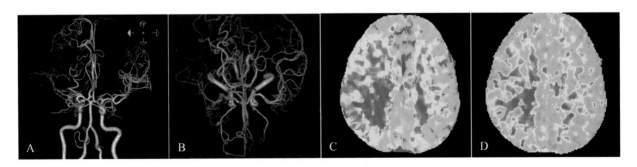

图 9.2.1　头部 CTA 示右大脑中动脉未见显影（**A** 和 **B**），CTP 示右侧额、颞、顶、岛叶低灌注（**C** 和 **D**）

Case 55 Direct and indirect extracranial-intracranial revascularization for the right middle cerebral artery occlusion

1. Clinical presentation and radiological studies

A 58-year-old male patient was admitted to the hospital due to sudden onset headaches and dizziness for two months.

The CT scans performed two months ago revealed the presence of cerebral hemorrhage. The CT angiography (CTA) indicated occlusion of the right middle cerebral artery. Furthermore, digital subtraction angiography (DSA) confirmed occlusion of the right middle cerebral artery.

The patient's medical history included cerebral infarction, cerebral hemorrhage, as well as postoperative radiotherapy for laryngeal cancer. In addition, he had been drinking and smoking for 30 years.

Physical examination showed dysarthria.

The CTA revealed occlusion of the right middle cerebral artery (Fig. 9.2.1 A, B). The CT perfusion showed hypoperfusion in the right frontal, temporal, parietal, and insular lobes (Fig.9.2.1 C, D).

2. Diagnosis

Symptomatic occlusion of the right middle cerebral artery.

3. Treatment schedule

After reviewing the patient's medical records and relevant radiological examinations, a diagnosis of right middle cerebral artery atherosclerotic occlusion-specifically, moyamoya syndrome with a hemorrhagic manifestation-was established. To reduce the abnormal compensatory dilation of the intracranial terminal vessels and minimize the risks of cerebral ischemia and re-bleeding, surgical intervention of right extracranial-intracranial arterial bypass was performed. Potential complications included cerebral infarction and hyperperfusion hemorrhage, which could lead to hemiplegia, aphasia, epilepsy, and in severe cases, even the highest-risk outcomes of comatose states and mortality.

4. Treatment and follow up

Under general anesthesia, the patient was supine with the head tilted to the left. After disinfection, the posterior and anterior branches of the superficialtemporal artery were exposed and isolated by cutting the scalp with a Y-shaped incision along the superficial temporal artery. The flap was retracted and turned to both sides. The temporalis fascia and temporalis muscle were cut open in a T-shape and were retracted to both sides to expose the skull. Two holes were drilled into the skull, and the bone flap was cutted about 6 cm×5 cm. The middle meningeal artery and its branches were exposed. The dural was cut along the arc. A middle cerebral artery M4 branch with a diameter of about 1.0 mm was isolated from the lateral fissure and covered with a papaverine tampon. The anterior branch of the superficial temporal artery was dissociated, the proximal end was temporarily blocked, and the distal end was ligated. The diameter of the anastomotic end was about 1.2 mm. After the outer membrane was peeled off, the lumen was washed with heparin saline, and the target M4 branch was blocked with two temporary blocking clips. The branch of the middle cerebral artery was longitudinally cut about 1.4 mm, the lumen was washed with heparin saline, and the anterior branch of the superficial temporal artery was anastomosed with the branch of the middle cerebral artery end-to-side by 10-0 suture (10 intermittent stitches). The blocking clips of the middle cerebral artery branch were removed, and the middle cerebral artery and superficial temporal artery were filled. Then the blocking clip of the superficial temporal artery was removed. There was a small amount of bleeding at the anastomotic site and no active bleeding after being covered with hemostatic fiber. The artery pulsated well. The posterior branch of the superficial temporal artery was applied to the surface of the brain tissue, and the dura was reversed and applied. The dura was not sutured, and covered with the suture-free artificialdura. After sufficienthemostasis, the bone flap was reduced and fixed. The temporalis muscle, musculofascia, subcutaneous tissue, and skin were sutured layer by layer. The operation was successful.

The follow-up CTA performed after eight months revealed the patency of the bypass vessels within the region of the right craniotomy bone flap (Fig. 9.2.2 A, B). The CTP demonstrated a noteworthy enhancement in the hypoperfusion observed in the right frontal, temporal, and parietal lobes (Fig. 9.2.2 C, D).

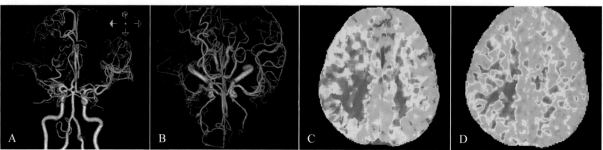

Fig. 9.2.1 The CTA showed occlusion of the right middle cerebral artery (**A**, **B**), and CT perfusion revealed hypoperfusion in the right frontal, temporal, parietal, and insular lobes (**C**, **D**)

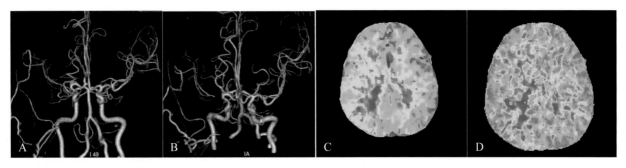

图 9.2.2　术后 8 个月复查头部 CTA 和 CTP 如下：CTA 示右侧开颅骨瓣区搭桥血管通畅（**A** 和 **B**），CTP 示右侧额、颞、顶区缺血较前明显改善（**C** 和 **D**）

（五）讨论

本例患者为颅内动脉粥样硬化性闭塞所致脑出血，针对该部分患者，血管内介入治疗诱发再次脑出血的风险较大，经神经介入与神经外科联合诊疗，决定行直接＋间接血运重建手术，预防再出血的风险，同时改善病变血管供血区域的低灌注。

（王嵘　秦舒森）

病例 56　左大脑中动脉闭塞颅外-颅内直接＋间接血运重建术

（一）临床病史及影像分析

患者，男性，51 岁，主因"发作性左侧肢体麻木 3 年，言语不利 1 年"入院。

患者在药物保守治疗下仍有多次脑缺血症状发作，影像学检查提示左大脑中动脉狭窄，为行进一步治疗转入我院。

既往史：高血压病史 2 年。吸烟、饮酒 30 年。

查体：神经系统查体未见明显异常。

入院后完善头部 CTA ＋ CTP：CTA 提示左大脑中动脉闭塞（图 9.3.1 A 和 B），CTP 提示左侧额、颞、顶、枕叶可见大片低灌注区域（图 9.3.1 C 和 D）。

MRI：左侧放射冠、基底节区、侧脑室旁多发小片状梗死灶（图 9.3.2）。

术前 DSA：左大脑中动脉 M1 段闭塞，伴局部烟雾样穿支血管增生，可见同侧大脑前动脉通过软脑膜支向大脑中动脉代偿（图 9.3.3）。

（二）诊断

症状性左大脑中动脉闭塞。

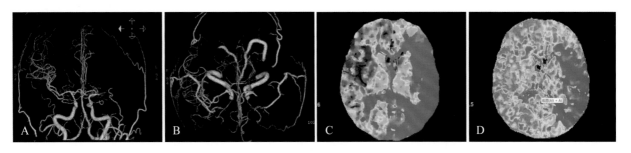

图 9.3.1　**A** 和 **B**. 头部 CTA 提示左大脑中动脉闭塞；**C** 和 **D**. 头部 CTP 提示左侧额、颞、顶、枕叶可见大片低灌注区域

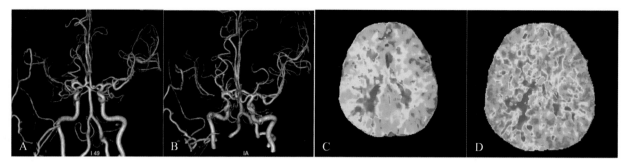

Fig. 9.2.2 (**A**, **B**) The follow-up CTA performed after eight months revealed the patency of the bypass vessels within the region of the right craniotomy bone flap. (**C**, **D**) Additionally, the CTP demonstrated a noteworthy enhancement in the hypoperfusion observed in the right frontal, temporal, and parietal lobes

5. Comments

In this particular case, the patient suffered from cerebral hemorrhage caused by occlusion resulting from intracranial arteriosclerosis. Given the heightened probability of recurrent hemorrhage associated with endovascular treatment in this specific population, a multidisciplinary approach combining neuro-interventional and neurosurgical disciplines was employed. The consensus was to proceed with a comprehensive direct and indirect vascular reestablishment surgery, aiming to not only mitigate the risk of potential reoccurrence but also enhance the perfusion in the affected vascular territory.

(Translated by Shusen Qin, Revised by Zhikai Hou)

Case 56   Left-side combined bypass surgery for the left middle cerebral artery occlusion

1. Clinical presentation and radiological studies

A 51-year-old man was admitted to the hospital due to recurrent episodes of transient numbness in the left limbs for 3 years and dysarthria for 1 year.

Despite undergoing medical intervention, the patient's manifestations of cerebral ischemia persisted. Furthermore, imaging analysis indicated the presence of stenosis in the left middle cerebral artery.

The patient had a 2-year history of hypertension. Moreover, he had been a smoker and drinker for 30 years.

He was neurologically intact on admission.

The CT angiography (CTA) showed the presence of occlusion in the left middle cerebral artery (Fig. 9.3.1 A, B). The CT perfusion indicated significant hypoperfusion in the left frontal, temporal, parietal, and occipital lobes (Fig.9.3.1 C, D).

The MRI result showed multiple small infarctions in the left corona radiata, basal ganglia, and periventricular region (Fig. 9.3.2).

The digital subtraction angiography (DSA) revealed the occlusion in the M1 segment of the left middle cerebral artery, accompanied by moyamoya collateral vessel proliferation. The ipsilateral anterior cerebral artery provided the compensatory blood flow to the territory of the middle cerebral artery through the pial arteries (Fig. 9.3.3).

2. Diagnosis

Symptomatic occlusion of the left middle cerebral artery.

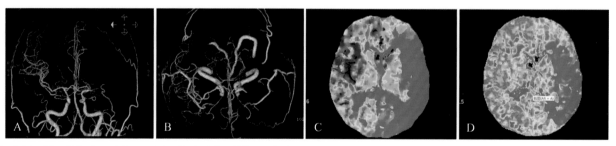

Fig. 9.3.1   The CTA showed the occlusion in the left middle cerebral artery (**A**, **B**). The CT perfusion showed significant hypoperfusion in the left frontal, temporal, parietal, and occipital lobes (**C**, **D**)

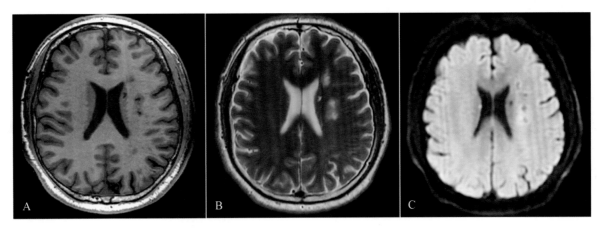

图 9.3.2　头部 MRI 提示左侧放射冠、基底节区、侧脑室旁多发小片状梗死灶

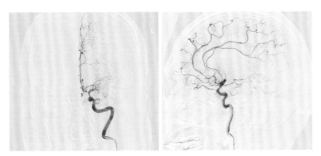

图 9.3.3　术前 DSA 提示左大脑中动脉 M1 段闭塞，伴局部烟雾样穿支血管增生，可见同侧大脑前动脉通过软脑膜支向大脑中动脉代偿

（三）术前讨论

患者左侧大脑中动脉 M1 段闭塞，相应供血区有明显低灌注，结合患者临床症状及梗死灶分布特点，考虑左侧大脑中动脉 M1 段为责任动脉，可行左侧血管吻合术改善颅内供血，进而降低缺血发作及脑梗死复发风险。相关并发症包括新发脑梗死、高灌注出血等导致的偏瘫、失语、癫痫等，极其严重者可能导致昏迷、死亡等极端风险。

（四）治疗过程及随访

患者全麻后仰卧位头右偏，常规消毒后铺巾。沿颞浅动脉的走行直行切开头皮，暴露颞浅动脉后支及前支。进一步游离颞浅动脉后支及前支备用。牵开皮瓣翻向两侧，T 型切开颞肌筋膜及颞肌，牵向两侧，暴露颅骨。颅骨钻 2 孔，铣刀铣下骨瓣

约 5 cm×4 cm，显露脑膜中动脉及分支。弧形剪开硬脑膜，于外侧裂颞侧脑沟分离出一大脑中动脉分支，直径约 1.0 mm。分离处理颞浅动脉前支，临时阻断近端，结扎远端，吻合端直径约 1.2 mm，处理外膜后，用肝素盐水冲洗管腔，2 枚临时阻断夹阻断暴露的大脑中动脉分支。用玻璃刀纵行切开大脑中动脉分支约 1.2 mm，用肝素盐水冲洗管腔，10-0 线将颞浅动脉前支同大脑中动脉分支行端-侧吻合间断缝合。先取下大脑中动脉分支的阻断夹，大脑中动脉及颞浅动脉充盈，然后取下颞浅动脉的阻断夹，吻合口未出血。颞浅动脉后支贴附于脑表面。术中吲哚氰绿造影示搭桥血管及颞浅动脉后支血流通畅。止血纤维覆盖后无活动性出血，动脉搏动好。硬脑膜翻转贴敷，未缝合，外覆免缝人工硬脑膜防止脑脊液漏，充分止血后骨瓣复位、固定。逐层缝合颞肌、肌筋膜、皮下组织及皮肤。手术顺利。

术后 3 个月行 CTA + CTP 复查，见左侧开颅骨瓣区搭桥血管通畅，左侧额、颞、顶区低灌注情况较前明显改善（图 9.3.4）。

（五）讨论

本例患者左大脑中动脉闭塞，伴局部烟雾样穿支血管增生，考虑诊断为单侧颅内动脉粥样硬化性闭塞所致的烟雾综合征。针对该部分患者，直接＋间接血运重建手术可改善症状，降低脑梗死复发等风险。

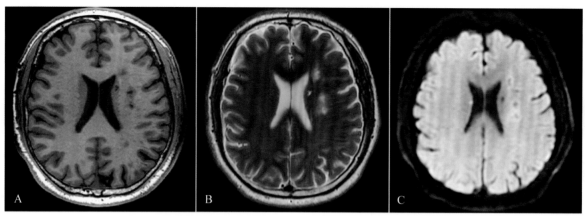

Fig. 9.3.2 The MRI results showed multiple small infarctions in the left corona radiata, basal ganglia, and periventricular region

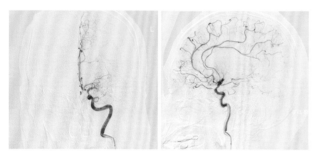

Fig. 9.3.3 DSA revealed the occlusion in the M1 segment of the left middle cerebral artery, accompanied by moyamoya collateral vessel proliferation. The ipsilateral anterior cerebral artery provided the compensatory blood flow to the territory of the middle cerebral artery through the pial arteries

3. Treatment schedule

The occlusion of the M1 segment of the left middle cerebral artery in the patient resulted in obvious hypoperfusion in the corresponding supply region. Based on the clinical symptoms and the distribution characteristics of the infarct lesions, the left middle cerebral artery was identified as the responsible artery. A left-side vascular anastomosis procedure may improve intracranial blood supply, thereby reducing the risk of ischemic attacks and recurrent cerebral infarctions. Potential complications include new-onset cerebral infarction, hemiplegia, aphasia, and epilepsy caused by hyperperfusion bleeding. In severe cases, it could lead to extreme risks such as coma and even death.

4. Treatment and follow up

Under general anesthesia, the patient maintained a supine position with his head tilted to the right side. The operation field was disinfected. A linear cut along the course of the superficial temporal artery was adopted to expose and separate both posterior and anterior branches of the superficial temporal artery. After the skin flaps were elevated, the temporalis was cut in a T-shape and retracted to expose the cranium. Two holes were drilled into the skull and a bone flap about 5 cm×4 cm was cut with a milling cutter. The dura mater was opened in an arc fashion. Separate a

branch of the middle cerebral artery (diameter about 1.0 mm) from the temporal sulcus of the lateral fissure. The anterior branch of the superficial temporal artery was separated and processed, the proximal end was temporarily blocked, and the distal end was ligated. The diameter of the anastomotic end was about 1.2 mm. After the adventitia was peeled off, the lumen was flushed with heparin saline. The recipient artery, the M4 branch of the middle artery was blocked by two temporary blocking clips. The M4 branch was cut longitudinally about 1.2 mm with a glass knife, the lumen was flushed with heparin saline. The anterior branch of the superficial temporal artery was anastomosed end-to-side with the M4 branch using an interrupted suture technique with a 10-0 Prolene suture. Blocking clips of the middle cerebral artery branch were removed first, and then the blocking clip of the superficial temporal artery. Filling of the middle cerebral artery by the superficial temporal artery can be seen. The posterior branch of the superficial temporal artery was then attached to the surface of the brain. Intraoperative indocyanine green angiography was used to ensure the patency of the bypass vessels. After careful hemostasis, the dura flap was turned over and attached to the brain. The dura mater was left un-sutured but covered with a seam-free artificial dura to prevent leakage of cerebrospinal fluid. The bone flap was reset and the temporalis muscle, muscle fascia, subcutaneous tissue, and skin were closed layer by layer.

The CTA after three months of the operation showed the patency of the bypass vessels. The CTP indicated a significant improvement in the hypoperfusion within the left cerebral hemisphere (Fig. 9.3.4).

5. Comments

In this case, the patient presented with occlusion of the left middle cerebral artery, accompanied by moyamoya collateral vessel proliferation, leading to a suspected diagnosis of hemodynamic syndrome caused by unilateral intracranial atherosclerotic occlusion. For such cases, direct and indirect revascularization surgeries can be performed to improve symptoms and reduce the risk of recurrent cerebral infarctions.

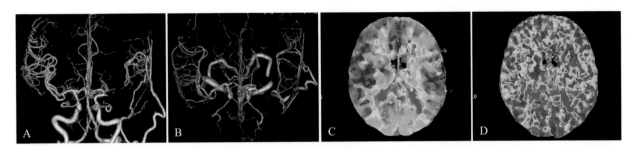

图 9.3.4　术后 3 个月复查头部 CTA 提示左侧开颅骨瓣区搭桥血管通畅（**A** 和 **B**），头部 CTP 提示左侧额、颞、顶区低灌注情况较前明显改善（**C** 和 **D**）

（王嵘　秦舒森）

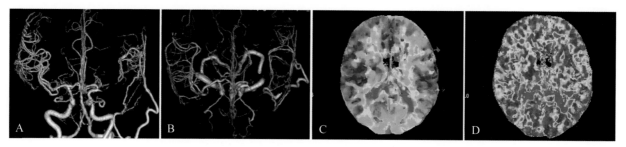

Fig. 9.3.4 The CTA after three months of the operation showed the patency of the bypass vessels (**A**, **B**), and the CTP indicated a significant improvement in the hypoperfusion within the left cerebral hemisphere (**C**, **D**)

(Translated by Shusen Qin, revised by Zhikai Hou)

索　引（**Index**）